A Time To Heal

Missionary Nurses in Churches of Christ,
Southeastern Nigeria (1953-1967)

*to my colleague
Kathryn Webster!*

Martha E. Farrar Highfield

*Martha "Marty" Highfield
September 2021*

*May your research adventures be
many! "How much better to get
wisdom than gold, to choose
understanding rather than silver."
— The writer of Proverbs 16:16*

SULIS
ACADEMIC
PRESS

An Imprint of Sulis International Press
Los Angeles | Dallas | London

A TIME TO HEAL: MISSIONARY NURSES IN CHURCHES OF CHRIST, SOUTHEASTERN NIGERIA (1953-1967)

Cover photograph: Iris Hays, RN, teaching injection technique, 1966. Author collection.

ISBN (print): 978-1-946849-82-3
ISBN (eBook): 978-1-946849-83-0

Published by Sulis Academic Press
An Imprint of Sulis International
Los Angeles | Dallas | London

www.sulisinternational.com

Contents

Foreword..i

Preface..iii

Abbreviations..x

Selected Correspondents...xi

Professional Missionary Nurses and Their Tenures in Nigeria (1953–1967)..xii

List of Illustrations..xiv

Timeline...xviii

1 Entering In: The Mission Begins 1

2 Nursing: Lauded, Costly, Uncompensated...9

3 Going to Nigeria, Come What May 23

4 Nursing Spreads Into Igboland 33

5 Controversy, Diaspora, and Duty...43

6 Transitions: Theology in Action..53

7 Steps and Missteps: A Nurse Unplanned 61

8 The Evolution of Nancy Petty..75

9 The Revolution of Iris Hays...85

10 Advice: Strife, Snakes, and Sheets..93

11 Active Waiting..99

12 Course Corrections..105

13 Making a Start: The Nurses Arrive 117

14 Becoming "The Nurses" 125

15 Goodwill Ambassadors 133

16 Watershed Moment: Decision to Stay...145

17 Recruiting, Repercussions, and Redemption 151

18 "Nigerian Christian Cracker-Box"...163

19 Opening the "Cracker-Box"...169

20 "Many Colors Together" 179

21 Revolutionaries 187

22 Keeping the Mission Alive..193

23 United By NCH..199

24 Out with the Old; In with the New..207

25 Walls Up; Missionaries Down; Nigeria Uncertain 215

26 The Wider Workforce..225
27 Saving Evangelism...231
28 Joining Forces and Families...237
29 Launching the Hospital 245
30 Growing Pains..255
31 Replacement-less 267
32 Fully Engaged: "Boots Feel Better Than Shoes"...........275
33 Walking Away: End of Their Beginnings 289
Epilogue 301
Works Cited 309
Index 325

To "Mama Grace"
Nne-amaka

Foreword

I knew Dr. Highfield before I knew her! When I was 6, I visited her at the missionary compound at the Nigerian Christian Hospital at Onicha Ngwa and in the company of my parents and my older siblings. But for a long time neither of us knew this nor did we know each other at that time.

It will be another 40 years before we will meet again—this time knowing ourselves and catching up on old times! Now, I am very honored to recommend *A Time to Heal* to all students and lovers of missions, history, anthropology, and even the occasional and casual student of cultural confluence!

In an easy, narrative, and reader-friendly style, Dr. Highfield brings the reader face to face with the uncertainties, doubts, struggles, frustrations, victories, joys, and accomplishments of these early missionaries as they strove to serve their Nigerian hosts.

Reading *A Time to Heal* is like taking a trip into the past! Dr. Highfield meticulously and delicately unwraps the intricate but intriguing life of pioneer Church of Christ missionary families as they play this dog-on-dog game with the Nigerian recipients of their Christian charity. As the Igbo says: *Egwu nkita l'ibe ya bu idaram m'adaraghi!* ("Dog's play is you fall for me, and I fall for you!")

The book reads like a time-encapsulated-movie, seamlessly weaving in and out of the missionaries' lives, breathing life into their actions and interactions; while holding missionary and local interests together by their common goals to serve and be served.

Historical books are often dry, lack luster, boring, and difficult to enjoy! But Dr. Highfield has masterfully infused life, humor, and a freshness that is rare into chronology, places, dates, and the piecemeal accounts of events into one seamless narration that keeps one wanting to know what happened next! Simply inviting!

Chi Ekwenye Hendricks, PhD
Director of Right Steps, Inc.
June 22, 2020
Obuzor, Nigeria

Preface

"It is from a small seed that the giant Iroko tree has its beginning." So reads the Nigerian proverb. In the same way, it was from the scarcely noticed backdoor clinics of a few incidental nurses that an enduring healthcare mission grew.

The nurses came to Nigeria's rural rainforests as missionaries first, and nurses second. Yet as first-hand witnesses to the physical suffering of their Nigerian neighbors, these women determined to chart a new mission course from the field, and their volunteer, uncompensated nursing care was quickly embraced by church of Christ (COC) evangelists in the field. Local demand grew, and missionary men lauded nursing's "untold value" to the evangelistic mission itself.[1]

Glenna Peden, RN, was first among them. She moved from Tennessee to the remote southeastern Nigerian village of Ikot Usen in 1953 with her family and evangelist husband, Eugene Peden, as they answered Nigerians' persistent pleas for US COC preachers. An energetic Nurse Peden began a robust, uncompensated practice "on the side."[2] She delivered care from her home, educated locals, and apprenticed lay missionary women colleagues who started their own backdoor clinics. Thus, wherever new COC mission points sprang up, nursing followed.

As waves of new COC missionaries followed, other women took up nursing as an expected part of their daily work. The nurses were diverse: professional and lay, married and single, adult and teen, enthusiastic and reluctant. Working alone or in small groups, they rendered first aid using a few medications and bandages, applied their general or professional knowledge of health and hygiene, and drove miles in their own cars to deliver the sickest to distant hospitals. Without a broader COC vision, however, their nursing work waxed and waned as individual missionaries came and went.

In 1958 missionary views of the sustainability of such ad hoc nursing reached a tipping point. When evangelist Rees Bryant's best efforts failed to save a man's life, the missionaries began to see their backdoor care as theologically, fiscally, and professionally inadequate. Incidental nursing

---

[1]Horton, quoted in Goff, *Great*, 23.
[2]Peden, Interview.

used resources intended for other purposes, inadequately met the needs of underserved locals, and failed to fulfill the missionaries' growing sense of a Christian duty to heal physically. No longer were physical and spiritual care juxtaposed as dichotomous; Jesus had provided both, and so would they. No longer was it enough to bring people to a hospital; they needed to bring a hospital to the people. No longer was it acceptable to limit healthcare to voluntary women's work; they felt obligated to recruit qualified professionals. COC missionaries' new perspective flowed back into the US: "Come over to Nigeria and help us," they wrote to every COC nurse and physician they knew.

Their Macedonian call was heard, and by 1965 Henry Farrar, MD, Grace Farrar, RN, Iris Hays, RN, and Nancy Petty, RN, moved to Onicha Ngwa in order to establish a COC hospital. These professionals' religious convictions both drove and freed them to do what they could. None possessed experience or education to begin such a work, yet in less than eighteen months they overcame political hurdles, funding shortages, government bureaucracy, and their own acknowledged weaknesses to complete, equip, staff, and open the Nigerian Christian Hospital (NCH) at Mile 11 on the Aba-Ikot Ekpene Road. There they sought to embody their informally adopted motto: "We dress the wound. God heals it."[3]

Almost as soon as NCH opened, however, its fortunes changed along with those of Nigeria itself, as missionaries fled in the face of 1967 civil war. Yet their past achievements were not undone. An all-African staff assumed the work of NCH, treating the sick and saving lives, and when the Nigeria-Biafra conflict ended in 1970 with the country's reunification, US COC physicians and nurses returned to help in resurrecting a looted and gutted—but still standing—NCH.

But those post-war stories are for another time. This book is about beginnings.

The Challenge

My interest in COC missionary nurses to Nigeria began long ago. As a daughter of 1960s missionaries Henry and Grace Farrar, I knew many actors in this story, but only as a child knows them: heroes and a few villains. My interest became professional after a chance meeting with nurse historian Dr. Sonya Grypma, who inspired me to record the work of Iris Hays and Nancy Petty, neighbors from my Onicha Ngwa childhood.

---

[3]From Harvard's Aesculapian Club motto that itself was adapted from 16th century, French surgeon Ambroise Pare who wrote, "I bandaged him and God healed him."

I learned quickly that the COC nursing story in Nigeria was broader and more fascinating than I imagined but less documented than I hoped. From Nigeria's late colonial era forward, a series of COC women quietly restored health and saved lives. Faith, family, and the COC community inspired them, strengthened their resilience, provided context for their experiences, and brought their personal and professional identities together in new ways. Each played her part in a team that moved the COC toward professionally delivered care in a creditable hospital.

Yet despite their remarkable pioneering roles in COC medical benevolence—now called healthcare missions—these nurses received scant attention, and my efforts to remediate this situation proved no easy task. No COC mission society or related archive existed to preserve records, so documentation was left to congregations and missionaries themselves. Few public documents described their work, perhaps because US COC members were more interested in the activities of their paid evangelists than in those of incidental nurses. Moreover, COC doctrinal controversies about whether congregations should fund hospitals, physicians, and nurses complicated intra-church conversation.

Fortunately, however, not all who knew the nurses were silent. Evangelist colleagues drew attention to the merit of the women's practices, and key supporters published limited accounts to the COC at large. Moreover, missionaries themselves preserved thousands of documents, including business and personal correspondence, news clippings, church bulletins, and many rare materials. Others later self-published memoirs, and COC-affiliated universities began developing relevant archives.

Gathering sources became a work itself, and I delighted in the privilege of compiling materials from the boxes, bags, basements, and memories of the nurses and those who knew them. Many individuals generously shared private collections and provided new oral history that yielded insights found nowhere else. This book would have been impossible without those gifts.

The Aim

My purpose is to describe missionary nurses' leadership in COC healthcare in Nigeria, and I hope that my account will inspire and add to an understanding of missionary nurses, Christian missions, COC women, Restoration churches, West African healthcare, and Nigerians' agency. Using a narrative approach viewed through a religious lens, I describe these nurses' work as shaped by their contexts and choices, and I make every effort to understand the women's stories as lived and narrated.

Their stories illustrate many complexities of 20th century missions—complexities that sometimes confirm and sometimes defy current perspectives on West Africans and expatriate missionaries. Additionally, although my goal is not to provide a history of NCH, other missionaries, or the entire COC mission project in Nigeria, I have of necessity included much about those things.

I confess freely that the project is enabled and constrained by its timing, its author, and its sources. It represents what Hegel described as "original" history—that is, a history in which the author seeks to document events and actors within her own time and thereby lays a foundation on which others can build reflectively, critically, and philosophically.[4] Only a still-unfolding future will reveal the full historical significance of the actors in this story and allow a chorus of other voices to join in. Moreover, many Nigerians—in ways great and small—made these missionary nurses' work possible, and alas, I can include only those who are known to me. Too, like every other writer, I cannot escape my own personal history. Thus, as I finish this manuscript, I am forced to conclude that attempting a book is perhaps one of the best ways to shine a light on my own limitations, and I eagerly anticipate others' help in deepening our combined understanding.

Clarification

I offer several notes to promote reader clarity. First, the majority of my sources come from private collections, including papers, personal communications, correspondence, diaries, interviews, photographs, or limited-publication documents (e.g., church newsletters). Many were donated or loaned to me as originals or copies, and I inherited much of my parents' collection. For correspondence, unless otherwise noted, I use the date a letter was started, even if the writer occasionally added a subsequent date and material to the same document. Additionally, much of Rees and Patti Bryant's correspondence is preserved only as transcribed by Patti Bryant, and many letters from Nancy Petty are lost. Too, for clarity in footnotes, I include some first initials along with correspondents' surnames. Moreover, I have often grouped multiple sources into single footnotes when each provided various or confirmatory details. I also provide known spelling iterations of individuals' names, and permit in-

---

[4]Inwood, *Hegel*, 119–20.

formants to speak in their own sometimes colloquial language with minimal or no correction of spelling and grammar.

Moreover, I have taken the liberty of using sometimes unstated, but discoverable sender and recipient identities or dates in citations. In most cases, the letter writers or recipients' full names are clear based on nicknames, letter content, handwriting, transcriber attribution, or letter collection. For example, Grace Farrar knew that her letters would be shared among her parents and siblings, and so sometimes addressed them broadly to "Dear Folks" and signed them with her childhood nickname, "Dit."[5] Beyond correspondence, it was impossible to identify full citation information for some clippings and other personal collection materials.

I offer also a few points about oral history notations and websites. First, in interview citations, Iris Hays is designated as Hays-Savio and Nancy Petty as Petty-Kraus for reader clarity. Second, Hays-Savio preferred to read from her diary rather than allow direct review, and that selective reading is included in her summer 2009 oral history—a transcribed interview comprised of three sessions in two days and cited as a single source. Third, my one-day interview with Rees and Patti Bryant is also cited as a single interview, despite the transcript's division into three parts related to a recorder glitch. Additionally, unless otherwise specified, all references to Henry Farrar in text and footnotes are to Henry Cheairs Farrar Jr., MD (not his father, Henry C. Farrar Sr., or his son, Henry C. Farrar III, MD). Too, pages from the Find A Grave website appear in footnotes only, while other websites and webpages are listed in bibliography.

All correspondence and most interviews were unpublished and obtained directly from missionaries. My intention is to move materials in my possession to the Center for Restoration Studies, Abilene Christian University (ACU), Abilene, Texas; most informants have already granted written permission for this. Nancy Petty-Kraus, John Morgan, and Betty Peden hold important original collections; papers from Rees and Patti Bryant were moved to ACU with some on DigitalCommons@ACU. Finally, numerous photographs were widely shared among concurrent missionaries and are part of numerous individual collections; I include date and photographer attribution when known.

---

[5]Farrar, *Stand*, vii.

Appreciation

To the extent that this book is accurate, I thank my remarkable sources and reviewers. To the extent that it is in error, I accept responsibility. The project was possible only through the generous sharing of memories and materials by many Nigerians, missionaries, and their supporters and families, including Patti Mattox Bryant, Rees O. Bryant, Dorothy Buice, Jeanie Nicks Crocker, Chi Ekwenye-Hendricks, Henry C. Farrar Jr. (deceased), Grace Johnson Farrar (deceased), Henry C. Farrar III, CeLeste Fraga, Barbara Oteka Kee, Joyce Massey, Donna Morgan, John Morgan, Rose Ngwakwe, Eno Otoyo, Ida Palmer, Betty Jo Peden, Nancy Petty-Kraus, Iris Hays-Savio (deceased), and Jane Doe (pseudonym; name withheld per request). These and other "detectives" helped me to ferret out important details of the story—among them Monday John Akpakpan, Tom Childers, Rebecca Dorfmueller, Eunice Uzuegbu Uche, Hank Farrar, Paul Farrar, Don Harrison, Mac Ice, Carol Kaplan, Fleta Mooney, Jane Petty, Pat Palmer Pleasant, Wanda Talley, Patty Wilson, Annette Whitaker, and CSUN librarians Marcia Henry, Lynn Lampert and Susana Eng-Zisken. My thanks also go to those who published memoirs of Nigeria. Without each of these, much would be lost to time and war.

A host of colleagues, friends, and family also supported me—my "book village." First among them is my husband, COC theologian Dr. Ron Highfield, who has been a reliable, meticulous, and kind encourager, listener, questioner, and advisor. Dr. Chi Ekwenye-Hendricks, one of my dearest sisters, has also given me strength for the book journey through her enthusiasm, gentle prodding, unwavering friendship, and insider perspectives and connections. I especially thank Betty Peden, Dr. David Baird, Dr. Carolyn Hunter, Dr. Rees Bryant, Patti Bryant, and Jane Doe for reading full or partial drafts. My thanks also to Mark Horton, who patiently scanned pictures and listened encouragingly, and to photographer Ron Hall, who assisted with the image gracing the book's cover. Moreover, I would not and could not have done the work without historian and writing mentors, Drs. Baird and Grypma, who together inspired me, asked questions, and gave direction and critique. I am grateful, too, for a thoughtful reading of the manuscript by Assistant Professor McGarvey "Mac" Ice, for editorial and proofing help from Tammy Ditmore and Bonnie Miller, and to Dr. Markus McDowell for publishing assistance. Special recognition for small grant funding during early days of the project is due to Gamma Tau Chapter at-Large of Sigma Theta Tau International Nursing Honor Society, California State University/Northridge, and Kaiser Permanente of Southern California.

Most of all, I thank my parents: nurse and homemaker extraordinaire Grace Farrar (1924–2013) and compassionate, determined physician-preacher Henry C. Farrar Jr. (1926–2010), who moved our family to Nigeria in 1964. Throughout their lives, they modeled at home and abroad what it means to keep promises, to believe, to hope, and above all to love. To them, I owe whatever measure I have of the beginning of wisdom.

Abbreviations

ACC	Abilene Christian College, Abilene, TX (now University)
AUTH	Martha E.F. Highfield (author) private collection
BJP	Betty Jo Peden private collection
BTC	Bible Training College in Ukpom or in Onicha Ngwa, Nigeria
COC	Church of Christ/church of Christ
HGF	Henry and Grace Farrar private collection in author collection
IHCF/ACH	International Health Care Foundation/African Christian Hospitals
JD	Jane Doe private collection
JNC	Jeannie Nicks Crocker private collection (includes Bill and Gerry Nicks papers)
JRM	John R. Morgan private collection
KJV	King James Version of the Bible
LA-COC	Lawrence Avenue Church of Christ, Nashville, TN
LCC	Lubbock Christian College, Lubbock, TX (now University)
LPN/LVN	Licensed Vocational (or Practical) Nurse [US]
MMM	Medical Missionaries of Mary in Urua Akpan and Anua, Nigeria
NCH	Nigerian Christian Hospital
NCSF	Nigerian Christian Schools Foundation
NCSS	Nigerian Christian Secondary School, Ukpom, Nigeria
NPK	Nancy Petty-Kraus private collection
NRN	Nigerian Registered Nurse
PH	Port Harcourt, Nigeria
QEH	Queen Elizabeth Hospital, Umuahia, Nigeria
RN	Registered Nurse [US]
RPB	Rees and Patti Bryant private collection
RPB:N	Bryant file, "Nigerian Newsletters (1958-1967)" in author collection
USAID	United States Agency for International Development
W-COC	West End Church of Christ, Nashville, TN
WEV	*West End Visitor*, mimeographed church bulletins, West End COC

Selected Correspondents

E. Bryants	Emmett and Nell Bryant (Rees Bryant's parents)
P. Bryant	Patti Mattox Bryant
R. Bryant	Rees O. Bryant
G. Farrar	Grace Farrar (nickname "Dit")
G.B. Farrars	George and Evelyn Farrar family (H. Farrar's brother; W-COC elder)
H. Farrar	Henry Farrar Jr.
Mrs. H.C. Farrar	Nina Ellen Farrar (Henry Farrar Jr.'s mother)
M. Johnson	Martha Thayer Johnson (Grace Farrar's mother)
Johnsons	Elva and Martha Johnson (Grace Farrar's parents)
Mattoxes	F.W. and Mildred Mattox (Patti Bryant's parents)
McInteers	Jim Bill and Betty McInteer family (W-COC preacher and family)
Spann(s)	Diane (Nancy Petty's sister) and Raymond Spann family, including nephew J. Spann and niece N.B. Spann

Professional Missionary Nurses and Their Tenures in Nigeria (1953–1967)

Glenna Shifflett Peden, RN (1953–1955, 1957–1959)
Mary B. Rogers Kelton, RN (1957–1958)
Letty Sermanoukian (1961)
Grace Johnson Farrar, RN (1964–1967)
Iris Fay Hays, RN (1965–1967)
Nancy Corinne Petty, RN (1965–1967)

List of Illustrations

MAPS

1. Nigeria, artist Henry Farrar Jr., 1964. HGF.
2. Onicha Ngwa mission compound, artist Nancy Petty, 1965. NPK.
3. Republic of Biafra, artist Henry Farrar Jr., 1967. HGF.

PHOTOGRAPHS

1	Peden family passport photo, 1953.
2.1	Glenna Peden, RN, holding newborn Pamela Rose Johnson, 1953.
2.2	Glenna Peden, RN, delivering backdoor care in Ikot Usen, Ibibioland, ca. 1954.
3	Mary Buel Rogers, RN, BA, ca. 1957.
4.1	"Our first hospital:" Gerry Nicks delivering Igboland backdoor care, ca.1959.
4.2	Gerry Nicks, Patti Bryant, and Glenna Peden, RN, in Igboland backdoor clinic, 1958.
7	Nurse Letty Sermanoukian formally welcomed to Onicha Ngwa, 1961.
13	First meeting of Nancy Petty and Iris Hays, Port Harcourt, Airport, April 7, 1965.
14	Church of Christ mission compound, Onicha Ngwa, 1965.
15	Women's village health class, Summer 1965.
16	Iris Hays, RN, and Patti Bryant's Sunday afternoon Bible Class, ca. 1965.
17	"Founding Nurses:" Farrar, Petty, and Hays, ca. 1965.
18	Healthcare team, Summer 1965: Morgan, Petty, Farrar, Hays, 1965.
19	NCH Staff on Clinic opening day, August 29, 1965.
24	Iris Hays, RN, at NCH, ca. 1966.
26	Grace Farrar, RN, with children, packaging USAID supplements for NCH, June 1966.
28	Nancy Petty with foster daughter, Virginia, ca. 1966.
29.1	First NCH couplet, August 29, 1966.

29.2   Iris Hays, RN, capping Eunice Ukegbu, BTC, Onicha Ngwa, August 29, 1966.

30   Hazel Buice, RMT, with lay technicians Peter Uhiara and Sylvanus Nwagbara, ca. 1966.

31   NCH auxiliary graduates from 1966 and 1967, Onicha Ngwa, February 15, 1967.

32.1   Henry Farrar MD, Gertrude Mbong, and Nancy Petty RN, 1967.

32.2   Patience, Nigerian Christian Hospital, 1967.

33   Nigerian Christian Hospital, ca. late 1966.

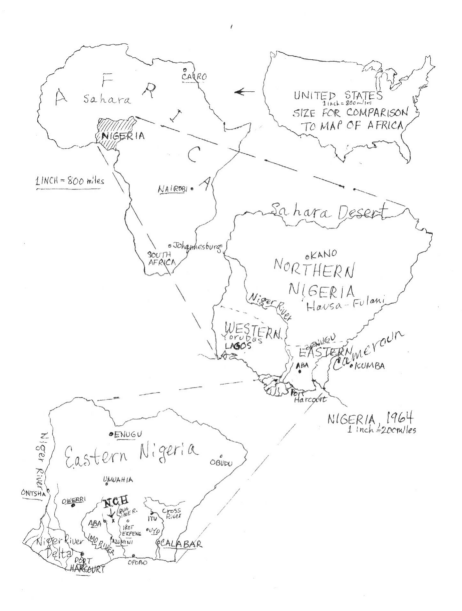

Map 1. Nigeria. Artist Henry Farrar Jr., MD. 1964. Author collection.
(Scale altered for print)

Timeline

1942

May 3   Mary Buel Rogers graduates from Methodist Hospital School of Nursing, Dallas, TX

1943   Glenna Jean Shifflett graduates Kanawha Valley Hospital School of Nursing, WV

1943–46   Mary Rogers, RN, serves as 1st Lieutenant in US Army Nurse Corps

1945

Aug 26   Glenna Shifflett, RN, and Eugene Peden wed in Belle, WV

Feb 19   Grace Johnson graduates Bethesda Hospital Nursing School, Cincinnati, OH

1950

Aug 8–17   Boyd Reese and Eldred Echols make exploratory trip to Nigeria

Dec 2   Grace Johnson, RN, and Henry Farrar wed in Searcy, AR

1952

May 26   Mary Rogers graduates from Abilene Christian College, Abilene, TX

Nov 24   First COC family arrives in Ikot Usen: Jimmy and Rosa Lee Johnson

Nov 27   Second family arrives in Ikot Usen: Howard and Mildred Horton

1953

Apr 10   Mary Rogers, RN, and Tom Kelton wed

Oct 12   Third COC family arrives in Ikot Usen: Eugene and Glenna Peden

Oct 21   Birth of first COC missionary child in Nigeria: Pamela Rose Johnson

Dec 4   Fourth COC family arrives in Ikot Usen: Elvis and Emily Huffard

1954

Feb 1	Ukpom Bible Training College (BTC) begins
Mar 22	Henry Farrar graduates from UT College of Medicine, Memphis, TN
Jul 15	Jimmy and Rosa Lee Johnson family furloughs
Oct 20	Fifth COC family arrives at Ikot Usen: Lucien and Ida Palmer
Dec 7	Horton family furloughs

1955

Apr 16	Huffard family furloughs
Jul 23	Nigerian government officially recognizes the Church of Christ
Aug 6	Peden family furloughs
Oct 5	Bill and Gerry Nicks family arrives in Ukpom

1956

Aug 10	Palmer family furloughs
Aug 25	Sewell and Caneta Hall family arrives in Ukpom

1957

Jan	Finney and Nicks families begin new mission point in Onicha Ngwa
Jul 12	Tom and Mary Kelton family arrives in Ikot Usen
Nov 12	Pedens return to Nigeria; this time in Onicha Ngwa
Dec 9	Nicks family furloughs

1958

Mar 13	Rees and Patti Bryant family arrives in Onicha Ngwa
Mar 24	Pedens move to Ukpom
Apr 24	Finney family furloughs
Jun 12	Nicks family returns to Onicha Ngwa
Jun 21	Hall family furloughs
Dec	Mary Kelton and daughters return to US

1959

Jan 6	Tom Kelton returns to US
Jun 30	Leslie and Sarah Diestelkamp family arrives in Nigeria
Jul 26	Pedens depart permanently
Sep 23	Bryant family furloughs
Nov 30	Diestelkamps move from Ikot Usen to Lagos

Dec 7   Jim and Joyce Massey family arrives in Onicha Ngwa

1960
Apr 5   Bryants return to Onicha Ngwa
Apr 13   Nicks family furloughs
Oct 1   Republic Day—Nigerian independence from Great Britain
Sep 15   Halls return to Nigeria; this time in Lagos
Dec 15   Doug and Charla Lawyer family arrives in Onicha Ngwa

1961
Jan 20   Letty Sermanoukian arrives in Onicha Ngwa from Tripoli,
         Libya
Jul 19   Bryants begin premature furlough
.   Petty graduates Mid-State Baptist Nursing School, Nashville,
         TN
         Hays graduates Lubbock Christian College, Lubbock, TX
         Sermanoukian work terminated with missionaries

1962
Spring   Masseys return to Onicha Ngwa
Dec   Lawyer family furloughs

1963
Jun   Lawyers return to Onicha Ngwa
Sep 13   Henry Farrar, MD, begins three-week, exploratory visit to
         Nigeria
Dec   Sermanoukian court settlement with missionaries

1964
Jul 25   Henry and Grace Farrar family arrives in Onicha Ngwa
Aug 1   Bryants return to Onicha Ngwa
Aug   Hays graduates Methodist Hospital School of Nursing,
         Lubbock, TX
         Sermanoukian immigrates to US

1965
May 18   Lawyers depart permanently for US
Mar 24   Iris Hays, RN, arrives in Onicha Ngwa
Apr 7   Nancy Petty, RN, arrives in Onicha Ngwa
Aug 18   Hays begins classes for first cohort of seven nursing auxil-
         iary students

Aug 21   Grand opening of Nigerian Christian Hospital (NCH) Out-
          patient Clinic
Aug 23   NCH Outpatient Clinic opens to patients
Oct 18   Land lease signed for NCH inpatient buildings

1966
Jan 16   Military coup d'état in Nigeria
Mar 28   Hays begins classes for second cohort of seven nursing aux-
          iliary students
Jul 29   Military counter coup d'état in Nigeria
Summer   NCH hires first Nigerian Registered Nurses/midwives
          (NRNs)
Aug 23   Grand opening of NCH inpatient units
Aug 29   Hospital opens to patients. First NCH birth attended by Far-
          rar
Aug 29   First auxiliary class graduation ceremony
Sep 4   First NRN midwife-attended NCH birth.
Sep 9   First NCH surgery: a C-section in the delivery room

1967
Feb 5   First NCH surgery in new operating room
Feb 15   Second auxiliary graduation ceremony
Feb 22   Bryant family furloughs
Mar 29   Hays and Petty furlough
May 30   Republic of Biafra (Eastern Nigeria) declares independence
Jun 6   Grace Farrar and children evacuate to Lagos
Jul 6   Nigeria–Biafra civil conflict begins
Jul 19   Remaining Onicha Ngwa missionaries, including Henry Far-
          rar, evacuate

1967–1970 West African staff and the Red Cross operate NCH during
          the war

1970
Jan 15   Nigeria-Biafra war ends. Nigeria reunifies under military
Sep 2   Henry Farrar returns to Nigeria to rehabilitate NCH

1972
Jul 20   African Christian Hospitals Foundation incorporated (now
          IHCF/ACH)

2020   NCH staffed by Nigerians and governed by on-site Nigerian Policy Board

1
Entering In: The Mission Begins
(1948–1953)

Try the Lawrence Avenue Church of Christ
—Anna-Maria Braun

On Monday, October 12, 1953, Glenna Jean Shifflett Peden, RN, stepped onto the village soil of Ikot Usen, Nigeria. She arrived with evangelist husband, Eugene, in response to years of Nigerian pleading for missionaries from US churches of Christ (COCs); her nursing expertise was incidental to the cause.[1] Still, Glenna registered as a nurse with the British Protectorate of Nigeria, perhaps because of encouragement to do so by missionaries already there.[2]

The Pedens traveled to Africa by air with young daughters Betty Jo and Dinah from the US through war-damaged London.[3] Entering Nigeria through its western port city of Lagos, they flew on to southeastern Port Harcourt (PH) in the Niger Delta, and then completed "a slow, rough drive over a hundred miles to the east"[4] on coal-tar (asphalt) roads followed by seven plus miles of bumpy dirt ones.[5] Their new Ikot Usen home in Ibibioland was deep in the rainforest, forty miles past the railroad's end.[6]

---

[1]Horton, quoted in Goff, *Great*, 23; Peden, Interview; Peden, "Chronology."
[2]Ida Palmer, quoted in Pat Pleasant, email to author, September 6, 2014; Peden, Interview.
[3]Peden, Interview.
[4]Echols, "Beginning," 9.
[5]P. Bryant to Mattoxes, February 7, 1959.
[6]Reese and Echols, *Report*, 6–8. The Ibibio include six subcultures with three major language groups: Annang, Ibibio, and Efik. Ikot is an Ibibio prefix related to ancestral origins and means "village of…," "house of…," or "the people of…." Hence Ikot Usen is the village, people, or house of Usen.

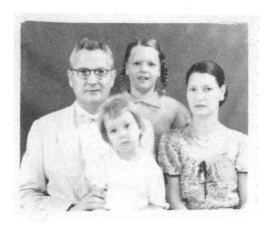

Photograph 1. Peden family passport photo: Eugene holding Dinah with Betty Jo and Glenna. 1953. (Peden collection with permission)

In Ikot Usen the Pedens were enthusiastically welcomed by families already there: Jimmy and Rosa Lee Johnson and Howard Patrick and Mildred Gladney Horton (1917–1991) with young daughters Ann and Angela.[7] The Johnsons and Hortons, who arrived a year earlier in November 1952, were the first resident COC missionaries to join the *Great Nigerian Mission*, and Howard Horton lauded the Pedens' 1953 coming as "a day of rejoicing…[that] accelerated the work greatly."[8]

Continents Together

For COC members, the arrival of the Pedens, Johnsons, and Hortons in Nigeria was confirmation of God's providence. In the 1940s a curious set of post-World War II coincidences connected Africa, Europe, and North America and swung wide Nigeria's door to the COC. In Nigeria, Efik-speaking, Christian evangelist Coolidge Akpan Okon Essien (1915–1960) was eager to study English and the Bible;[9] in Germany, Anna-Maria Braun (1913–missing) established the postwar *Internationales Korrespondenz-Buro* to promote language learning; and in the US, the Lawrence Avenue

---

[7]Goff, *Great*, 23; Harp, "Howard Patrick Horton (1917-2000);" Mildred G. Horton, February 3, 2014, findagrave.com no. 124585606.
[8]Goff, *Great*, 17–18; Horton, quoted in Goff, *Great*, 23.
[9]Burger, "God's Providence;" Owolabi, *New*, 7–11.

COC (LA-COC) in Nashville, Tennessee, was distributing a twenty-six-lesson, English-language Bible correspondence course.[10]

Braun bridged this continental triad between Essien and the LA-COC,[11] although no one—even Braun herself—was sure how she learned about LA-COC's Bible course.[12] George Turner, course author and LA-COC minister and elder, asserted that missionaries to Germany told Braun about it when inviting her to their evangelistic meetings.[13] In competing stories, Turner's wife speculated that Braun's German students informed her,[14] others maintained that Braun received a flyer advertising the LA-COC course,[15] and still others suggested that she heard about it through a recorded sermon of Reuel G. Lemmons's South African radio program.[16] Whatever the case, Braun enrolled in LA-COC's course in 1947,[17] and on June 19, 1948, she acknowledged receiving small, gummed stickers by which she could promote it.[18]

About that same time, Nigerian preacher Essien enrolled in Braun's *Internationales Korrespondenz-Buro* and "purely on impulse" wrote on a return lesson, "Do you know of anybody who has a correspondence course on the Bible?" The marked lesson came back with the note, "Try the Lawrence Avenue Church of Christ in Nashville, Tennessee."[19] Essien did so, and "his unusual return address Ibiaku, Ikot Usen, Ibiono, Itu, Nigeria, West Africa" garnered immediate staff attention.[20]

Essien, like US COC members, wanted to practice Christianity as he saw it described in the Bible's New Testament. Baptized into the reformed Presbyterian Church of Scotland in Itu, he attended Hope Waddell Presbyterian School in Calabar.[21] Soon, however, Essien rejected the Scottish Church for not following the Bible strictly enough and was subsequently rebaptized by immersion for forgiveness of sins into the Pentecostal Assemblies of the World (PAofW). He was promptly ordained as

---

[10]Goff, *Great*, 1–6.

[11]Burger, "God's Providence;" Goff, *Great*, 6; Owolabi, *New*, 8. Goff records that Essien was misquoted or misspoke his tutor's name as Eva Braun—a mistake that gave rise to persistent COC rumors that his tutor was Hitler's former secretary.

[12]Goff, *Great*, 5.

[13]Echols, "Beginning," 7–11.

[14]Goff, *Great*, 5.

[15]Farrar and Hood, "The Beginning."

[16]R. Bryant, "Nigerian Highlights–1959;" Bryant and Lawyer, "Opportunities."

[17]Goff, "There Stood."

[18]Goff, *Great*, 5.

[19]Essien, quoted in Echols, "Beginning," 7.

[20]Goff, *Great*, 6.

[21]Farrar and Hood, "The Beginning."

a PAofW pastor, but then rejected the PAofW for the same reasons he had rejected the Presbyterians. Unable to find a denomination that believed as he did, Essien established at least fifty congregations of his own church: the Apostolic Church of Christ (ACOC). Essien completed LA-COC's Bible correspondence course in 1949 and convinced other Nigerians to enroll. Moreover, he changed ACOC practices to match US COC ones, including taking the name "church of Christ," singing a cappella, and discontinuing interpretation of dreams and prophecy.[22] Essien also began a persistent stream of letters to LA-COC "pleading for white missionaries.... "We can teach our own people," he argued, "But we need more teaching ourselves. Send men to teach us, and we shall take Nigeria for the truth.""[23]

In the absence of a COC-wide mission society, LA-COC elders responded to Essien's request by asking two trusted men to evaluate the dual possibilities of recognizing Essien's churches as COCs and of sending missionaries. Thus, in 1950, Boyd Reese, US missionary in Southern Rhodesia, and Eldred Echols, US missionary in South Africa, spent a week evaluating Essien's work in Nigeria and created the skillfully detailed, inspirational, and sometimes humorous, how-to manual for future missionaries and their supporters: the *Reese-Echols Report on Nigeria*. Furthermore, despite pre-visit skepticism, Reese and Echols declared Essien's COCs as compatible with US congregations.[24]

The *Report* addressed issues that potential missionaries would face, from geography to government, salaries to shopping, leasing land to visas, missionary health to homemaking, churches to challenges, and social life to schools. The authors concentrated on practical concerns that missionary families would face in Nigeria's rural rainforests and outlined the role of supporting congregations.[25] They did not call for physician or nurse missionaries and offered scant details useful to such, an unsurprising gap given their roles as preachers, the brevity of their visit, LA-COC's focus on evangelism, and Essien's request for preachers and teachers.

Reese and Echols did list common diseases and Western prevention practices but never suggested that locals might seek healthcare from mis-

---

[22]Goff, *Great*, 6–8; Owolabi, *New*, 7–11. Owolabi called PAofW the Pentecostal Assemblies of World Missions. The lower case "c" in "church of Christ" was an assertion that congregations were autonomous gatherings of Christians like those in the New Testament and not a human-designed denomination. COCs arose from within the US Restoration Movement.

[23]Essien, quoted in Goff, *Great*, 8.

[24]Goff, *Great*, 9; Reese and Echols, *Report*, 8–10; Echols, "Nigerian Diary," August 13, 1950.

[25]Reese and Echols, *Report*.

sionaries. The authors recommended that missionaries boil water, hydrate, wear cool clothing, get immunizations, take antimalarials, use mosquito nets, wear shoes to avoid parasites, and take both African vacations and US furloughs for mental health. Additionally, Reese and Echols identified sources of missionary care as "clinics in most of the larger towns…a hospital in Aba and a large white hospital at Lagos (6 hours from Ikot Usen by car and plane)."[26] Unmentioned were hospitals in PH, Uyo, Umuahia, Anua, and Urua Akpan, where early COC families typically sought care.[27]

The two Americans left Nigeria exhausted but enthusiastic, impressed that "several thousand native Africans have, without the presence of a single white man…found the church of God."[28] They wrote of an immense eagerness for Bible teaching and verified that Essien's churches, like US COCs, were seeking to restore nondenominational, first-century Christian practices and doctrine. Nonetheless, they found the Nigerians untaught. "They are all very much in favor of 'speaking where the Bible speaks,' but they are not very sure about what it says," Echols penned.[29]

Reese and Echols also made two recommendations: Empower Essien's churches through temporary financial support of local preachers and send at least "two white families."[30] Echols reasoned that the correspondence course had done its "indirect" evangelistic work well but that face-to-face relationships were now needed to facilitate "a strong, active, and independent church in Nigeria."[31] Their recommendation to send white missionaries was unsurprising given colonial-era Essien's call for whites and 1950s US COC racial segregation.

LA-COC's response to the *Report* was positive but fiscally cautious. Congregational elders thought their less-than-five-hundred-member church too small to begin this "vast" work. Thus, in order to recruit both missionaries and financial backers, LA-COC distributed the forty-four-page *Reese-Echols Report* widely to US COCs, along with promises to help provide salaries, Bibles, and church literature.[32] Whether the *Report* went to black US COCs is unclear.

---

[26]Ibid., 5, 13–18.

[27]Bryant and Bryant, Interview; Farrar, *Stand*, 121; Palmer, "Narrative."

[28]Reese and Echols, *Report*, 44.

[29]Ibid., 9. Common sayings within the COC, reflecting the US Restoration Movement intentions, included "Speak where the Bible speaks; be silent where the Bible is silent," and "Christians only, but not the only Christians."

[30]Ibid., 20.

[31]Ibid., 19.

[32]Goff, *Great*, 15.

Dream Realized

The response to LA-COC's call was silence. No congregations or evange-lists stepped forward. Undaunted, LA-COC elders started financial sup-port of Nigerian evangelists C.A.O. Essien and P.A. Alfred. Then, as "a further stop-gap, holding action," they paid Echols to return to Nigeria from July through October 1951.[33] This allowed Echols to keep a prom-ise "extracted" from him by a determined "Brother Essien" to teach in Essien's Preacher Training School.[34] During his stay, Echols' health dete-riorated under primitive living conditions,[35] but his enthusiasm remained.

Nigeria's mission opportunity is "'red-hot,' and won't wait," Echols de-clared,[36] and it didn't. Three months later, in February 1952, Howard Horton, preacher at Ridgedale COC in Chattanooga, Tennessee, and his wife, Mildred, committed to go to Ikot Usen. James E. "Jimmy" and Rosa Lee Johnson, young members at LA-COC, also volunteered. With the recommended two-evangelist-family quota met, LA-COC pledged to send them. Jimmy Johnson was just graduating from David Lipscomb College in Nashville, and the elders assumed that his "courage and devo-tion" would overcome his preaching inexperience.[37]

Fundraising for these first families proved easier than anticipated. Nu-merous COC members and congregations donated money for salaries, travel, housing, supplies, and materials, and LA-COC elders delegated the "staggering volume of details" to their new Nigeria Committee assisted by the church treasurer and secretary. Nine months later, all logistics were in place, and in fall 1952, the Hortons and Johnsons moved to Ikot Usen, where they occupied a mud and thatch house prepared for them by Essien, hung mosquito nets, uncrated a stove and beds, ate some of their canned food, and boiled drinking water.[38] A delighted Essien rejoiced: "The dream has…come true. The brethren we had long been expecting have…arrived."[39]

---

[33]Ibid., 16; Echols, "Nigerian Diary," July 3–October 29, 1951.

[34]Echols, "Beginning," 7. COC members addressed each other in family terms as "Brother [last name]" and "Sister [last name];" these titles were not religious offices. During 1951, Echols wrote on August 23, 1951 in his "Nigerian Diary" that Essien and others were baptized about this time, but Owolabi in *New* recorded credible details of Essien's COC baptism months later on March 12, 1952 (11).

[35]Echols, "Nigerian Diary," October 23–29, 1951.

[36]Echols, quoted in Goff, *Great*, 16.

[37]Goff, *Great*, 16.

[38]Ibid., 17–19; Reese and Echols, *Report*, 10–11. Reese and Echols earlier initiated lease proceedings with local Nigerians for the compound in consultation with the British District Office. Goff joined the LA-COC Nigeria Committee in 1953.

[39]Essien, quoted in Goff, *Great*, 1.

A year later, the Pedens joined the effort, and their 1953 arrival brought not only the first COC missionary nurse, but also the significant engagement of a second US congregation: the Sixth Street COC in Port Arthur, Texas, who salaried and supervised Eugene Peden. The three families shared two cars, two new concrete block houses, and one evangelistic mission.[40] Like other missionary women, Glenna Peden was a fulltime homemaker who relied on her husband's salary, but she was also a licensed nurse who wanted to use her skills.[41] Thus, without role model, professional colleague, or precedent, Peden began a COC nursing practice in Nigeria—to the delight of those around her.[42]

Conclusion

Essien's dream of welcoming US COC evangelists brought more than preachers to Nigeria. His imagination facilitated the incidental birth of a new, unformed vision: COC missionary nursing. An unexpected network brought Glenna Peden to Ikot Usen where she began to lay a nursing foundation for those who followed. The coming of a nurse was unintended, but Glenna intended her coming to count.

---

[40]Goff, *Great*, 23.
[41]Peden, Interview.
[42]Goff, *Great*, 23, 25.

2
Nursing: Lauded, Costly, Uncompensated
(1953–1955)

Sister Peden...too has been of untold value to the work.
—Howard Horton

Glenna Jean Shifflett was born July 18, 1920, to "French-Indian Chero-kee" coal miner Hezekiah Shifflett and wife, Della. As fourth of ten chil-dren, Glenna grew up in a log cabin without running water or utilities in mining camp #9 in Mammoth, West Virginia. After attending Cabin Creek High School, Glenna borrowed $100 from an uncle to attend Kanawha Valley Hospital (KVH) School of Nursing in Charleston, West Virginia. She graduated in 1943, then provided patient care and nursing student supervision at KVH and repaid the loan with her first paycheck.[1]

Despite avowed plans to buy a red convertible and never marry a coal miner or minister, Glenna wed COC evangelist Eugene "Gene" Peden (1920–1997) in 1945, six months after they met in Belle, West Virginia. Gene continued preaching, including the Sunday evening of their wed-ding day, and Glenna continued nursing.[2] Her self-described life priorities were to love Christ, then husband, then family.[3] Glenna Peden always assumed that she would follow Eugene in his work, and her cooking, singing, sewing, and nursing skills complemented his construction, car-pentry, engine repair, gardening, and public speaking proficiencies. Childhoods with limited means prepared both for rural Ikot Usen, and their marriage was a happy one.[4]

---

[1]Peden, Interview; "Glenna Jean Shifflett Peden," December 11, 2012, findagrave.com no. 102036166; "Robert Eugene Peden," December 11, 2012, findagrave.com no. 102035956; Peden, "Chronology;" Peden, email to author, October 22, 2019.
[2]Peden, Interview.
[3]Washington Street, "Glenna Jean Shifflett Peden."
[4]Peden, Interview.

In Nigeria, the Pedens worked as a team within a team.[5] Eugene's evangelism took center stage, and Glenna's four-part nursing practice flourished "on the side."[6] Glenna cared for missionaries, treated locals, taught backdoor nursing to other missionary women, and instructed Nigerian women in basic hygiene and health practices.[7] Writing to his supporters, colleague Howard Horton applauded Glenna Peden's nursing as of "untold value to the work:...Lives have been saved, eyesight preserved, pain eased, [and] loathsome disease halted by her patient and efficient service. Her counsel and her very presence here makes us all feel more secure concerning the welfare of our own children and wives."[8] Perhaps the Johnsons especially appreciated a nurse as housemate when they welcomed their first child, Pamela Rose, only nine days after the Pedens arrived. Pamela's birth site was a Port Harcourt (PH) hospital ninety miles and a three-and-a-half hour drive from Ikot Usen.[9]

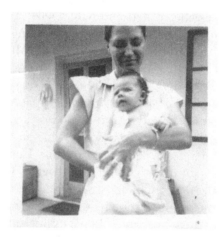

Photograph 2.1. Glenna Peden, RN, holding newborn Pamela Rose Johnson, Ikot Usen. 1953. (Peden collection with permission)

[5]Ida Palmer attachment to Pat Pleasant, email to author, September 4, 2014; Peden Interview.

[6]Peden, Interview.

[7]Ibid.; Bryant and Bryant, Interview; Horton, quoted in Goff, *Great*, 23, 25.

[8]Horton, quoted in Goff, *Great*, 23.

[9]Goff, *Great*, 21–22; Chi Ekweyne-Hendricks, personal communication, May 6, 2012. In a Florida meeting, Pamela Rose Johnson told Ekwenye-Hendricks that she was born in a PH hospital.

Missionary Healthcare

Nurse Peden's on-site care freed missionaries from unnecessary, health-care-seeking adventures that could devour time and dollars.[10] In her own family, she successfully treated daughters Dinah for filariasis and Betty for onchocerciasis (river blindness), keeping her in a dark room for two weeks and "dousing" her with antibiotics.[11] Still, Nurse Peden's skills were not always enough, as illustrated by Patsy Palmer's hospitalization.

In October 1954, one week after new missionaries E. Lucien Palmer (1921–2004) and Ida Coates Palmer (1922–) arrived to replace the fur-loughing Johnsons, their four-year-old daughter Patsy developed a severe head-to-toe rash.[12] Her concerned family first took her eleven miles over bumpy, bush roads to the closest facility, a "small Catholic hospital in Uyo [where] the 'Sister Nurse-Doctor'" referred them to PH. The physician sealed her orders in an envelope but withheld from Palmers her tentative diagnosis of smallpox because of a local outbreak. The next day with Mildred Horton as guide, the Palmers drove to PH in the missionaries' only working car and left Ida and Patsy there in order to return the vehicle to Ikot Usen.

The PH hospital offered no accommodations for family members and no communications with Ikot Usen. As a still jet-lagged Ida Palmer recalled,

> Patsy was put in a room (open to a veranda on both sides) with three other people and tightly tucked in with mosquito nets. The traffic through the room was constant since it was a throughway from one side of the hospital to the other…I had no chair, nothing to read or to do and no place to go, so I stood by Pat's bed all night on the cement floor. There were no windows or doors—her room was just open to everyone and everything. They brought Pat a little supper and eventually I had a cup of tea and piece of toast.[13]

Fortunately, the next day doctors diagnosed Patsy's rash as relatively harmless sand fly fever; unfortunately, they discharged her to nowhere. Thus, Ida and Patsy abruptly found themselves on their own for three

---

[10]Echols, "Beginning," 9; Goff, *Great*, 23.

[11]Peden, Interview.

[12]Goff, *Great*, 28; Brewer, *Missionary*, 160; "Edward Lucien Palmer," June 3, 2010, findagrave.com no. 53216354; Palmer, "Narrative," 14.

[13]Palmer, "Narrative," 14.

nights with little money, scrambling for a bed and meals in an unfamiliar West African world. When Lucien Palmer returned to PH, the relieved family made the long drive home to Ikot Usen only after completing PH shopping lists for all mission families.[14] It was not the last time that frightened COC missionaries rushed their own to distant, inhospitable hospitals.[15]

Caring for Locals

Nurse Peden also started a backdoor clinic within an Ibibio milieu of animist traditions, self-care, and sparse Western care. Traditional juju medicine of native doctors centered on charms, amulets, and the spirit world with a primary focus on finding out who (not what) caused the illness. Practitioners used purging and cutting to rid patients of fevers or disease and beatings to rid the mentally ill of demons. Additionally, locals exercised self-care, such as purchasing medicines like anti-malarial quinine in village markets[16] and maintaining good dental health with wooden "chewing sticks."[17] A British government doctor visited occasionally, "trained" locals ran scattered dispensaries, and nuns delivered care in a Roman Catholic hospital near Uyo,[18] accessible via miles of paths "littered with fallen trees" and the occasional snake.[19]

As word of Peden's clinic spread, local demand grew.[20] As Ida Palmer remembered, Nigerians called her "Sis nurse doctor," and she "was always cheerfully on call, hospitable...organized and ready to serve."[21] Peden triaged patients from the walkway between her house and outdoor kitchen and barred her daughters from the area for fear of contagion. Some patients she treated, others she sent to hospitals, and the imminently dying she sent home out of concern that missionaries would be blamed for their deaths.[22] If Peden kept clinic records, they are lost.

14Ibid., 14–15.
15Bryant and Bryant, Interview; Farrar, *Stand*, 113.
16H. Farrar, Interview 1; Nau, *We Move*, 14–19, 181–85, 349.
17Peden, Interview.
18Nau, *We Move*, 18; Palmer, "Narrative," 14.
19Golightly, "Medicine."
20Peden, Interview.
21Ida Palmer attachment to Pat Pleasant, email to author, September 4, 2014.
22Peden, Interview.

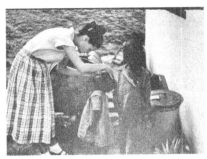

Photograph 2.2. Glenna Peden, RN, delivering backdoor nursing care on Ikot Usen COC mission compound in Ibibioland. ca. 1954. (Peden collection with permission)

Familiar and unfamiliar diseases and injuries confronted her, yet she hesitated to use indigenous treatments, such as herbal postpartum medicines and floating someone in water during spinal realignment.[23] Nurse Peden likely treated common problems of "yellow fever, malaria, typhoid, dengue fever, bilharzia, hook worm and filariasis...leprosy and yaws,"[24] bed bugs, snake and spider bites, diarrhea, tetanus, tropical ulcers, accidents, unhealed tribal scarification, tuberculosis, rabies, eye infections, difficult deliveries, and newborn tetanus caused by cutting the umbilical cord with a dirty knife. Starvation was common,[25] and infant mortality approached fifty percent.[26]

Like other Westerners, Glenna Peden tried to prevent twin killing. Yet, despite Pedens' explanations that Eugene had a twin sister and Glenna, identical triplet sisters,[27] locals remained convinced that twins were a punishment for some taboo violation or the result of the mother's intercourse with an evil spirit. Thus, despite a 1915 British law outlawing the practice, locals might promptly kill one or both twin infants and murder or ostracize the mother in order to protect their communities from supernatural disaster. Infants born feet first, with extra digits, or demonstrating anything else judged out of the ordinary were also killed.[28] One mother brought Peden her infant, who had been exposed in the forest to

[23]Ibid.

[24]Reese and Echols, *Report*, 5.

[25]Peden, Interview.

[26]H. Farrar, Interview 1.

[27]Barnes, *Rough*, 247–48; Basden, *Niger Ibos,* 183; Livingstone, *Mary Slessor*; Nau, *We Move*, 304–15; Peden, Interview.

[28]Asindi et al., "Brutality;" Basden, *Niger Ibos,* 59–61, 180–84, 262–63, 405–06.

die, and Peden amputated the child's sixth finger and used coals from her wood cook stove to warm the child in Betty and Dinah's doll basket.[29]

Most of Peden's patients were women and children, who came in defiance of native doctors, although Ibibio men also sought her care,[30] perhaps a sign that they had elevated her to the status of the occasional powerful woman admitted to men's circles among neighboring Igbos.[31] Some perhaps sought advice on whether or not a child's death was inevitable, so they could parse limited family resources,[32] others may have identified "Europeans"—their moniker for all white expatriates—as a source of education and knowledge, and still others may have attributed special healing power to white, Christian missionaries. Whatever their reasons, locals came and kept coming.[33]

Not everyone, however, was pleased with Peden's patient care. Unhappy with the new competition, native doctors put a hex on her—a curse they later withdrew when they needed her services themselves. Peden remained unafraid and "feisty," chasing machete-wielding, secret society men off missionaries' leased property with a broom when they threatened women who came to see her.[34]

Workforce Expansion

Glenna Peden also cultivated both a present and future healthcare workforce. Reports of her work from Lawrence Avenue COC's (LA-COC) pulpit drew nursing student Nancy Corinne Petty and physician Henry Farrar toward their own missionary futures.[35] Meanwhile, in Nigeria, she apprenticed missionary women colleagues as lay nurses, building on their knowledge of health, hygiene, and first aid.[36] That Peden-empowered cadre soon shared patient care, continued nursing during the Pedens' furloughs, passed on skills to new missionaries, and saved lives in new COC mission points. They gave aspirin for fever and chloroquine or quinine for malaria, used Vaseline-covered strips of torn bedsheets for dressings,

---

[29]Peden, Interview.
[30]Ibid.; H. Farrar, Interview 1.
[31]Chuku, *Igbo Women*, 19–24.
[32]Farrar, *Stand*, 77–78.
[33]Echols, "Beginning," 10.
[34]Peden, Interview.
[35]H. Farrar, Interview 1; Petty-Kraus, Interview 1.
[36]Peden, Interview.

and taught patients wound care and how to rehydrate infants using cooled, boiled water with salt and orange juice.[37]

Their volunteer nursing, however, came at a cost.[38] LA-COC provided in-kind support through shipped bandages and expired medications,[39] although we do not know when this began, its duration, and whether supply met demand. Moreover, each time missionaries drove someone to the hospital, they used costly petrol (gasoline), increased wear and tear on a vehicle, and engaged a mission car for a half day or more.[40] Ibibios sometimes brought dashes (gifts) of eggs or produce that defrayed missionaries' expenses, but the Americans charged no fees, an approach that worked to their advantage on at least one occasion. On that night when a menacing crowd with machetes and torches barricaded the road and demanded money, a nonthreatening Eugene Peden gained safe family passage by reminding them of Nurse Peden's gratis work.[41]

Nevertheless, evangelist men had raised US COC funds for travel, living, and preaching, not for nursing and makeshift ambulances. Thus, any dollar converted to shillings and pounds for healthcare came either from discretionary personal salaries or from carefully accounted business expense funds.[42] We know little of how the missionaries coped with financial and time demands, but we do know that more and more Nigerians sought care.[43] Perhaps to these first families, caring for the sick simply seemed another inevitable task of what it meant to be a missionary in that time and place. Shopping was different, roads were different, the climate different, and loving their neighbors as instructed by Jesus (Matthew 22:36-40) turned out to be different as well. Missionaries witnessed great need, incurred related costs, and praised backdoor nursing's "untold value."[44] For Glenna Peden nursing was not only "the right thing to do;" she "wanted to do" it, and she did it.[45]

No records suggest that missionaries solicited direct funding for their medical benevolence. Perhaps they feared that supporters would object to diverting resources from the COC priority of evangelism and worried that any ensuing controversy might halt their clinics. Such concerns were

---

[37] H. Farrar, Interview 1.
[38] Echols, "Beginning," 10.
[39] Peden, Interview.
[40] Ibid.; Goff, *Great*, 36.
[41] Peden, Interview.
[42] Ibid.; Bryant and Bryant, Interview.
[43] Echols, "Beginning," 10.
[44] Horton, quoted in Goff, *Great*, 23.
[45] Peden, Interview.

not unreasonable, for while COCs accepted caring for the sick as an appropriate, unpaid role for women, they summarily rejected the "social gospel"—good works devoid of direct efforts toward Christian conversion.[46] Thus, in the 1950s, COC women's nursing remained lauded, costly, and uncompensated.

Women's Work

Missionary women's nursing was remarkable given the rigors of life in Nigeria's deep bush. Both men and women worked hard, and the setting shaped their lives in ways that sometimes resembled America's frontier more than a 1950s middle-class lifestyle. Tasks of daily living necessitated personal responsibility and teamwork. Modern conveniences and utilities were absent, American-compatible schools nonexistent, and appliances and cars imported. Although by 1953 missionaries had upgraded their houses from mud and thatch to concrete block with screened windows, families still built cabinets and furnishings on site.[47] Moreover, as Reese and Echols projected for potentially homesick Americans: "Even with two families, it will be lonely and there is no social life except what you make for yourselves." The nearest known Westerners were miles-away Lutherans and a Church of Scotland family.[48]

This situation required adapting familiar roles and adopting new ones. Thus, in a gendered division of labor that mirrored US work, missionary men altered their public roles of preaching and teaching, and women adjusted their more private homemaking and childrearing work. In both US and Nigeria, the men preached, taught church members, and guided local congregations as they developed into communities that modeled a COC understanding of first-century worship. In Nigeria, however, missionaries encountered polygamy and other unfamiliar practices affecting Christian churches: household gods, fetishes, ancestor veneration, secret societies, cannibalism, and more as manifestations of an animistic worldview in which the physical and spiritual were one.[49] A Western-like division of sacred and secular was meaningless; spirit and matter instead were "interwoven… bound up in the bundle of life and as intimately related as the fibre to the tree."[50]

---

[46]H. Farrar, Interview 1.
[47]Goff, *Great*, 30–33; Echols, "Beginning," 8–10; Reese and Echols, *Report*, 14–18.
[48]Reese and Echols, *Report*, 18.
[49]H. Farrar, Interview 1; Nau, *We Move*; Peden, Interview.
[50]Basden, *Niger Ibos*, 33–53.

US evangelists also engaged in new work: preaching in open-air markets, educating preachers, constructing schools, managing government-funded primary schools where Bible was taught alongside other subjects, and launching a two-year Bible College preacher training school (BTC).[51] Their work was intense and complicated by poor (or no) roads, bridgeless river crossings, tropical weather, language and literacy barriers, and car breakdowns with limited repair options. The men also assisted with shopping, transportation, gardening, and building their houses.[52] After dark, when malarial mosquitos and other dangers emerged, they spent time at home with families.[53]

Missionary women faced perhaps a sharper contrast between their expected roles in the US versus in West Africa. Each was still a homemaker providing support to husband, children, and church, but enacting homemaking in rural Nigeria differed. Instead of overseeing teacher-assigned homework, the women became homeschool educators. Electricity was missing, and drinking water boiled. Cooking, cleaning, obtaining water, and caring for the grounds were so labor-intensive that they required the women to train and manage multiple household staff—a colonial solution that also created jobs. Wash water was heated over an open fire, food was cooked on wood stoves in separate kitchen buildings, and laundry was scrubbed by hand and pressed with a charcoal-heated iron. Workers hand-cut grass back from houses with a machete. Water flowed by gravity into houses from large metal shipping drums that were mounted on steps outside kitchen and bathroom—barrels alternately fed by roof run-off in rainy season and worker-fetched stream water in dry season. The women sewed clothes and curtains, corresponded with US family and friends, and provided healthcare to family members inside and locals outside their homes.[54] At least one wrote a short piece for a US church publication.[55]

Missionary women also shopped and planned meals differently to achieve results that satisfied American palates. The cost and "continual scarcity of food" necessitated creativity.[56] "Crackers are 70 cents per pound but bananas make it equal out by being five cents per dozen," wrote Emily Huffard (1920–2000), who arrived two months after the Pedens did and in the company of evangelist husband Elvis Huffard and

---

[51]Horton, quoted in Goff, *Great*, 22–27; Huffard, "Christian," 218–20.
[52]Echols, "Beginning," 9–10; Goff, *Great*, 27–28, 32.
[53]Broom, "Typical."
[54]Bryant, *Divine*; Farrar, *Stand*; Peden, Interview.
[55]Broom, "Typical."
[56]Echols, "Beginning," 9.

children Joyce, Sue, and Hy.[57] Perhaps this balancing act resulted in meals resembling Reese and Echols's 1950 supper of "pineapple, bananas, and limeade."[58] Moreover, while Eugene Peden wrote home enthusiastically about his prolific vegetable garden, purchasing meat in PH, and having "everything but Tennessee smoked sausage,"[59] his contemporary, Ida Palmer, wryly observed that it would take a book to document frustrations of their two-day PH resupply trips made every six weeks.[60]

Food preparation gained new complexity as well. A simple peanut butter sandwich required buying, shelling, roasting, winnowing, and grinding the peanuts as well as driving miles to buy bread ingredients to be kneaded and baked.[61] Although later missionary Patti Bryant said she did not believe the Lord expected any more of a wife on the mission field than a wife in the US,[62] running a household in mid-century Africa was a time-consuming venture, complicated by language differences. The Americans did not pursue language study, perhaps because of the eagerness of missionaries and Nigerians alike to start Bible instruction, the large number of local languages and dialects, and the teaching of Oxford English in colonial schools. Nonetheless, new missionaries struggled to understand Nigerian-accented British English, and Nigerians wrestled with missionaries' American English.[63] US COCs mandated no language learning for missionaries, and missionaries expected only minimal English proficiency from their staff.

Mirroring other US roles, missionary women also taught women and children's church classes. Prohibited by COC doctrine from leading public worship when men were present, women seized the opportunity to educate society's most vulnerable. By late 1954, five women engaged in this outreach: Emily Huffard led the work alongside Mildred Horton, Rosa Lee Johnson, Glenna Peden, and Nwa A. Ukpong Essien (C.A.O. Essien's wife). Their classes differed from the men's not only in audience, but also in content, with Nurse Peden teaching health as requested by locals. The other women focused on Bible instruction.[64] Thus, despite COC restrictions on their church speech, missionary women began to

---

[57]Goff, *Great*, 24, 61; Huffard, quoted in Goff, *Great*, 28; "Elvis Henry Huffard," March 20, 2010, findagrave.com no. 49977737; "Emily Ann King Hufford," January 4, 2014, findagrave.com no. 122768294.

[58]Reese and Echols, *Report*, 42.

[59]Peden, quoted in Goff, *Great*, 28.

[60]Palmer, "Narrative," 15.

[61]Farrar, *Stand*, 136.

[62]G. Farrar, Interview.

[63]Echols, "Beginning," 9; Farrar, *Stand*, 15, 26–27.

[64]Echols, "Beginning," 9–10; Horton, quoted in Goff, *Great*, 23, 25.

shape the entire Nigerian church-to-come by teaching all children, as well as the women.

Like their husbands, US women lectured in English with sentence-to-sentence translation by Nwa Essien or others. Christian songs, however, were a different matter, and missionaries used the Efik language in the participative, community act of COC a cappella singing. Variable spoken words could be translated piecemeal in real time, but fixed hymn lyrics required translation in advance. Consequently, US supporters shipped 10,000 Efik-language hymnals to Nigeria, while Nwa helped missionary women translate US Christian children's songs into Efik—an effort well-received by audiences "ages 4 to 84."[65] Perhaps singing in their heart language facilitated locals' adding a new Christian identity without rejecting their Ibibio one.

Missionary men greeted the women's classes with enthusiasm, and evangelist Horton wrote to supporting churches that the COC mission would fail without their work. In 1954, he placed their classes as fifth on his list of seven mission highlights. Nwa Ukpong, "a well-trained Nigerian lady," he reported, assisted missionary women in teaching large, eager groups in villages of Ikot Usen, Use Ndon, and Ikot Adaidem. In the Ikot Adaidem Friday classes,

> Mrs. Huffard teaches the women, Mrs. Horton and Mrs. Johnson teach the children, and Mrs. Peden...gives the women elementary instructions in hygiene, food care, simple first aid, care of children, etc. Womanhood is tragic in this country. The women are many times no more than chattel property, serving the husbands almost as slaves. Few can read. Ignorance, superstition and almost tragic resignation hold them down. The church can never be really strong until the women and children are reached.[66]

For Horton, elevating the status of local women through education was critical to achieving functioning church communities, and he delighted in their desire to learn. He, of course, expected US supporters to join in his enthusiasm for Bible classes, while he may have been concerned that some might see health instruction as stealing time from Bible study. Perhaps this is why he was careful to explain that Glenna deliver health edu-

---

[65]Horton, quoted in Goff, *Great*, 25.

[66]Ibid. Barnes in *Rough* describes mid-1950's existence of both powerful Efik women's societies from which men were excluded and the formidable economic control of some women lorry owners and traders.

19

cation on Fridays, not Sundays, the COC day of worship. Additionally, Horton noted that Glenna Peden's classes were by "special request of the village,"[67] placing her work solidly within the raison d'etre for the entire Ikot Usen project. It was Essien's pleading that brought COC missionaries to Nigeria, and Horton's audience knew that story well. Finally, in 1950s etiquette, Horton's use of each woman's formal married name conferred power by association with her better-known husband yet highlighted how the women made missionary work their own.

Vocation Embraced

Ida Palmer, the Pedens' housemate for six months,[68] wrote decades later of Glenna Peden's work and character. Eugene Peden was seldom home during the day while Glenna provided backdoor care, planned meals, directed the family's "1 cook, 2 stewards, 2 yardmen, a laundry man and one or two night watchmen," and homeschooled their children. Nurse Peden, she mused, was like the biblical, worthy woman in Proverbs 31, who—rather than being a domestic prisoner—was wise and virtuous, honored her husband, and attended successfully to her own business, land, and family. Glenna Peden's caring, "love for the Lord and concern for the people of Nigeria was evident in every phase of... daily living."[69] She "fully embraced" nursing and took her and Eugene's "'calling' very seriously."[70] Such intentional engagement suggested that her enthusiasm for the Nigeria work was equal to her husband's[71] and revealed a contrast between her mid-twentieth-century views and those of mid-nineteenth-century Florence Nightingale, who rejected marriage for herself so that she might fully follow her nursing calling to serve the sick and poor.[72] Glenna Peden found marriage, her practice, and patients' gratitude satisfying, and she enjoyed laughter, vacations, and teammates. Nonetheless, slow trans-Atlantic communications were painful, and her worst day in Nigeria was when she received mailed news of her mother's unexpected death and pictures from the funeral six weeks earlier.[73]

---

[67]Ibid.

[68]Palmer, "Memories," 16–17.

[69]Ida Palmer attachment to Pat Pleasant, email to author, September 4, 2014.

[70]Ida Palmer, quoted in Pat Pleasant, email to author, September 6, 2014.

[71]Peden, Interview.

[72]Cook, *Life*, 99–104.

[73]Peden, Interview.

Conclusion

The explicit aim of the Pedens and this first wave of COC missionary families was to support Nigeria's indigenous Christian restoration movement. To that spiritual purpose, Glenna Peden added physical care. Her four-part Nigerian operationalization of missionary nursing garnered positive attention, perhaps because of its status as supererogatory, voluntary women's work "on the side."[74] Still, even that modest clinical practice soon competed with evangelism for human, time, transportation, and funding resources.

---

[74]Ibid.

3
Going to Nigeria, Come What May
(1955–1958)

And so we came…sight unseen.
—Patti Bryant

Volunteer nursing practice soon became a daily routine. Thus, when the Pedens furloughed in 1955 after two years in the field, a second and then third wave of missionary women inherited local expectations of care.[1] Among the second wave was Lou Anna McNeil Bawcom (1917–1986), who moved to Ikot Usen in 1954 alongside her evangelist husband, Burney Eli Bawcom, and their three young sons. LA-COC sponsored the Bawcoms, and Lou Anna likely learned lay nursing from Glenna Peden during their overlapping nine months.[2]

Other eager workers arrived just three weeks after the Pedens left in August 1955. Unmarried June Hobbs accompanied novice missionaries, Wendell Wright and Betty Madge Billingsley Broom (1924–) and their four young children,[3] and Broom later summarized his family's preparation for Nigeria as "one notch above zero."[4] Several northeastern US congregations supported Hobbs, and the Brooms were sponsored by the Tenth and Francis Street COC in Oklahoma City.[5]

Housemates Hobbs and Betty Broom staffed the morning clinic, and Lou Anna Bawcom handled the afternoon one. Together they treated "a constant stream of sick people… [with] appalling …wounds and illnesses…: extensive burns, deep tropical ulcers, badly infected cuts, [and]

---

[1]H. Farrar, Interview 1; Goff, *Great*.
[2]"Burney Eli Bawcom," September 30, 2008, findagrave.com no. 30204463; "Lou Anna McNeil Bawcom," April 10, 2013, findagrave.com no. 108277741; Goff, *Great*, 30, 61.
[3]Brewer, *Missionary*, 38–39; Goff, *Great*, 31; Granberg, "Wendell Broom," 3–18; Wendell Broom Sr., findagrave.com no. 176516725.
[4]Granberg, "Wendell Broom," 2.
[5]Goff, *Great*, 31.

fevers of all descriptions." Missionaries still transported worst cases to distant hospitals because locals didn't trust the eight-mile-away ambulance, and Betty Broom concluded that "a registered nurse would be worth her weight in gold."[6]

The next year, the number of lay nurses rose to four. The furloughing Bawcoms were replaced in 1956 by Calvin Leonard and Bernice Cagle Johnson (1911–2010) with their teenage daughter, Janice.[7] The Johnson women likely took over afternoon clinics, and Janice drove the ill to hospitals, served as a secretary to the evangelists, taught women's Bible classes, distributed medications during late afternoons, and treated wounds at the back door until summer 1957 when she left for the US with Hobbs. June exited because of poor health, and Janice left to begin college. The Johnsons were supported by Sunset Ridge COC in San Antonio, Texas, with assistance from LA-COC,[8] and no records suggest that Janice's parents completed more than a single two-year tour in Nigeria. (Leonard Johnson, however, did co-lead a group of short-term missionaries to Nigeria during summer 1966.)[9]

In Nigeria Leonard Johnson took up Lucien Palmer's mantle of managing eleven village schools and their approximately seventy-five teachers, but soon concluded that COCs should discontinue that work. Locals and US missionary colleagues disagreed with him, and the majority won the day. Nonetheless, Johnson's concern galvanized Palmer and others to establish the US nonprofit Nigeria Christian Schools Foundation to manage and fundraise both for the village schools and for a planned COC Nigerian Christian Secondary School (NCSS). Another purpose of the Foundation (later renamed African Christian Schools Foundation)[10] was likely to minimize COC debate over whether direct congregational funding of schools was biblically permissible.

Mary Kelton, RN

On July 12, 1957, during the middle of the Johnsons' tour, a second COC US registered nurse arrived in Ikot Usen: Mary Buel Rogers Kelton,

---

[6]Broom, "Typical."

[7]Goff, *Great*, 32; Harp, "Calvin Leonard Johnson (1910-1994);"
Bernice Cagle Johnson," August 5, 2010, findagrave.com no. 55919070.

[8]Goff, *Great*, 32, 34–36.

[9]Chronicle News, "Month-long."

[10]Church of Christ Nigeria, "Church History;" Goff, *Great*, 32, 40–41; Huffard, "Christian," 219–21.

RN, with her evangelist husband, Tom, and preschool daughters.[11] Born August 14, 1921, to Clinton and Stella Rogers in Caddo, Oklahoma, Kelton graduated from high school in 1938 in Caldwell, Kansas, where her father's postal service job had taken them. After earning her nursing diploma at the Dallas Methodist Hospital School of Nursing in 1942, she served during WWII as first lieutenant and flight nurse in the Army Nurse Corps at Randolph Field in San Antonio, Texas (1943–1946).[12]

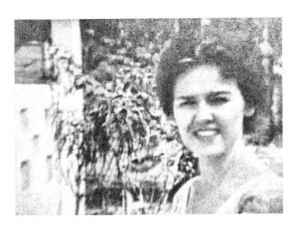

Photograph 3. Mary B. Rogers Kelton, RN. Ikot Usen mission compound. ca. 1957 (private collection with permission).

Following her honorable discharge, Rogers relocated to Abilene, Texas, to attend Abilene Christian College (ACC) on the GI Bill. There she experienced a self-described life-changing Christian baptism in the COC, worked as an ACC school nurse,[13] completed her BA in Greek magna cum laude in May 1952, and received the Dean's Award for her achievements as an outstanding student.[14] From Abilene, Rogers moved to Florida Christian College (FCC) in Temple Terrace, Florida, where she taught Greek and worked as school nurse. There she met and married FCC student, Tom Kelton, who was ten years her junior. This was his first marriage and her second.[15] Tom began preaching in COC congregations, and

---

[11]Goff, *Great*, 34, 62.

[12]Abilene, "Experiences," 77; Doe and Fraga, Interview; Mary Buel Rogers, Nursing Diploma, Dallas Methodist Hospital, May 3, 1942 (private collection); Wofford, "Resume."

[13]Doe and Fraga, Interview; Wofford, "Resume."

[14]McGarvey Ice, email to author, July 29, 2019.

[15]Kelton, *More*, 22; "Mrs. Mary Kelton Wofford," Obituary.

the couple soon delightedly welcomed daughters CeLeste and Starr.[16] During Tom's tenure in Odessa, Texas, Mary Kelton taught at Mary Meek School of Nursing, Hendrick Memorial Hospital in Abilene (1954–1957).[17]

Meanwhile, Tom became interested in Nigeria because of its flourishing COC growth. He enthusiastically reported on those COC successes in his *Nigerian Torch* newsletter and convinced the Southside COC in Odessa, to sponsor his family as missionaries. After difficult visa acquisitions,[18] the Keltons boarded a New York freighter in June 1957, and a month later cleared Nigerian customs with their "'57 Chevrolet pick-up, a kerosene refrigerator, an iron cook stove, a gasoline clothes washer, and all…personal belongings."[19] Their July 12 arrival at the newer COC compound in Ukpom surprised resident missionaries, and the four Keltons likely moved in with the soon-to-depart six Brooms in Ikot Usen eighteen miles away. Tom's sponsoring congregation purchased the Brooms' Ikot Usen house from LA-COC for the Keltons; Leonard and Bernice Johnson became Keltons' next door neighbors.[20]

Meanwhile, planned missionary furloughs were already shrinking the volunteer nursing workforce at Ikot Usen. Janice Johnson and June Hobbs left before the Keltons came, and two weeks after the Keltons' arrival, the Brooms set sail for the US.[21] This left only Mary Kelton and Bernice Johnson to provide backdoor care, and when the Johnsons, too, furloughed a few months later, Nurse Kelton became the only missionary woman at Ikot Usen. There, for about six weeks, she managed a solo practice that was previously covered by four women, until finally novice missionaries Joe and Dorothy Cross arrived with young Scott and Melody.[22]

Meanwhile, COCs added two new mission compounds in Ukpom (est. 1954) and in Onicha Ngwa (est. 1957), and where evangelists went, COC nursing followed. Ukpom compound families included returning Palmers and Brooms as well as the novice Sewell and Caneta Hall family with preschoolers Gardner and Cherry. The Finney and Nicks families relocated from Ukpom to Onicha Ngwa, and the returning Pedens and inexperienced Bryants joined them there, as detailed in Chapter 4. Jimmy and

---

[16]Kelton, *More*, 22–23.

[17]Wofford, "Resume."

[18]Goff, *Great*, 34; Kelton, *More*, 23–24.

[19]Kelton, *More*, 24.

[20]Eno Otoyo, email to author, May 3, 2018; Goff, *Great*, 34, 62; Kelton, *More*, 24–25.

[21]Goff, *Great*, 36, 62.

[22]P. Bryant to Family, May 28, 1958.

Rosa Lee Johnson, C. Leonard and Bernice Johnson, the Huffards, the Hortons, and June Hobbs furloughed permanently.[23]

"Swamped"

When the Keltons first arrived, Betty Broom and Bernice Johnson likely mentored Mary in new routines, and soon she was running backdoor clinics, managing a nanny, cook, and laundryman, shopping in local markets, buying bananas by the stalk, and using groundnuts (peanuts) as the family's major protein source. She later joked about her "running water" —water fetched by her yardman on foot from the stream. The Kelton family healthcare routine included taking antimalarials, installing mosquito nets, boiling water, and ironing laundry to kill parasites. In addition, Mary needed an emergency appendectomy, which was probably performed at a Medical Mission of Mary (MMM) hospital.[24]

Nurse Kelton was as proud of her Nigerian practice as of her WWII service,[25] and she later described her African patients as "humble and grateful" with "poise and confidence."[26] Nonetheless, the clinic workload was heavy, and Wendell Broom wrote that during her first days Kelton was "swamped with patients anxious to be treated by the 'new nurse.'"[27] Those who couldn't or wouldn't travel the miles of bush paths for hospital care lined up at dawn for Kelton's attention[28] with problems including "malaria, tropical ulcers...worms...malnutrition, and hernias from carrying very heavy loads on their heads."[29]

Kelton did what she could with what she had. She removed parasitic (probably Guinea or Loa loa[30]) worms from the skin by gradually winding them onto an applicator, treated wounds, and administered expired medications shipped by US friends, who occasionally included toys and shoes for her delighted daughters. Additionally, her household staff helped to tear and roll cloth strips for bandages, and Kelton cleaned and sharpened her own reusable glass syringes and needles. She spent long hours teaching patients about nutrition and hygiene and probably contin-

---

23Goff, *Great*, 61–63; Nicks, "Unexpected," 77–79.
24Doe and Fraga, Interview; Golightly, "Medicine." Golightly mis-records the nearest hospital as Enugu.
25Jane Doe, email to author, July 31, 2017.
26Golightly, "Medicine."
27Broom, quoted in Goff, *Great*, 31.
28Doe and Fraga, Interview; Golightly, "Medicine."
29Golightly, "Medicine."
30H. Farrar to Massey, November 18, 1965, W-COC file.

ued taking the most ill to nearby hospitals; there, providers delivered ether anesthesia for some procedures by dripping it onto cloths covering patients' faces.[31]

Alike, Yet Different

In many ways, Mary Kelton was much like her RN predecessor, Glenna Peden. Born respectively in 1921 and 1920, both were in their thirties when they arrived in rural 1950s colonial Nigeria. Each accompanied an evangelist husband, was a US-educated RN, and had two young daughters. Peden nursed uncounted locals; Kelton reportedly served "10,000."[32]

In other ways, they differed. Unlike Peden, Kelton did not register as a nurse in Nigeria, and she initially hesitated to go. As Tom Kelton wrote later, "the Nigeria idea was more mine than Mary's...After I talked more and more about this new venture, Mary did not object and finally agreed that it was a good idea." Furthermore, Glenna Peden proactively began a backdoor nursing practice, while Mary Kelton inherited local expectations of the same.[33] The pioneering Peden, J. Johnson, Horton, and Huffard families built their missionary roles while they learned, so that the work matched their knowledge, interests, energies, and talents. In the second missionary wave, the Palmers, Brooms, Bawcoms, L. Johnsons, and Hobbs continued to develop initiatives while maintaining existing work. As part of a third wave, the Keltons inherited five years of established group efforts.

Moreover, while earlier Ikot Usen missionaries formed a close-knit team, the Keltons' relationships with immediate missionary neighbors were sometimes strained. Neither the Johnson nor Cross families were happy in Nigeria, and so may have provided little social support to the Keltons.[34] Still, the Bryants in Onicha Ngwa and Keltons rendered mutual care during difficult times. Tom Kelton and Rees Bryant had been college classmates, and Tom's "fiery" *Nigerian Torch* newsletter triggered the Bryants' decision to move to Nigeria in 1958.[35] In the field, Rees Bryant described Tom as "zealous and able," and Bryant's daughter enjoyed the

---

[31]Doe and Fraga, Interview; Golightly, "Medicine."

[32]Doe and Fraga, Interview; Kelton, *More*, 25; Peden, Interview.

[33]Kelton, *More*, 25.

[34]P. Bryant to Mattoxes, February 7 and July 3, 1959.

[35]Bryant, *Divine*, 3; Bryant and Bryant, Interview.

Kelton girls.[36] Patti Bryant found Mary Kelton "a real blessing....a 'life-saver'"[37] in treating Patti's personal health problems, and the families met together for meals, visits, and collaborative work despite the thirty miles of bad roads between them.[38]

Additionally, the Keltons' intrafamily support seemed less robust than that enjoyed by other missionary families. Betty Broom, for example, wrote that their Ikot Usen work typically ceased after sunset, allowing the family to spend quiet evenings together at home.[39] The Keltons did not follow this pattern, and although missionary contemporaries admired Tom Kelton's evangelistic fervor, they grew increasingly concerned about the Kelton family as they witnessed Tom's "extreme highs" and nonstop work to evangelize "all Nigeria." He loved preaching in distant towns like Abakaliki, Enugu, and Onitsha, leaving his wife and daughters alone for days with no communications and no knowledge of his whereabouts.[40] Only years later did Kelton acknowledge how his behavior damaged family cohesion.[41]

Reese and Echols had anticipated challenges to Ikot Usen missionaries' physical and emotional health, and thus recommended stationing "not less than two white families" together.[42] But without strong support between those families, Reese and Echols's precaution proved inadequate, and as her second year in the field began, Mary Kelton prematurely started packing for home. She was exhausted by loneliness, bouts of malaria, her appendectomy, one six-week period as the only Ikot Usen missionary family, and lack of privacy from Nigerian evangelist men working out of her home. New theological questions troubled her, and novice missionary Dorothy Cross, who needed encouragement herself, likely provided little support to Mary.[43] In early December 1958, these challenges became "too much for her,"[44] and when Mary Kelton again fell ill with malaria, she returned to the US with her daughters. US colleagues offered to

---

[36]R. Bryant to E. Bryants, April 9, 1958; P. Bryant to Mattoxes, October 31, 1958.
[37]Bryant and Bryant, Interview.
[38]Ibid.; P. Bryant, email to author, February 14, 2012; P. Bryant to Family, August 25, 1958; R. Bryant to Mattoxes, April 5, 1958; R. Bryant to E. Bryants, April 9, 1958; R. Bryant, "Newsletter No. 3" May 1, 1958, in Bryant letters.
[39]Broom, "Typical."
[40]P. Bryant to Mattoxes, February 7, 1959; R. Bryant, "Nigerian Highlights–1959;" Bryant and Bryant, Interview; Kelton, *More*, 25.
[41]Kelton, *More*, 23.
[42]Reese and Echols, *Report*, 20.
[43]P. Bryant to Mattoxes, April 15, 1958 and February 7, 1959; P. Bryant to Family, May 28, 1958; Salmon to Bryants, March 15, 1961.
[44]Bryant and Bryant, Interview.

cover Tom Kelton's Nigeria responsibilities and urged him to return with his family, but he insisted on staying in Nigeria and furloughed a month later on January 6, 1959, only after he learned of his wife's hospitalization in the US.[45] During these difficulties, Mary Kelton struggled to remain positive, attributing her difficulties "to worry" and expressing no public animosity toward Tom. Nothing, however, suggested that she shared his view that "family life 'in the bush' had been good for" their marriage.[46] Six months after Keltons left, the Crosses also departed Ikot Usen earlier than planned, when they, too, were overwhelmed by isolation, illness, and homesickness.[47]

Soon, the Keltons moved to Abilene where Mary resumed hospital nursing and Tom completed his undergraduate degree at ACC with straight "A" grades. After graduation, he returned to fulltime preaching in the Texas towns of Pharr and then Sharpstown, where, in his words, he "pushed Mary very hard." After a serious disagreement, she and the girls returned to Abilene. Tom followed them, but the marriage dissolved as his behavioral health issues grew.[48]

In Abilene, Mary Kelton earned her master's of education at Hardin-Simmons University (1970) and remarried in 1973, assuming the surname Wofford.[49] She worked in a variety of care and leadership nursing roles in Texas, including at the Abilene State School, Hendrick Memorial Hospital, and Tarrant County Junior College.[50] In 1977, her chapter of the American Business Women's Association selected her as Woman of the Year, and in 1996 Mary returned to Nigeria for a two-year tour at the Nigerian Christian College near Ukpom, where she delighted in teaching first aid, hygiene, and nutrition to ninety-three attentive students. Unfortunately, ill health compelled her US return after only a few months, and she eventually retired in Abilene, then moved to Colleyville, Texas, near daughter CeLeste. Kelton remained active in the COC until her death at age ninety-one, and she is buried in the Dallas-Fort Worth National Cemetery.[51]

Tom Kelton never returned to Nigeria. After successful psychiatric treatment for his cyclic mania and depression (1963–1971), he married

---

[45]Ibid.; P. Bryant to Mattoxes, February 7, 1959; R. Bryant to Folks, January 5, 1959.
[46]Kelton, *More*, 26.
[47]P. Bryant to Mattoxes, July 3 and July 4, 1959.
[48]Kelton, *More*, 28.
[49]Doe and Fraga, Interview; Master of Education Diploma, May 18, 1970, JD.
[50]Golightly, "Medicine;" Wofford "Resume."
[51]Doe and Fraga, Interview; "Mary B. Rogers Wofford," December 28, 2014, findagrave.com no. 140587203.

Betty Jane Wortham Walker in 1985.[52] Motivated both by a desire to help others and his physician's encouragement, Kelton detailed his mental health struggles in a 1995 autobiography, in which he expressed gratitude for "the army of friends that stood by me." Kelton preached in the COC until his 1998 death, that was precipitated by the lithium that kept him functional.[53]

Conclusion

COC missionaries enjoyed neither the benefits nor the restrictions of a church-wide mission society that might assist or constrain them; COCs argued that such societies were not biblically authorized. Instead, families developed work that matched both their capabilities and the expectations of supporting congregations. Preparation for many was informal counsel from returning COC missionaries.[54] For most missionary families, that counsel sufficed, but others found their best intentions undermined by isolation, personal frailty, demanding work, and inadequate preparatory guidance. The result was trial and error learning in the field, and in 1959 Wendell Broom wrote to US supporters that intending COC missionaries should prepare more systematically. Reflecting on his own experience, Broom argued that novice COC missionaries could learn much from recorded experiences of their COC predecessors and "denominationalists" with decades of experience.[55]

Given the COC 1950s state of affairs of mission education, it is perhaps less remarkable that a few missionaries experienced personal crises in Nigeria, than that so many flourished. As Patti Bryant later reflected, none of them knew about culture shock or studied culture, missions, or language: "We were the untrained Have-Bible-Will-Travel kind of missionaries...We...heard from the other missionaries that the Nigerians were asking for missionaries to train their preachers....and so we came... sight unseen, *come what may*."[56]

---

[52]"Tom Kelton," July 10, 2010, findagrave.com no. 54744592.

[53]Ibid.; Kelton, *More*, 108.

[54]Bryant, *Divine*, 3–8, 23–24; Farrar, *Stand*, 12–15, 186–87; Lawyer, untitled questionnaire, ca. 1961, RPB:N; Nicks, "Our First," 6–7. See also Chapter 10.

[55]Broom, "Newsletter, No. 36," August 16, 1959, RPB:N.

[56]Bryant, *Divine*, 23.

4
Nursing Spreads Into Igboland
(1957–1959)

People were coming day and night.
—Gerry Nicks

Incidental nursing soon took root alongside evangelism in Igboland.[1] While June Hobbs, Betty Broom, and Bernice Johnson delivered care in Ikot Usen and others did so in Ukpom, Geraldine "Gerry" Nicks (1924–2012),[2] began a practice at Onicha Ngwa on the newest COC compound. She was not a registered nurse, and she did not intend a clinic. The ill and injured simply came.[3]

Gerry Nicks's family came to Igboland through Ukpom in Ibibioland. Mid-century accounts of rapid church growth in Nigeria had inspired Proctor Street COC in Port Arthur, Texas, to look for "the right man" to send as an evangelist. This they found in Gerry's husband, John William "J.W." (or "Bill") Nicks. Concurrently Howard Horton's vision for a new work among Ibibio neighbors, the Igbos, resonated with the couple, and Horton lent them his advice and fundraising help.[4] After landing in Port Harcourt (PH) in October 1955, they asked Lucien and Ida Palmer if they could share the Palmers' two-bedroom home in Ukpom, where Lucien served as Bible College (BTC) principal. The Palmers were gracious, and the families compatible. Gerry and Bill Nicks took one bedroom, and the Palmers kept the other, while part of the living room was cur-

---

[1]Basden writes that "Igbo" and "Ibo" are used interchangeably by westerners to refer to a people, land, and language. "Ibo" may be Anglicized Igbo (*Niger Ibos*, xi-xxii).
[2]"Geraldine May Petty Nicks," January 28, 2013, findagrave.com no. 104292616; Goff, *Great*, 34–36.
[3]Nicks, "Unexpected," 77–79.
[4]"John William 'Bill' Nicks," January 22, 2013, findagrave.com no. 104003629; Nicks, "Our First," 6–8; Summerlin to R. Bryant, October 18, 1961.

tained off for school-aged Becky, Jeanie, and Sue Nicks.[5] "The five Nicks and...four Palmers" shared expenses and chores and built a friendship that lasted a lifetime.[6]

Ten months later, James and Mary Louise Finney, with sons Joe, Timmy, and Mark, also arrived in Ukpom. Then in January 1957, both the Finney and the Nicks families relocated to Onicha Ngwa to begin a BTC modeled after the Ukpom one.[7] With colonial government permission, the Nicks became housemates for almost a year with the numerous gecko occupants of a nonelectrified, plumbing-less, abandoned British building at Mile 11 Aba-Ikot Ekpene road.[8] The location was along the missionaries' PH-to-Ukpom and PH-to-Ikot Usen routes. Bill Nicks and James Finney leased fifteen acres from Chief Ebere (also Ibere) of Ntigha Onicha Ngwa on July 6 for thirty years at $30 per year, selected forty Igbo preaching students, and began building two missionary houses and other BTC buildings.[9] Locals leased the tribal battleground acreage to the Christian missionaries to see whether they could deal with the feared spirits of the dead inhabiting it.[10] Missionaries at the time were likely unaware.

"Part-time Nurse"

Homemaking still required hiring and directing staff to launder clothes, cook, and clean—all without running water, electricity, or modern appliances—and so Gerry Nicks noted multiple advantages to having staff when "you're not rich." Locals needed jobs, and workers freed her time for teaching and provided insight into local culture. The Nicks hired Christians who "were...brothers [...] more than servants," and she later wrote that Mark Apollos became "a real friend....[who] could cheer us up when we were down and encourage us to go on when we felt like giving up." As staff became part of the Nicks family, likewise, were missionaries drawn into confidences about the ups and downs of their workers' lives, and Igbo-American relationships prospered.[11]

[5]Nicks, "Familiarity," 9–11; Goff, *Great*, 31.

[6]Palmer, "Memories," 16.

[7]Bryant, *Divine*, 10; Goff, *Great*, 36, 41; Nicks, "Narrative."

[8]Bryant, *Gently*, bk. 3, 83; Bryant, "Newsletter No. 8," August 5, 1959, RPB:N; Nicks, "Okorobeke," 22; Nicks, "Narrative."

[9]Walker, "Summary," 170; Echols, "Beginning," 11; Goff, *Great*, 33;

[10]Farrar, *Stand*, 71.

[11]Nicks, "Why?," 67–69. See also Wilson, "Biography."

Gerry Nicks declared herself a "full-time teacher and part-time nurse."[12] Her nursing, which likely began in Ukpom and continued in Onicha Ngwa, was triggered more by local demand than missionary plan. Household staff translated during clinics held in a shed behind her home in order to minimize the impact on her homeschooling, household chores, and Bible classes. Unlike Glenna Peden, Nicks allowed her daughters access to the clinic, at least for one photo opportunity, and people came at all hours with dysentery, malaria, tropical ulcers, belly pain, headaches, accidental injuries, difficult deliveries, tetanus, and more. Missionaries drove serious cases to the hospital, and Nicks "gave out so many aspirin during the Asian flu epidemic that they called it 'the white man's ju-ju.'"[13]

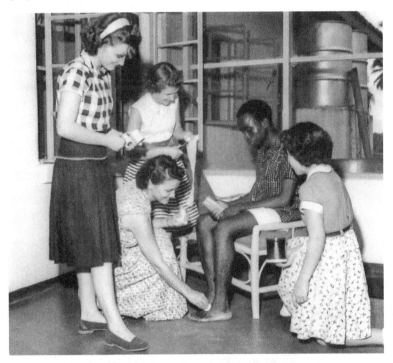

Photograph 4.1. "Our first hospital:" Gerry Nicks delivering care in shed behind her house, Onicha Ngwa. Daughters Becky, Jeanie, and Susie Nicks looking on. ca. 1959. (Nicks-Crocker collection with permission.)

---

[12]Nicks, "Why?," 67.
[13]Jeannie Nicks Crocker, Facebook Messenger to author, March 29, 2020; Nicks, "Healing Prophet," 45; Nicks, "Unexpected," 77–79.

Gerry Nicks's only home visit was to a woman who was unable to walk to the mission compound because "the flesh [of her leg] was eaten away to the bone." Gerry daily washed the malodorous wound with hydrogen peroxide and applied Terramycin powder until the woman could ambulate again. The Terramycin, she wrote, came from Batsell Barrett Baxter, a name likely used as proxy for the Nashville, Tennessee, Hillsboro COC where he preached.[14]

Changing of the Guard

That same year, the Pedens arrived in Onicha Ngwa for their second two-year tour (1957–1959), instead of returning to Ikot Usen where the Johnsons and Keltons occupied both houses.[15] The Pedens moved in with the Nicks family, who soon furloughed, and shortly thereafter the Pedens gained new housemates: Patti Nell Mattox Bryant (1933–), her evangelist husband, Rees Odeil Bryant (1930–), and their toddler Sara Jo and infant Billy. Proctor Street COC financially supported Rees, while Glenna Peden and Mary Louise Finney morally supported a delighted Patti. Patti thus became Peden's newest student in tropical nursing.[16]

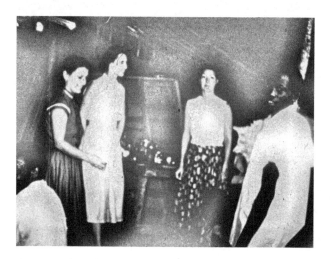

Photograph 4.2. Gerry Nicks, Patti Bryant, and Glenna Peden, RN, in backdoor shed clinic, Onicha Ngwa. 1958. (Author collection of slides.)

---

[14]Nicks, "Unexpected," 77–79; Harp, "Batsell Barrett Baxter (1916–1982)."
[15]Goff, *Great,* 62.
[16]Bryant, *Divine,* 3–12; Brewer, *Missionary,* 39; P. Bryant to Mattoxes, March 16, 1958; Bryant and Bryant, Interview; Peden, Interview.

Patti Bryant's nursing apprenticeship, however, was short-lived. In Ukpom the Palmers' ten-year-old son developed tuberculosis, necessitating his family's abrupt return to the States, and the Pedens immediately relocated to Ukpom to fill BTC duties vacated by Lucien Palmer. Thus, within a month of arrival, Patti Bryant inherited Glenna Peden's practice, and Rees became heir to Eugene's ambitious preaching and teaching schedule. The effects of having inadequate healthcare for missionaries rippled through the COC compounds.[17]

Meanwhile, Glenna Peden continued nursing in Ukpom, so that by the time the Pedens left Nigeria permanently in 1959, Glenna had provided care from all three COC compounds: Ikot Usen, Onicha Ngwa, and Ukpom. In the US Glenna Peden continued working alongside Eugene during his preaching jobs in Michigan, Tennessee, Kentucky, and Indiana. They fostered children from 1967 to 1979, and she cared for Eugene during his final years. Glenna kept her RN license active, but in shyness refused an invitation to teach about tropical diseases in Vanderbilt University's nursing program in Nashville. She actively volunteered in a variety of organizations until her death at age ninety-one in 2012.[18]

Pivot Point

Within the first twenty-four hours of the Bryants' arrival in Onicha Ngwa, their thinking about COC-delivered healthcare was transformed. On the morning of March 14, 1958, as twenty-seven-year old Rees Bryant walked down to observe BTC classes he was met by a bicyclist with his injured brother on the back luggage carrier. The injured man had ruptured a hernia while hoeing yams that morning, and the bicyclist begged Rees to take his brother to the hospital.[19]

For Bryant, the choice was clear. If he planned to preach about loving his neighbor as himself, he must act accordingly. He borrowed a car and drove the men eight miles on the unfamiliar, left side of the road to a place he had never been: the Medical Missionaries of Mary (MMM) hospital in Urua Akpan. There the injured man "was rushed into surgery" while Rees returned home. That afternoon, MMM staff sent a note via a bicycle messenger: "I'm sorry to inform you, Mr. Bryant, but the man

---

[17] P. Bryant to Mattoxes, March 14, 16, and 25, 1958; Bryant and Bryant, Interview.
[18] Peden, Interview; Peden, "Chronology."
[19] P. Bryant to Mattoxes, March 16, 1958; Bryant, "Reflections," 20; Bryant and Bryant, Interview.

you brought to us today died on the operating table."[20] Rees Bryant was stunned; his prior inattention to medical missions gone. Abruptly, the Bryants found they could no more ignore Nigerians' physical needs than they could ignore the spiritual ones that brought them to Igboland.[21]

Ten days later, on March 23, their attention was riveted to missionaries' own physical needs. The Bryants had just seen the Palmers return to the US for medical care, and now the day after Glenna Peden, their health-security-blanket, left for Ukpom, two-and-a-half-year-old Sara Bryant developed a 104-degree fever, vomiting, and diarrhea. As self-labeled "inexperienced parents and new, scared missionaries," her parents rushed her to Urua Akpan MMM for medication.[22] When Sara was no better the next day, they drove her forty miles to the larger MMM in Anua. There, Patti Bryant held down her screaming daughter while providers started intravenous (IV) rehydration fluids. Meanwhile, a worried Rees Bryant drove forty miles home to check on six-month-old Billy, who had been left in their cook's care. Determining that Billy was fine, he drove forty miles back to Anua. Sara was still crying, and Rees Bryant demanded that staff remove the IV. Fortunately, Sara had tonsillitis, not the malaria they feared, and while her physical healing was swift, she experienced nightmares for weeks.[23]

Moreover, only four weeks later the Finneys unexpectedly left to obtain urgently needed medical care in the US—a shuffling of missionaries that, alongside the Johnsons' Ikot Usen furlough, left the Bryants alone at Onicha Ngwa and the Keltons solo at Ikot Usen[24] as described in Chapter 3. It was during this time that the families coped by joining forces, and Tom Kelton drove to Onicha Ngwa twice a week to assist with BTC teaching.[25] Seven weeks later, the relieved Bryants welcomed the returning Nicks family in Onicha Ngwa, and Gerry Nicks proved a welcome comfort to Patti Bryant, mentoring her in every aspect of missionary women's work.[26]

---

[20]Bryant, "Reflections," 20; Bryant and Bryant, Interview; Medical Missionaries, "Milestones."

[21]Bryant and Bryant, Interview.

[22]Bryant, *Divine*, 13–14.

[23]Ibid., 13–14, 78; P. Bryant to Folks, March 31, 1958; Bryant and Bryant, Interview.

[24]Bryant, *Divine*, 13, 18–19; P. Bryant to Mattoxes, April 7, 1958; R. Bryant to Mattoxes, April 5, 1958; Goff, *Great*, 62.

[25]R. Bryant, "Newsletter No. 3," May 1, 1958, RPB:N; R. Bryant to Mattoxes, April 5, 1958.

[26]P. Bryant to Mattoxes, March 16 and June 16, 1958; R. Bryant to Proctor Street, July 1, 1958.

Sara Bryant's illness would not be the last health scare for her family. Often when family members became ill, they would start driving to the hospital, not knowing how sick the person might become. In one case, they arrived at the hospital with little time to spare. When Rees Bryant developed bacillary dysentery that didn't improve with medicine from Urua Akpan MMM, Bill Nicks and Patti Bryant took him to the more distant Anua MMM. Although the hospital had no beds "for a white man," the physician insisted Rees would not live long enough to get to a PH hospital, and so they moved a Nigerian to a porch mat, put Bryant in the bed, and started IV fluids. After four days of antibiotics and pain medications, a grateful Rees returned home to Onicha Ngwa. West Africa "wasn't called white man's graveyard for nothing," Patti reflected.[27]

Stop-Gap Care

Before long Gerry Nicks and Patti Bryant divided their labor so that Bryant ran the backdoor clinic while Nicks homeschooled. In her nursing clinic, Patti Bryant cared for ten to thirty patients daily using a Merck Manual, her college education, and what she had learned from Glenna Peden.[28] Mrs. Isong Uyo, the wife of a BTC teacher, translated.[29] Bryant treated persons with illnesses and injuries so severe that if they had been family members, she would have taken them to a physician. But because she thought her patients could not or would not go unless they were dying, Bryant did what she could. Patients waited behind her house until she could break from parenting, housekeeping, and grading hundreds of Bible correspondence course papers.[30] She handed out Paludrin for malaria to everyone, removed thorns, dispensed aspirin, used Terramycin powder to bandage and rebandage tropical ulcers (possibly yaws), and saw "the tremendous need for medical care."[31] She soon charged a penny for bandaging and a penny for five aspirin with the dual intent of instilling self-respect and sorting out the sick from attention seekers. Fees weren't always paid in money, and Bryant passed one woman's payment of "a bowl full of hot peppers" along to her delighted yardmen.[32]

---

[27]P. Bryant to Mattoxes, May 7, 1959; Bryant and Bryant, Interview.
[28]P. Bryant to Mattoxes, July 2, July 21, and September 10, 1958; Peden, Interview.
[29]P. Bryant to Mattoxes, July 10, 1958.
[30]P. Bryant to Mattoxes, August 4 and September 10, 1958.
[31]Bryant and Bryant, Interview.
[32]P. Bryant to Mattoxes, May 7, May 8, and July 21, 1958.

She was relieved that Gerry Nicks engaged in morning homeschooling rather than patient care because Nicks thought clinic treatments should be free. Nonetheless, by September Bryant asked Nicks to share the load, and each woman saw patients on three different afternoons per week.[33] There is no record of how the issue of fees was resolved. In the clinic Nicks shared both "white man medicine" and the Christian message with one native doctor who sought only the first for his daughter, while Bryant was exasperated that so many promised to join the COC if she would give them a Bible.[34]

Patti Bryant was also frustrated by Nigerian's avoidable injuries. For example, blood from one young woman's "facial markings (cuttings)" beside each eye was "caked in her hair, down her bare breasts, down her leg. And she was holding a dirty rag to the cut." Unable to deal with this on an empty stomach, Bryant breakfasted and dressed before cleaning and closing the wound with a butterfly bandage. She was angry that a dirty instrument was likely used to make these tribal or beautifying cuts.[35] Additionally, she was disturbed by patient injuries from "chemist" injections of river water or other liquids, from other injurious native doctor treatments, and from skin slashes to let out evil or pain from wherever the patient reported it was "biting."[36]

Other situations she found rewarding. For one little boy with tropical ulcers between his toes, she "piled on the Terramycin powder" and created a gauze sock and tape shoe to keep the dirt out; she was happy when such wounds would "die," as Nigerians said.[37] She sent some with more intimidating problems to the hospital, including a tiny baby with an ear-to-ear abscess and a man with a stick through his wrist.[38]

Aware that contact with disease created risks for her family, Bryant reassured her own mother that she always washed her hands thoroughly after clinic. And Patti didn't scrub only her hands. When infant Billy became the center of physical affection at church, Bryant did her best to make sure no germ survived. After their first Nigerian Sunday morning worship service, "an old, wrinkled *ma* took him… and passed him around in a circle of women eagerly waiting their turns to hold him, kiss him, and hug him." Ready to "share the gospel," but not Billy, Patti tried to

---

[33]P. Bryant to Mattoxes, July 21 and September 15, 1958.

[34]P. Bryant to Mattoxes, September 10 and 28, 1958.

[35]P. Bryant to Mattoxes, March 31, 1958. See details of gender-specific cutting in Basden's *Niger Ibos,* 331-33.

[36]Bryant and Bryant, Interview.

[37]P. Bryant to Mattoxes, July 21, 1958.

[38]P. Bryant, quoted in Bryant, "Reflections," 21.

smile, and then once home "scrubbed that little fellow from head to toe with a strong solution of Dettol, the antiseptic" that missionaries added to their stream bathwater.[39]

Her concerns about infectious disease were not wholly unwarranted. Their own cook required hospital care for amoebic dysentery, prompting all Onicha Ngwa missionary families to have blood tests for themselves and household workers. The missionaries were declared healthy, but the wife of the cook for the Nicks family required treatment for parasites. The Bryants paid for their own cook's hospitalization and treatment but then dismissed him permanently as a precaution.[40]

Too, rabies was common, and most victims died at home. One night Rees Bryant transported a feverish girl, who jumped "with the light" and bit her mother. Bryant touched her to see if she was feverish, then touched shaving nicks on his face. The girl's eventual diagnosis of rabies necessitated sixteen daily vaccinations at MMM for both him and the mother.[41]

After months of backdoor clinic, transporting patients to the hospital over poor roads at all hours, and sometimes paying patients' medical bills, Patti Bryant paused: "Why don't we have some medical missionaries?"[42] COC religious competitors, the Roman Catholics and protestant denominations, had them, but the COC did not, she noted aloud, yet even her own family included two physicians.[43] Moreover, no hospital existed in Eastern Ngwa.[44] In answer to their own question, the Bryants decided it was not enough to ameliorate healthcare access; they needed to revolutionize it. It was not enough to bring people to distant health professionals; they needed to bring health professionals to the people. With little idea of where they were going or how they would get there, the Bryants (and soon Nicks[45]) began a stream of letters sounding an urgent Macedonian call for COC physicians and nurses to "come over to Nigeria and help us."[46]

---

[39]Bryant, *Divine*, 16.
[40]P. Bryant to Mattoxes, June 3, 1959.
[41]R. Bryant to Mattoxes, August 21, 1959; Bryant and Bryant, Interview.
[42]Nicks to R. Bryant, February 26, 1960; Bryant, "Reflections," 21.
[43]Bryant and Bryant, Interview.
[44]Bryant to Dickson, September 2, 1960.
[45]Nicks to R. Bryant, February 26, 1960.
[46]Bryant, "Reflections," 21.

Conclusion

Missionaries in the field led evolutionary change in COC healthcare. Glenna Peden's start-up nursing clinic developed into an ongoing expectation for all COC missionary women, and now the Bryants shifted perspectives even further. Rees and Patti Bryant began to call on the COC to take its place among other churches in providing professional care to locals and missionaries for whom there was otherwise little access. They could no longer imagine their evangelism without professional healthcare.

5

Controversy, Diaspora, and Duty

(1959–1960)

Christ's example of healing compelled us.
—Rees Bryant

Historically, COC missionaries had often complemented their evangelism with healthcare. Some trained to that end, either treating individuals or running small, mostly informal clinics in Africa and Asia, but no COC hospital existed in 1960.[1] One significant barrier to establishing official COC healthcare missions was the contentious, intra-church debate about whether or not the Bible authorized congregations to establish para-church organizations like Christian colleges, orphanages, or hospitals. COCs that forbade congregational funding of such institutions reasoned that because first-century congregations did not do so, then neither should twentieth-century ones. Called noninstitutional churches, they neither prevented individual Christians from voluntary provision of healthcare nor forbade congregations to help their own members. In contrast, institutional COCs favored church funding of healthcare and argued that Christians should conform to Jesus's example of physical and spiritual healing. Each side grounded their theological arguments in the same criteria for Biblical interpretation: Church actions are legitimate if supported by biblical command, apostolic example, and/or necessary inference.[2]

This US controversy soon spilled over into Nigeria via missionaries when noninstitutional adherents arrived on each of the three COC compounds: James and Mary Louise Finney in Onicha Ngwa, Leslie and Sarah Diestelkamp in Ikot Usen, and Sewell and Caneta Hall in Ukpom.[3] No one documented any backdoor nursing by women in these families, and although Leslie Diestelkamp admitted that financial support of a

[1]Boyd, "Historical;" Eichman, *Medical.*
[2]Williams et al., eds., *Stone-Campbell*, Chapter 8.
[3]Bryant and Bryant, Interview; Goff, *Great*, 62; Nicks, "Fellow Workers," 14.

COC physician was scripturally allowed, he viewed it as "unwise"—the first move down a slippery slope.[4] Diestelkamp had persuaded the Halls to adopt noninstitutional doctrine.[5]

Diaspora

Conflict emerged in 1959 shortly after Leslie Eugene and Sarah Alice Wright Diestelkamp arrived with young son Roy for two years in Nigeria. Sponsored by the Thomas Boulevard COC in Port Arthur, Texas, Diestelkamp promptly asserted his opposition to medical missions,[6] and neither he nor Rees Bryant hesitated to preach to the other. When Diestelkamp argued that "the church is not in the hospital business," Bryant agreed that "the church is not in any business." When Diestelkamp argued that "individuals can do this but the church can't," Bryant countered that the church is composed of individuals.[7]

This doctrinal split quickly widened into a geographic one. Only five months after arriving in Nigeria, the Diestelkamps relocated to Lagos, six hundred miles to the west, in order to avoid working with colleagues who approved of medical missions.[8] The advantages of this move were that each could preach as he believed, southeastern evangelists could pursue a medical mission, and a new COC mission point began in Lagos. Those gains were amplified when the Finneys and Halls joined the Diestelkamps in Lagos after their furloughs and were replaced by institutional missionaries in the southeast. Too, the Finneys' house was sold to the Bryants' sponsoring church, with the money going to Diestelkamps' work.[9] Meanwhile, correspondence between Onicha Ngwa and Lagos missionaries remained peppered by active debate that convinced south-

---

[4]Diestelkamp to West End, May 31, 1961. Harding College professor James D. Bales wrote to R. Bryant on March 7, 1960 proposing a medical missionary model to circumvent noninstitutional objections: Increase missionary income "so that the group can support their own M.D.," who could teach and care for missionaries and others. Also Nicks in *Missions* extensively discusses his own theology of church cooperation in "benevolence" work (96–104).

[5]Bryant and Bryant, Interview.

[6]Ibid.; P. Bryant to Mattoxes, February 7, 1959; R. Bryant to Mattoxes, July 27, 1959; Goff, *Great*, 41; "Leslie Eugene Diestelkamp," January 18, 2006, findagrave.com no. 13062678; "Sarah Alice Wright Diestelkamp," May 8, 2006, findagrave.com no. 14228295.

[7]Bryant and Bryant, Interview.

[8]Bryant, "Reflections," 23–24; Goff, *Great*, 62.

[9]R. Bryant to Summerlin, June 9, 1960; Bryant and Bryant, Interview; Nicks, "Fellow Workers," 14.

eastern missionaries more than ever of the rightness of their healthcare cause and perhaps likewise strengthened convictions of those in Lagos.[10]

As in the US, the controversy advanced into an enduring split between Nigerian COCs. Still, Diestelkamp and Bryant's letters reflected an often-surprising cordiality, as they pragmatically communicated with one COC voice to the Nigerian government on legal, tax, and missionary quota issues. Additionally, they sometimes collaborated in evangelistic work.[11] Although Bryant found Diestelkamp's letters increasingly "war-like," he later wrote that Diestelkamp was a "good Brother"—dissonant descriptions reflecting their complex relationship and Bryant's self-described "lack of malice."[12]

Rees Bryant long tolerated these missionary differences. Later in the 1960s, when he served as missionary-elected Secretary of the government-recognized Registered Trustees of the COC, he did not use support for Christian hospitals as a litmus test for missionaries.[13] Instead, Bryant allowed both noninstitutional and institutional missionaries to use the COC immigration quota, while still fighting to gain new slots for healthcare professionals, teachers, and preachers.[14] Bryant saw his unpaid Secretary position as a political necessity and stewardship, not as a church office with authority to say who was and was not a COC member. Still, decades later he wondered what his stance contributed to ongoing intra-COC conflict.[15] Bryant's sharing of the immigration quota meant the balance of power between institutional and noninstitutional evangelists in Nigeria rested not on strategic planning, but instead on an individual Secretary's disposition and on which contingent could recruit more missionaries.

Duty

The vision of a COC medical mission grew despite both the controversy and the utter lack of healthcare experience in the Bryant and Nicks fami-

---

[10]R. Bryant to Hall, January 24, 1961; R. Bryant to Nicks, May 4, 1961; Lawyer to Summerlin and Elders, February 28, 1961; Nicks to R. Bryant and all, April 1, 1961. Per R. Bryant, personal communication, July 19, 2010: Bryant invited Hall to speak in BTC chapel in hopes of changing his mind.

[11]Diestelkamp to R. Bryant, May 21 and September 13, 1960; H. Farrar to McInteer, February 24, 1967.

[12]Bryant, "Reflections," 23; R. Bryant to Nicks, May 4, 1961.

[13]R. Bryant to Mattoxes, Lawyers, and Masseys, May 20, 1966; Bryant and Bryant, Interview.

[14]R. Bryant to Elders, March 4, 1965; R. Bryant to Friends, April 20, 1965.

[15]Bryant and Bryant, Interview.

lies. The Bryants later described themselves as "naïve...ignorant," and confident. Starting a facility and recruiting missionary nurses and physicians seemed simply "the right thing to do"[16] given their faith and financial means.

All COC missionaries understood that they were wealthy by rural Nigerian standards, and their relative affluence both caught them off guard and created a sense of Christian duty.[17] In the US, Rees Bryant thought himself poor, wearing "Uncle Rupert's hand-me-down suits" and earning less money preaching with his master's degree than did his cousin working in a shoe factory. Now he found himself richer than almost everyone around him and thus subject to biblical directives regarding the obligation of the rich to the poor.[18] Missionaries lived in concrete block houses with indoor bathrooms, concrete flooring, and screened windows. They received dependable salaries, paid full-time household staff, possessed stoves and refrigerators, owned cars, and could purchase petrol (gasoline). In contrast, most rural Igbos were subsistence farmers who lived in palm thatch and mud homes with outdoor latrines, walked or bicycled everywhere, and trekked to the stream for baths, laundering, and drinking water. Later evangelist Douglas "Doug" Lawyer said his "greatest shock in personal adjustment" to Nigeria was learning to work alongside those who owned so little.[19]

Thus, missionaries "soberly" counted their economic blessings.[20] Patti Bryant reflected at length on how to use their comparative wealth to benefit Nigerians, and Lawyer reported that he "learned to be rich" by acting in love. Although he turned down constant appeals for financial aid—requests that he likely lacked resources to meet—he responded to those requests "by friendly conversation and letting petitioners know what love isn't and who it is." Material goods ("what love isn't"), Lawyer argued, could never meet spiritual needs. Real prosperity was to be found within God's love ("who it is").[21]

To such words, missionaries added moral action. As Rees later wrote, "Desperate physical needs continued to trouble us. We could not ignore the great suffering all around us. Christ's example of healing compelled us" to render first aid, recruit health professionals, drive the ill to hospi-

---

[16]Ibid.
[17]Ibid.; P. Bryant to Folks, May 1, 1958; Lawyer, untitled questionnaire, ca. 1961, RPB; Nicks, "Why?."
[18]Bryant and Bryant, Interview.
[19]Ibid.; Bryant, *Divine*; Lawyer, untitled questionnaire.
[20]Lawyer, *Nigerian Newsletter*, April 30, 1961, RPB:N.
[21]P. Bryant to Fine, June 7, 1958; Lawyer, untitled questionnaire.

tals when locals with cars refused, and ask US supporters to be more conscious of their own relative wealth and so more generous.[22] COC missionaries could not have taken such action without relative wealth and would not have done so without a sense of religious obligation. Their motivation to bring healthcare to their corner of Nigeria was from the Bryants' perspective a duty "to obey the Lord," and not to increase baptisms or please the government. Christian conversions were already plentiful, locals begged missionaries to preach in their villages, and Nigeria had officially recognized the COC since 1955.[23]

Aid versus Influence

Almost one year to the day after Rees Bryant's encounter with a dying man, Bill Nicks wrote home to US supporters about locals' continuing burden of illness and evangelists' corollary burden of care. The time for a Christian physician and facility has come, and Nigerians are ready, he penned. "I hope someone reads this who will help make our dream a reality!" One Nigerian man, Bill Nicks reported, was asking Nicks to recruit a US physician for him and declared having $6,000 ready for hospital construction.[24] How much the request was related to a scarcity of Nigerian physicians versus a village desire to gain prestige by finding an "European" healer was unknown.

Five months later, Bill Nicks penned another, more urgent plea to Proctor Street COC. In the final paragraph of a typed, two legal-sized-page letter on evangelism, Nicks abruptly changed the subject to the "critical...doctor situation." The nearest eye hospital was over nine hundred miles away, and the nearest dentist, over two hundred. Medical facilities were "overcrowded and understaffed." Missionaries had sent one BTC student 110 miles to the closest eye clinic, and another had waited six months just to schedule surgery at a hospital thirty-two miles away.[25] Nicks's message was clear: Students suffered, and each incapacitated BTC evangelist-in-training deprived the COC of another preacher.

While Bryant primarily framed the need to provide healthcare as a Christian duty, Nicks often described healthcare as a means toward spiri-

---

[22]Bryant, "Reflections," 22; Bryant and Bryant, Interview; Salmon to Bryants et al., February 8, 1961.

[23]R. Bryant *Newsletter No. 6* to Friends, October 1, 1958, RPB:N; Bryant and Bryant, Interview; Goff, *Great*, 31.

[24]Nicks to [missing], March 13, 1959.

[25]Nicks, "News From Nigeria," August 7, 1959, RPB:N.

tual healing and expansion of COC influence. Adamant that "something" must be done, Nicks called on US partners: "Pray that we may... relieve suffering to the end that we may more effectively reach their souls by our living, loving faith. Nothing short of trained doctors and nurses with proper equipment will do this work."[26] At the same time, all missionaries remained cautious about "medical converts." They understood a hospital as a two-edged evangelistic sword; healthcare might advance evangelism either properly—when received as a demonstration of Christian compassion—or improperly—as a material inducement to join the COC.[27] The risk was real given an Igbo history of seeking economic gain via Christian missionary education, and missionaries already avoided driving people to streams for baptism, fearing that the desire for a car ride might be a more powerful motivator than religious conviction.[28] "We don't want people following just for the loaves and fishes," Bryant asserted in biblical reference to John 6:26.[29]

Nevertheless, US evangelists welcomed at least two instances when their ad hoc ambulance service moved Nigerians toward the COC. In 1958, a concerned Bill Nicks drove a consenting, critically ill juju doctor to a hospital for successful treatment. When locals saw the doctor as unable to heal himself, Nicks believed their eyes were opened to both Western medicine and the Christian message.[30] In a second instance, Rees Bryant's car axle broke just as he drove a patient onto Anua MMM hospital grounds, and the transported man later became a COC member and thanked Rees for saving his life at the cost of a car.[31]

Working Furlough

In September 1959, the Bryants began an eventful, six-month, first furlough, sharing their medical mission vision with anyone who would listen. Rees Bryant's speaking itinerary sometimes included daily presentations in Texas, Oklahoma, New Mexico, Colorado, Alabama, Tennessee, Arkansas, and Louisiana.[32] His schedule was so full that it is no surprise

---

[26]Ibid.

[27]Ibid.; Bryant to Elders, August 3, 1961.

[28]Ayandele, *Nigerian*, 167–91; Lawyers to Friends, March 27, 1961, RPB:N.

[29]Bryant to Elders, August 3, 1961.

[30]Nicks, "Doctoring," 120–23; Nicks, *Missions*, 254.

[31]Bryant and Bryant, Interview.

[32]P. Bryant to Mattoxes, September 21, 1959; Nicks, "Rees Bryants."

he did not remember meeting college student Iris Hays—an encounter that inspired her radical transformation into missionary nurse.[33]

Both Bryants did remember their eventful telephone meeting with potential missionary physician recruit, Henry Cheairs Farrar Jr., MD, and his wife, Grace Angeline Johnson Farrar, RN. Patti Bryant already had written to Dr. Farrar from Nigeria, and now her father, LCC President Fount William "F.W." (or "Billy") Mattox, facilitated Rees Bryant's Nigerian invitation to Farrars in Kentucky from the Mattox dining room in Lubbock.[34] That phone call came as the Farrars were in a quandary. In China, 1940s revolutionaries had forced out all "white devils," making it impossible for Farrar to fulfill his long-planned dream of medical mission work at the Canton Bible School. Subsequently, they turned their sights toward India, but soon learned that only Commonwealth citizens were allowed entry.[35] In the face of these two closed Asian doors, the disappointed Farrars still affirmed their "plan and dream" to be medical missionaries,[36] although their next step was unclear.

Rees Bryant's call now opened an African door, but there the Farrar-Bryant conversation paused. The Bryants' furlough ended, and the family, now with three children, returned to Onicha Ngwa in April 1960.[37] In their US wake, surgeon-in-the-making Henry Farrar and nurse-in-the-making Iris Hays started their separate journeys toward Nigeria; neither yet knew of the other. The Bryants were the first to introduce the Farrars to the needs in Nigeria,[38] and Grace Farrar later identified Patti's "persuasive" letters as possibly the most influential factor in the family's ultimate decision to go.[39]

As the Bryants passed through New York, they were delighted by unexpected news. West End COC (W-COC) elder John S. Cayce, MD, in Nashville, Tennessee, called them to say that W-COC had "planned for years" to fund Dr. Farrar as "our boy;"[40] then in a separate call, elder Ike

---

[33]P. Bryant, email to author, February 14, 2012; Bryant and Bryant, Interview; Hays-Savio, Interview.

[34]R. Bryant to Summerlin, December 29, 1959 and January 4, 1960; Bryant and Bryant, Interview; Farrar, "Chronology."

[35]Grace Farrar, personal communication, 2012; Farrar, "Story;" H. Farrar, Interviews 1 and 2; Kharlukhi to Farrars, October 3, 1960.

[36]Henry and Grace Farrar to [annual Christmas card list], December 17, 1959.

[37]P. Bryant, email to author, February 14, 2012; R. Bryant to Summerlin, December 29, 1959; Bryant and Bryant, Interview.

[38]Grace Farrar, personal communication, April 15, 2012.

[39]Farrar, *Stand*, 18.

[40]P. Bryant to Mattoxes, March 25, 1960; Grace Farrar, personal communication, August 1, 2011.

Summerlin from Proctor Street COC told Rees Bryant that they would fund the Farrars.[41] Rees had proposed that Proctor Street support Farrar because he thought that W-COC was disinterested in supporting a medical mission. Now or perhaps later, the Bryants began to realize that W-COC wanted to support Henry Farrar as an evangelist, who also practiced medicine, but they didn't want to fund a hospital. The surprised Bryants left resolution of this rare double-support problem to the two congregations.[42] Still, only ten days later, Bryant wrote to Proctor Street suggesting that they prioritize funding of evangelist Douglas Lawyer, while hinting to leaders in both churches that perhaps one congregation might finance a second physician. "Wouldn't that be good?" he enthused.[43]

During their April return journey to Nigeria, the Bryants also visited the Lawrence Taylor family, longtime missionary friends, in Libya. The Taylors introduced them to two nurses. The name of the first went unrecorded in correspondence, but the second was "public health nurse" Letty (also Lettie, Letti, or Lucy) Sermanoukian (also Sermonoukian or Semonukin). Both nurses were members of the Tripoli COC, well-regarded by Taylor, and interested in the Bryants' hospital vision.[44] No one imagined the missionary role Sermanoukian would play in Nigeria.

Nineteen Trips in Eighteen Days

Arriving back in Onicha Ngwa just eight days before the Nicks family was to leave on furlough, the hopeful Bryants asked Bill Nicks to follow up with Farrars while he was in the US. "Be sure to get Henry to come," they insisted, and follow up Nicks did, within days.[45] Meanwhile, in Nigeria, the Bryants enjoyed reconnecting with their close friends, the Masseys, who replaced the Nicks. Evangelist James "Jim" Richard Massey (1930–1995) and Rees Bryant had been roommates at Harding College and then faculty colleagues at Alabama Christian College. Now Jim and

---

[41]P. Bryant to Mattoxes, March 25, 1960. In citation P. Bryant mistakenly referred to W-COC as LA-COC.

[42]Bryant, *Divine*, 106-07; R. Bryant to Summerlin, December 29, 1959; R. Bryant to Summerlin, January 4, 1960.

[43]R. Bryant to Summerlin, January 4, 1960; R. Bryant to Summerlin et al., April 16, 1960.

[44]Bryant, *Divine*, 107-08; P. Bryant to Mattoxes, December 31, 1960; R. Bryant to Elders, January 28, 1961; Taylor to R. Bryant, April 29, 1960.

[45]Bryant and Bryant, Interview; Nicks, "Narrative;" Summerlin to R. Bryant, May 8, 1960.

Joyce Brewer Massey (1934–) and young daughters, Carol, Beth, and Anne Marie, were the Bryants' neighbors. Masseys were sponsored by South Park COC in Beaumont, Texas.[46]

The two families shared round-the-clock ambulance duties. Often a messenger would knock on a bedroom window at night, and the missionary guided by an interpreter would drive "out these little dark paths that served as roads…through the jungle" to a village where they would gather up the ill person and drive to an MMM hospital. They avoided closer Aba and Ikot Ekpene government hospitals, judging their care as unacceptable.[47]

Such emergency situations stole time from other duties and were often difficult; yet some were filled with humor or even joy. On one occasion, interpreter Stephen Okoronkwo and Rees Bryant chuckled over two passengers arguing about whose pain was more severe. "Typical human beings" to judge our own problems worse, reflected Bryant.[48] Then, on another occasion, while transporting a woman in labor, Rees Bryant's interpreter first called out frantically in Igbo, then in English, "Go, sir! Go, sir! The baby is coming! Go, sir!" Bryant sped up, but the baby arrived in the van before the van arrived at the hospital. "They named the little boy Chibuzo, 'God is the way,' a good name for a baby delivered by God on the way," penned Bryant.[49] Why a midwife did not manage this seemingly uncomplicated delivery at home was unexplained.

Both men and women shared in these hospital drives. In one instance, Joyce Massey recorded her bewilderment at a husband's desperate efforts to leave his laboring wife behind at the hospital. In order to deliver their daughter safely, the woman needed surgical repair of work done the previous night by a juju doctor. Despite the physician's demand that the woman's much older husband must stay, the man pleaded to return with Massey, running behind her van until she pulled away.[50] Perhaps he was an Igbo afraid to be left on Ibibio land or perhaps he feared he would be asked to donate blood.[51]

The cost of these ambulance excursions was high, and after one stint of nineteen trips to the hospital in eighteen days, Rees Bryant spent a

---

[46]Bryant, *Divine*, 109, 162; Harp, "James Richard Massey;" Massey, "Rees Bryants," RPB; in correspondence; Joyce Massey, Facebook Messenger to author, June 24, 2020. See also R. Bryant, "Nigerian Highlights–1959."

[47]Bryant and Bryant, Interview; G. Farrar to author, July 2, 2010.

[48]Bryant and Bryant, Interview; Bill Nicks in "Okorobeke" tells the same/similar story as his own experience (25).

[49]Bryant "Reflections," 20; Bryant and Bryant, Interview.

[50]R. Bryant to Summerlin, June 9, 1960.

[51]Umeora, Onuh, and Umeora, "Socio-Cultural."

substantial £90:12 shillings from his working funds on the Volkswagen bus that the Nicks left for missionaries' use.[52] Shortly thereafter, missionaries began charging patients for petrol, a step designed perhaps to increase the value patients placed on the service, to balance missionary books,[53] and to tip the scales away from emergency transport as a status symbol or undue influence on Christian conversion. Scattered documents suggest that they otherwise recouped monetary expenses from designated donations, missionary discretionary salary dollars, or business expense accounts, but they could not regain their time.[54]

Conclusion

Such volunteer nursing and ambulance services continued on all three COC compounds,[55] albeit not at the new noninstitutional mission point in Lagos. Missionaries in southeastern Nigeria remained troubled by the theological, fiscal, and professional inadequacy of their efforts to meet their own and others' healthcare needs.[56]

---

[52]R. Bryant to Summerlin, August 18, 1960.

[53]Bryant and Bryant, Interview. R. Bryant to Massey, October 18, 1964, lists churches paying for car maintenance.

[54]R. Bryant to Summerlin, August 18, 1960; R. Bryant to Elders, August 3, 1961; R. Bryant to Massey, October 18, 1964; Bryant and Bryant, Interview; Doe and Fraga, Interview; Nicks, "Unexpected," 77; Peden, Interview.

[55]H. Farrar, Interview 1; Martin, quoted in Goff, *Great*, 45; Peden, Interview.

[56]Lawyer, "Narrative," 37.

6
Transitions: Theology in Action
(1959–1961)

If Christians will not help... who will?
—Douglas Lawyer and Rees Bryant

At the turn of the decade, local illness and injury were no different, but COC missionaries were. Previously the missionaries lauded backdoor healthcare as the supererogatory work of unpaid, mostly lay volunteers, but now they viewed providing professional care as a moral duty. Dr. Henry Farrar's potential coming to Onicha Ngwa presented a way to meet that Christian obligation. Yet it also raised pragmatic questions of where he would practice and theological questions of why. They pursued these issues in the context of Nigeria's final move to formal independence from Great Britain in 1960.

Practical Matters

During 1960, missionaries in southeastern Nigeria gathered information and brainstormed options. They wanted a setting that appealed to Dr. Farrar, maximized Nigerian financing, and minimized COC controversy. In a mostly one-way conversation with Nigeria's almost-independent Ministry of Health, Bill Nicks found Nigerians hesitant to admit more "'*Beke*' [whites] to manage affairs." Aware of government-COC collaboration in the operating of Ikot Usen village schools, he thus proposed to Bryant that a US COC-funded, maternity clinic under Nigerian District Council oversight might generate both a welcome for Dr. Farrar and government subsidies. Too, in a nod to the work of the African Christian School Board, Nicks recommended that a similar board, not a COC congregation, fundraise for the clinic. This, he wrote, might make it palatable for "really good men" of conscience, influenced by years of doctrinal

ꞏments against church-supported hospitals, to support a clinic.[1] Per-
ꞏps he had earlier been among them.

Bill Nicks's pursuit of a clinic halted with his spring 1960 furlough, and
Rees Bryant took up the torch, relaying what he learned to Farrar, Nicks,
and key supporters in the US.[2] Only ten days after his return to Onicha
Ngwa, Bryant and COC colleagues from Ukpom, Wendell Broom and
Glenn Martin, met with Dr. Mitchell. Mitchell was an experienced missionary physician in solo practice at the 140-bed, Qua Iboe Church Hospital (est. 1927) in Etinan. They learned from Mitchell that Nigeria welcomed preventive Health Centres or small rural hospitals that met national standards, that Centre operating costs could be covered by a combination of patient fees and government subsidies, and that existing
COC immigration quota categories accommodated entry of a physician.
Moreover, Bryant's fear of "too-much-local-support-too-much-local-con-
trol" was allayed when he learned that a COC missionary physician
would report to the senior medical officer in Aba and the regional minister of health in Enugu, "not to local politicians."[3] This information,
combined with Bryant's self-confessed naïveté and selective inattention to
the power of village politics, made hospital planning seem straightforward. Only later did he find the official government chain of command
cumbersome and discover the extent to which missionaries must still ne-
gotiate with traditional rulers and villages over hospital governance,
funds, land, and labor.

Mitchell complained that the size of the Qua Iboe Hospital "strangled"
his spiritual work, leading to Bryant's suggestion to Farrar that a smaller
Health Centre would allow more time for preaching in fulfillment of Farrar's childhood dreams and church expectations. Moreover, a Centre con-
formed to the preventive medicine interests that Farrar had developed
while completing his US military draft obligation in the US Public Health
Service. Rees Bryant expressed confidence that he and Bill Nicks could
raise any necessary funds.[4]

A few weeks later, however, Bryant changed his recommendation after
meeting with Dr. Amobi, the Senior Medical Officer in Aba. Amobi laid
out the cost of a twenty-bed hospital as £15,000 ($42,300), a price tag
that included a surgical suite, a ten-bed men's ward, a ten-bed women's

---

[1] Nicks to R. Bryant, February 26, 1960.

[2] R. Bryant to Summerlin et al., May 3, 1960; Bryant, "Reflections," 22–23; Bryant
and Bryant, Interview.

[3] Bryant, "Reflections," 22–23; Ottuh, "Church and Community."

[4] R. Bryant to Summerlin et al., April 16, 1960; G. Farrar to Johnson, January 29,
1957; Farrar, "Chronology;" Farrar, "Heroes" Interview.

ward, kitchen, laundry, and an outpatient clinic with an office, dispensary, and treatment rooms. Amobi also outlined two options for the government and church to share decision-making and costs, and he reassured Bryant that the COC would retain facility control.[5] Based on this new information, Bryant now endorsed building a hospital in Onicha Ngwa.[6] Such government underwriting of the construction costs of a hospital "for their indigent if the church would staff it…is exactly what…[Henry is] looking for," Grace Farrar wrote.[7]

Dr. Farrar's interest in surgery was growing, and he welcomed the hospital proposal. His physician mentor and W-COC elder John S. Cayce earlier suggested that Farrar complete surgical residency and board certification before going to Africa, and Farrar took Casey's advice. Thus, by 1960 he was finishing surgical residency requirements in Winston-Salem, North Carolina,[8] while continuing his beloved preaching and Bible teaching on Sundays off.[9]

Grace Farrar, RN, remained a supportive participant in her husband's plans. She also long intended to be a missionary and later began her spiritual autobiography by writing, "God chose good parents for me."[10] Born at home on December 13, 1924, with midwife grandmother Martha Thayer in attendance, Grace arrived as the third of four children to parents Elva "Pete" and Martha Olive Thayer Johnson. Elva was a farmer in the Northwest Township of Orange County, Indiana, and Martha was a lay nurse with an eighth-grade education and skills in all things domestic.[11] From her parents, Grace gained practical skills, self-discipline, thrift, creativity, healthy curiosity, and high integrity. She proudly lived by her dad's assertion, "My word is my bond."[12]

As Grace Johnson grew, so did her faith. She was baptized in the nearby Orangeville community church "on the Methodist Episcopal circuit" and became president of the church's teen group. Grace stood in pledge when a teen camp speaker asked who would promise to be a missionary. In 1942, after graduating from Orleans High School as valedictorian,

---

[5]R. Bryant to Summerlin et al., May 3, 1960.

[6]R. Bryant to Summerlin, June 9, 1960.

[7]G. Farrar to Johnson, February 27, 1963.

[8]Farrar, "Chronology;" Farrar, "Story," 41–42; "Biographical Sketches" (Farrar), 196–97; Nicks to R. Bryant, February 26, 1960; Farrars, personal communication, n.d.

[9]G. Farrar to Johnson, June 17, 1959; G. Farrar to Folks, August 1, 1958, September 18, 1958 and September 15, 1959.

[10]Farrar, "My Spiritual Journey."

[11]Farrar, "Chronology;" G. Farrar, untitled book ms.

[12]Author's recollection.

Johnson entered Reid Memorial Hospital Nursing School in Cincinnati, Ohio, but soon transferred to nearby Bethesda Hospital Nursing School so she could join the Cadet Nurse Corps. That decision was both financial and patriotic, but WWII ended before she could serve. Consequently, she began a 1945 job on night shift in Bethesda's newborn nursery and passed state nursing boards with the highest score in Ohio that year.[13]

Grace Farrar described her younger self as a "truth-seeker and voracious reader" who did not fit in well with progressive urban Methodists. When Cincinnati roommate Bettye Foreste invited her to attend Walnut Hill Church of Christ, Grace found her final church home in the COC and was "immersed to become a Christian not just a…Methodist."[14] The next year she began her bachelor's degree in home economics at Harding College, where she served as school nurse and met fellow student Henry Farrar. In 1948, she completed her undergraduate degree at unaccredited Harding, while he completed his at accredited University of Tennessee, Knoxville (UTK), in order to be eligible for admission into UT medical school.[15] Unable to afford medical education, Farrar went on to earn his master's degree in parasitology and considered replacing his medical mission dreams with a UTK teaching appointment, but a wiser Grace insisted that he pursue his lifetime goals.[16] They married December 2, 1950, in Searcy, Arkansas, and in January 1951, Henry started UT Memphis medical training.[17] Like Eugene and Glenna Peden, Henry and Grace Farrar became a strong team.

Grace Farrar was proud of her nursing preparation, and she used it to facilitate her husband's debt-free graduation from medical school in spring 1954. By then they were expecting their second child, and Grace was thrilled to begin pursuing her own lifelong ambitions of full-time motherhood and homemaking. The growing family moved often as Dr. Farrar practiced briefly in Tennessee, then consecutively completed his internship in Florida (1955), draft obligation in Texas and North Carolina (1957), surgical residency requirements in Kentucky and North Carolina

[13]Farrar, "Chronology;" Farrar, "My Spiritual Journey."
[14]Farrar, "My Spiritual Journey."
[15]Ibid.; Farrar, "Chronology;" H. Farrar, Interview 2.
[16]Grace Farrar, personal communication, February 2010.
[17]Farrar, "Chronology;" Farrar, "My Spiritual Journey."

(1962),[18] and a preceptorship in Tennessee (1964). That self-designed, mission-preparatory career path usurped plans to move to Nigeria in 1961, 1962, and 1963.[19] Instead, in fall 1963, Henry made a six-week exploratory visit to Onicha Ngwa, where W-COC elder, Bruce D. "Jack" Sinclair joined him for two weeks.[20]

Meanwhile, Grace Farrar maintained a solid commitment to homemaking and raising their five children—Paul, Martha (Marty), David, Henry III (Hank), and Lee—but her RN credential led others to expect different things from her. Rees Bryant anticipated Grace's working in the proposed hospital, while Dr. Farrar, two college presidents, and others used her nursing qualifications to market hospital plans.[21] Her reactions to this are unrecorded, but she never registered as a nurse in Nigeria. Nonetheless, once there she did use her nursing knowledge in ways she likely did not anticipate.[22]

Theological Justification

While missionaries were still planning for Dr. Farrar's coming, the Onicha Ngwa COC compound continued to grow. Sponsored by Proctor Street COC, Marion Douglas "Doug" Lawyer (1927–1998) and expectant wife Charla Rebecca Cranford Lawyer (1934–) along with young daughters Shauna and Tami joined the Masseys and Bryants in December

---

[18]Farrar, "Chronology." Per author's recollections and personal communication with Paul D. Farrar, and Henry C. Farrar III: Dr. Potter, Chief of Surgery in charge of Henry Farrar's residency at Miner's Hospital, asserted that no logical person could believe in Christianity, made Farrar take a course in logic, and raised Farrar's fears that he would fail Farrar. Dr. Farrar with the help of a friend—probably Dr. Ismael Goco MD—was able to transfer residencies to Winston-Salem City Hospital, who were originally hesitant, but later pleased.

[19]G. Farrar to Johnson, June 27, 1961; G. Farrar to Friends, December 1961; H. Farrar to Mission Committee, August 15, 1962, W-COC file.

[20]Gore USS telegram to Sinclair and Bergstrom, September 12, 1963; G. Farrar to Johnson, August 1963; G. Farrar to Folks, September 15 and October 26, 1963; Farrar to Mission Committee, September 12, 1963, W-COC file; H. Farrar to Sinclair, September 7, 1963; "Mission News," August 22, 1963, *WEV*. Per Carol Kaplan, email to author, August 1, 2016: John S. Casey was Henry Farrar's much older Nashville cousin by marriage, who attended Henry's birth. Casey's wife was the daughter of their paternal great-uncle. J.S. Cayce and Jack Sinclair "ran the [W-COC] mission committee and ensured" the Farrars' support.

[21]Benson, "Real;" R. Bryant to Summerlin, June 9, 1960; *Christian Chronicle*, "1–35,000;" *Christian Chronicle*, "99-Year;" Green Lawn, *Nigerian Evangelism*; Hillsboro, "Dr. Henry Farrar;" Mattox, "Nigerian Hospital."

[22]G. Farrar to Folks, August 24, 1965; Hays-Savio, Interview.

1960.[23] The Lawyers moved into the newest house that was constructed by Nigerian builder Anthony Agali using Lawyer-raised funds.[24] Patti Bryant and Joyce Massey completed its finishing details, and Patti later enthused that "we couldn't ask for better co-workers" than the quick-to-adjust Lawyers.[25]

Together, Doug Lawyer and Rees Bryant responded to theological questions of why Dr. Farrar should begin a medical mission. Absent a COC-wide statement, they argued for Christian exceptionalism in a four-page, undated paper, "Opportunities in Nigeria." Condemning past slavers and lauding Nigeria's growing economic, political, and intellectual achievements, they described this "vast, turbulent, changing country" as having five Christian opportunities: evangelism, preacher training, establishing self-supporting churches, Christian teaching, and benevolence.

Their benevolence section focused on medical benevolence and read in full:

> We are here in Nigeria to save souls. But those souls live in bodies; and in Galatians 6:10 Paul says, "So then as we have opportunity, let us work that which is good toward all men, and especially toward them that are of the household of the faith." Most Nigerians are poor, and they have little medical care. Often, someone comes to us saying, "My brother has fallen from a palm tree. He is dying. Please help us." Or another says, "My wife is trying to deliver her baby but there is trouble. Please take us to the hospital." They come with wounds, dysentery, rabies, malaria, strangulated hernia, infections caused by pagan witch-doctors, and many other ailments. What shall we do? Shall we turn our backs upon such unfortunate ones? Shall we tell them that we came to preach and not to doctor? No, by God's grace, we will do all that we can to help them—sometimes treating them at our door, sometimes using our automobiles as ambulances to make emergency runs to the hospital. In this way, we are able to alleviate human suffering and to prolong human life. We thus give many people an opportunity to hear the Gospel who otherwise would not hear it, and we seek to demonstrate Christianity in addition to preaching about it. If Christians

---

[23]Brewer, *Missionary*, 123; Bryant, *Divine*, 132; Harp, "Marion Douglas Lawyer."

[24]Farrar, *Stand*, 10; Nicks to R. Bryant, February 26, 1960; R. Bryant to Nicks, June 10, 1960.

[25]P. Bryant to Friends, February 4, 1961; Lawyers, "Douglas Lawyers."

will not help such unfortunate people, who will? If they can't turn to those who are followers of the Lord and who should have compassionate hearts, to whom can they turn? How often we have yearned for doctors and nurses to come into our area—men and women who are dedicated to the Lord and who have special training which would permit them to treat such unfortunate people.[26]

Bryant and Lawyer were clear. Their duty was not limited to care of immaterial souls, and they defended healthcare as both a Christian obligation in itself and as the means to an end of Christian conversion. They justified this stance using a common three-fold COC method of biblical interpretation, pointing to a biblical command from the Apostle Paul, alluding to the example of the Good Samaritan in Luke 10:25-37 (i.e., "shall we turn our backs?"), and making a necessary inference that Christians must act. The two argued that healthcare was an embodiment of the Christian message, asserted that extending people's lives created opportunities for them to hear the gospel, and presented themselves as witnesses of great need.

Conclusion

The turn of the decade was a time of change. Colonial Nigeria transitioned to an independent Federal Republic on October 1, 1960, and Onicha Ngwa missionaries increased their numbers and sought to transform their physical caregiving from lay to professional. Henry Farrar shifted his focus from China to India to Nigeria and from preventive medicine to surgery, while Grace Farrar held steady, having already switched her identity from Methodist to COC and her primary role from nurse to homemaker. Dr. Farrar now used newer terms of "medical missions" and "medical evangelism"[27] instead of benevolence work; his medical missionary plans had shifted from healthcare support of a Bible school in Asia to patient care delivery in a COC hospital in Africa. Meanwhile, missionaries in the field developed the physical, organizational, and theological structures needed to transition from entrepreneurial, incidental, volunteer-driven healthcare to infrastructure-supported professional care.

---

[26]Bryant and Lawyer, "Opportunities."
[27]Farrar to Mission Committee, July 13, 1963, W-COC file.

7
Steps and Missteps: A Nurse Unplanned
(1960–1963)

There was no time for a normal exchange of letters.
—Rees Bryant

Nurse Letty Sermanoukian answered the Bryants' call for COC health professionals. Although Patti Bryant later identified her as "Lebanese by nationality [and] Armenian by race,"[1] little else is recorded or remembered of her personal or professional history beyond some unclear connections to Beirut and Syria. Reportedly Sermanoukian worked about five years in maternal-child health in the Libyan American Joint Services (LAJS) in Tripoli, and when LAJS disbanded in 1960, she was forced to choose between returning to her Beirut home or beginning anew elsewhere. Thus, in November 1960, US evangelist Lawrence Taylor working with the Tripoli COC notified the Bryants that Sermanoukian wanted to come to Onicha Ngwa and work as a nurse. She would pay her own travel.[2]

Taylor offered to help raise her modest, monthly salary of $200 from the US[3] and penned that she "loved children," could teach childcare, and "was an excellent nurse" without any living relatives. Although not a nurse himself, Taylor expressed confidence that Sermanoukian would be a medical mission asset,[4] and only later admitted to second-hand knowledge of her nursing expertise.[5] As Taylor and Sermanoukian saw it, Onicha Ngwa needed a nurse, and Sermanoukian needed a job. Taylor's assessment seemed reasonable, and the Bryants invited her to stay with them "until a niche can be found" and salary raised. Bryant also consult-

---

[1]P. Bryant to Friends, February 4, 1961.
[2]Bryant, *Divine*, 130–31; R. Bryant to Elders, January 28, 1961; Lawyer, "Narrative," 37; Taylor to R. Bryant, April 29, 1960 and May 14, 1961.
[3]Taylor to R. Bryant, April 29, 1960.
[4]Bryant, *Divine*, 130; P. Bryant to Mattoxes, December 31, 1960.
[5]Taylor to R. Bryant, May 14, 1961.

ed with the now Nigerian District Officer, who welcomed Sermanoukian's coming,[6] and Bryant wrote to Taylor that the missionaries could use her skills, perhaps even with beginning a hospital.[7]

If Sermanoukian wrote any letters, they did not survive. Instead, Lawrence Taylor and Rees Bryant corresponded on her behalf. Taylor relayed that Sermanoukian wanted to bring her car and beloved, large dog, Ruff, but would not do so if this presented a problem. "Would Rees meet her in Lagos to drive her car across country?" Bryant responded promptly: "Do not bring the car. Do not bring the dog." Do not come without a visa. If she received these directives, Sermanoukian ignored them.[8]

The first notice of Sermanoukian's imminent arrival was a January 3, 1961, cable from Taylor to a surprised Bryant: Sermanoukian would leave Tripoli for Nigeria on January 7, despite the British embassy's refusal to issue a visa from newly independent Nigeria. Bryant cabled back that Sermanoukian should obtain a visa from Lagos before coming and then fly into Port Harcourt (PH). Taylor should cable her arrival time in PH, where Bryant could meet her. These instructions also went unheeded, and on January 14, the Bryants received a second, unexpected telegram from Taylor informing them that Sermanoukian would arrive in three days at 8:35 a.m. in Lagos—without a visa—and planned to travel to PH from there.[9] The Bryants knew that Sermanoukian would not make it out of Nigeria's arrival terminal without a visa. But convinced that she was coming, Rees Bryant reasoned that he needed to meet with immigration officials anyway, and so on January 15 the Bryants made the costly, "break-neck," twelve-hour drive to Lagos with their two older children, leaving at 4:30 a.m. on a Sunday.[10] Although no COC congregation had approved or financially supported Sermanoukian's coming, the Bryants' rescue mission seemed right at the time.

Bryant later reflected that he should have stayed on his malaria sick bed. Instead, in combined naïveté and eagerness to welcome a qualified nurse, the Bryants met Sermanoukian's plane and took immigration responsibility for her.[11] The COC had no nurse quota, but Rees posted her repatriation deposit, probably from his working funds, and helped her

---

[6]P. Bryant to Mattoxes, December 31, 1960.

[7]Bryant, *Divine,* 131.

[8]Ibid.; Bryant and Bryant, Interview.

[9]Taylor to R. Bryant, January 3, 1961; Taylor and Bryant, quoted in Bryant, *Divine,* 133–34.

[10]R. Bryant to Summerlin, February 1, 1961; R. Bryant to Taylor, April 28, 1961.

[11]Bryant and Bryant, Interview.

obtain a visa within forty-eight hours "thanks to a minor miracle in the immigration office."[12] Thus, a still-recovering Rees Bryant and family arrived back in Onicha Ngwa with Sermanoukian on Friday, January 20, exhausted by their six-day, 1,200-mile round trip over poor roads shared with lorry drivers who were "not generally responsible people," according to Patti Bryant. Their fatigue was not helped by an overnight stay in Benin at what she pronounced "the filthiest, rattiest, most roach-infested place we have ever endured."[13]

Their post-trip rest was short-lived. Doug Lawyer roused them all at 6:00 a.m. the next morning to announce that Charla was in labor. Sermanoukian accompanied the missionaries over the thirty-six miles of bush and paved roads to Queen Elizabeth Hospital (QEH) in Umuahia "not knowing whether … [the Bryants'] Opel would beat the stork to the hospital."[14] Fortunately, Sermanoukian's expertise was not required,[15] and Charla Lawyer later gave a glowing account of her uncomplicated delivery, lauding Nigerian nurses who were "courteous, clean and ever ready" to help. She enjoyed a faster postpartum recovery than she experienced in the US and praised QEH for allowing her husband to be present throughout their daughter's birth—"an experience we would not have missed…I was the only white woman in my curtained off corner of a 16 bed ward," she wrote, "but I wouldn't have traded places with anyone… Cindi was the only little 'white Nigerian' in the nursery."[16] Yet despite Charla Lawyer's positive experience and Sermanoukian's reassuring presence, Doug Lawyer continued to wonder why no COC hospital existed for missionaries.[17]

Crossing Paths and Swords

For the Bryants, the challenges surrounding Sermanoukian's arrival were eclipsed by both the warm hospitality of their Leslie and Sarah Diestelkamp and Sewell and Caneta Hall hosts in Lagos[18] and the excitement of having the first full-time missionary nurse at Onicha Ngwa. "She

---

[12]P. Bryant to Friends, February 4, 1961; R. Bryant to Proctor Street, July 1, 1961; Bryant to Massey, October 8, 1964; R. Bryant to Taylor, April 28, 1961.

[13]Bryant, *Divine*, 135; P. Bryant to Friends, February 4, 1961.

[14]R. Bryant to Summerlin, February 1, 1961.

[15]Masseys to Brethren, February 20, 1961, RPB:N.

[16]C. Lawyer to Friends, n.d., RPB:N.

[17]Bryant and Bryant, Interview; Lawyer, "Narrative," 37.

[18]Bryant, *Divine*, 135.

is well qualified to do the work," Patti Bryant wrote home confidently.[19] Nonetheless, Sermanoukian's arrival revived disagreements as well as friendship with the Diestelkamps and Halls, who helped to facilitate Sermanoukian's immigration but objected to her receiving a church salary. Even before the Bryants left Lagos, Leslie Diestelkamp wrote to all Onicha Ngwa evangelists that he agreed Nurse Sermanoukian could do good in Nigeria but that her arrival heralded "the beginning of a vast departure" from biblical practices. He anticipated that she would be only the first of "medical missionaries" paid from church treasuries and that her presence would heighten intra-COC discord.[20]

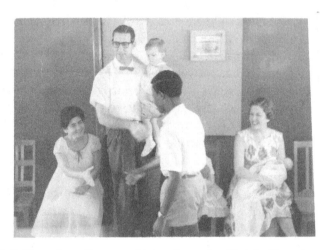

Photograph 7. Nurse Letty Sermanoukian welcomed to Onicha Ngwa by unidentified staff. Left to right: Sermanoukian, Douglas Lawyer holding daughter Tammy, with daughter Shauna seated behind staff, and Charla Lawyer holding newborn Cindi. 1961. (Bryant collection with permission.)

Rees Bryant responded to Diestelkamp within the week, thanking him profusely for his hospitality. "It was a joy to visit...and to discuss the Lord's work," Bryant reiterated, but it is "the *duty* of the church to do benevolent works for needy non-members." Similarly, he wrote to Sewell Hall, both expressing gratitude for the Halls' gracious assistance and making an optimistic defense of Sermanoukian that he later viewed as misplaced enthusiasm. While citing his awareness of her plans for eventual US immigration, Bryant expressed confidence to Hall that she was

---

[19]P. Bryant to Mattoxes, January 30, 1961; R. Bryant to Summerlin, February 1, 1961.
[20]Diestelkamp to Bryant, Massey, and Lawyer, January 18, 1961; R. Bryant to Summerlin, February 1, 1961.

worthy of financial support and that her coming to Nigeria was not "merely a 'stepping-stone'" to America.[21]

Investing

Within the week, Rees Bryant wrote to the elders at Green Lawn COC in Lubbock, Texas, asking them to salary "pioneer," Christian nurse Sermanoukian. She could have gone back to a "good job" in Beirut, he explained, but instead came to Nigeria to serve. He assured them that missionaries were cooperating with Nigerian health officials and planned to enlist a Nigerian preacher to interpret for her and teach patients about the faith, while she practiced in her anticipated maternal-child clinic. "I believe great good can be done in this way," Rees asserted.[22] In response, Green Lawn committed to half of the needed $200 per month; and Lubbock's Broadway COC and unnamed individuals, whom Bryant may have approached separately, also contributed.[23] No congregation, however, expressed willingness to assume legal, religious, or fiscal responsibility for Sermanoukian whom they did not know and whose work was initiated from the field.

Bryant also wrote to his sponsoring Proctor Street COC, using their own words as a measure of their willingness to take risks, asking only for their approval of (not funds for) Sermanoukian's work. He likely did not want to catch his own financial supporters off guard with his adding oversight of a nurse to an already full schedule of teaching, preaching, and gathering hospital information. Elder Ike Summerlin responded graciously on behalf of Proctor Street COC to "everyone, including Sister Letty" and wished her well in her mission work. Summerlin expressed hope that "Sister Letty will find open doors and rich rewards for her faith and service as she performs her errands of love in the Master's cause." He offered no funds.[24]

Bryant asked others for help as well. Among those responding with only moral support was John Dee Cox, preacher at the Sherrod Avenue COC in Florence, Alabama, where Rees Bryant's mother attended. While reporting that neither he nor Sherrod Avenue could help financially, Cox

---

[21]R. Bryant to Diestelkamp, January 24, 1961; R. Bryant to Hall, January 24, 1961; Bryant and Bryant, Interview.

[22]R. Bryant to Elders, January 28, 1961; R. Bryant to Brethren, February 20, 1961.

[23]R. Bryant to Brooms, May 6, 1961.

[24]R. Bryant to Summerlin, February 1, 1961; Summerlin to R. Bryant, February 15, 1961.

endorsed a theological justification of nurse and physician missionaries. Meanwhile, Lawrence Taylor sent well wishes from Libya, suggesting that Sermanoukian enjoyed work and Bryant should keep her busy. Additionally, Bill Nicks, who was back in the US raising mission funds, expressed hope that Sermanoukian could "lay some groundwork for Dr. Farrar."[25]

In Onicha Ngwa, Sermanoukian promptly began nursing practice from both the window of her room in the Bryant house and the same shed where Patti Bryant delivered care. Her work likely freed the Bryant, Lawyer, and Massey women from patient care, but because Sermanoukian was not yet registered as a nurse in Nigeria, her work was likely similar to theirs. Unlike the other missionary women, however, Sermanoukian practiced full-time, possessed formal nursing education, and left transportation of emergency cases to others.[26]

Missionaries invested in Sermanoukian's work as a platform to spread the Christian message. The recently organized COC congregation of staff and missionaries on the Onicha Ngwa compound purchased medical supplies and funded a salary for former BTC student, Wilson Agharanya, who translated for Sermanoukian, led daily devotionals, and distributed religious tracts during patient-care hours.[27] With government approval, missionaries and locals also prepared nearby abandoned, formerly British buildings for Sermanoukian's anticipated clinic[28] and waited impatiently for the arrival of her nursing credentials, so that in Doug Lawyer's view she could register with the government to "do the work that she is already doing." Lawyer wrote to Proctor Street COC of her "great work... [with] tremendous future possibilities," and Rees Bryant echoed those sentiments to Taylor in Libya.[29]

Disappointment

Unfortunately, disappointment followed optimism as the missionaries' best-laid healthcare plans were undercut by a combination of interper-

---

[25]Cox to R. Bryant, March 31, 1961; Taylor to R. Bryant, February 19, 1961; Nicks, "Narrative;" Nicks to Bryant and all, April 1, 1961.

[26]P. Bryant, email to author, July 26, 2016; R. Bryant to Brooms, May 6, 1961; R. Bryant to Taylor, March 6, 1961; Lawyer to Summerlin and Elders, February 28 and May 1, 1961; Joyce Massey, email to author, March 10, 2018.

[27]P. Bryant to Mattoxes, March 3, 1961; Lawyer to Summerlin and Elders, February 28, 1961.

[28]R. Bryant to Dickson, September 2, 1960; P. Bryant to Mattoxes, March 3, 1961; R. Bryant to Brooms, May 6, 1961.

[29]Lawyer to Summerlin and Elders, February 28, 1961; R. Bryant to Taylor, March 6, 1961.

sonal conflicts, unanticipated Nigerian requirements, and missing nursing credentials. Almost immediately, the Bryants found it difficult to host Sermanoukian, who voiced equal unhappiness at shared housing arrangements that she deemed "charity."[30] Although in the past whole missionary families amicably shared the same house for days, weeks, or months, the Bryant-Sermanoukian relationship quickly became strained.[31] The Bryants were also not comfortable with Sermanoukian's sense of personal space, particularly when she entered the couple's bedroom uninvited at night to comfort baby David, and the situation became so "unendurable" that Patti Bryant once ran to Joyce Massey's house pleading for "a bedroom where I can cry."[32]

Bryant and Lawyer quickly made different housing arrangements. They moved Nigerian household staff out of a small building in an upper corner of the compound and used Bryant's expense account to update it with paint and screened windows with plans to add an indoor bathroom later.[33] Sermanoukian's subsequent move into her own space improved the Bryants' family life, but to them, she seemed no happier.[34] Moreover, Letty soon collected her car and dog in PH, and although the Bryants appreciated Ruff's companionship to her, they and Masseys were dismayed that the dog ate better than many Nigerians.[35]

The insurmountable frustration, however, became Sermanoukian's inability to register as a nurse in Nigeria. When her nursing diploma arrived a few months after she did, Rees Bryant met in April with the Ministry of Health in Enugu for what he assumed would be a mere formality in her registration. Unfortunately, her diploma proved inadequate by itself, and the Ministry's Chief Matron informed Bryant that Sermanoukian could not work as a nurse in Nigeria without providing "a certificate of nursing competence from the Syrian government." Moreover, the Matron added, once registered, Sermanoukian could practice only in a hospital under a qualified physician. To the Bryants, the requirements seemed unnecessary bureaucracy that blocked services for desperate, local people, but a discouraged Rees Bryant suggested to Taylor in Libya that it might be "unwise" for Sermanoukian to stay in Nigeria. He asked for Taylor's prayers

[30]R. Bryant to Taylor, April 28, 1961; Bryant and Bryant, Interview.
[31]R. Bryant to Taylor, April 28, 1961; Farrar, *Stand*, 10; Goff, *Great*, 18; Nicks, "Familiarity," 9; Palmer, "Memories," 16.
[32]Bryant and Bryant, Interview.
[33]Ibid.; P. Bryant to Mattoxes, January 30, 1961; Bryants, personal communication, September 20, 2018; D. Lawyer to Friends, March 27, 1961, RPB:N.
[34]R. Bryant to Taylor, April 28, 1961.
[35]Bryant and Bryant, Interview; Joyce Massey, Facebook Messenger to author, March 10, 2018.

"for us and for Letty as we try to work out what has become an increasingly difficult situation."[36] No memories or documentation explained the Syrian competence certificate; perhaps it was an equivalent of a US RN post-degree license.

To missionaries, Sermanoukian was "*over* qualified to do ordinary dispensary work," but even if she were able to register with the government, they could not stomach sending a COC-funded nurse to practice in a hospital with Christian teachings that did not match their own or in a government hospital that represented no faith at all. An onsite COC physician was potentially years away, and Sermanoukian planned to move to the US in two years.[37] "It looks like we have rushed into a mess with the best intentions," lamented Patti Bryant.[38]

Interpersonal tensions escalated, for which Rees Bryant blamed both himself and Sermanoukian. He regretted his false assumption that her eagerness to come to Nigeria reflected a robust mission commitment, and he now thought that Sermanoukian demonstrated unhappiness about almost everything, possessed poor interpersonal skills, and showed "a lack of perspective about business and financial arrangements." Bryant conceded that Sermanoukian possessed "some good traits…[and] an unfortunate past," and he observed that the Americans recognized they were also imperfect. Nonetheless, he found Sermanoukian unprepared to be "an effective worker in a field which demands more maturity in the Lord."[39]

In ongoing correspondence, Bryant and Taylor affirmed respect for one another and recognized their joint responsibility in visiting this nurse-related challenge upon Onicha Ngwa. Taylor expressed surprise that Nigeria would not accept Sermanoukian's nursing qualifications[40]— although missing documentation blocked her practice, not qualifications per se. Taylor understood that Sermanoukian's colleague in Tripoli, a similarly credentialed nurse, had gained US employment. However, if the Nigeria situation remained untenable, he recommended Sermanoukian's termination, offered to help fund her travel back to Libya, and enclosed a check to reimburse Bryant for expenditures on her behalf. A still hopeful Taylor suggested that Bryant enact strict rules for Sermanoukian in any

---

[36]P. Bryant to Mattoxes, April 18 and May 5, 1961; R. Bryant to Taylor, April 28, 1961.

[37]P. Bryant to Mattoxes, March 3 and June 4, 1961.

[38]P. Bryant to Mattoxes, May 5, 1961.

[39]R. Bryant to Taylor, April 28, 1961.

[40]Ibid.; Taylor to R. Bryant, May 14, 1961.

work that they might find for her to do,[41] but nothing is recorded of her efforts beyond backdoor care.

Six months after Sermanoukian arrived in Nigeria, her Syrian competence certificate that was demanded by the Ministry of Health had not, and she informed missionaries that her papers were "destroyed in Beirut." She could never register in Nigeria.[42] Thus, in a sharp departure from their initial glowing assessment of possibilities, the Bryants now believed Sermanoukian was more interested in American immigration than in Nigerian service. Still, Patti Bryant acknowledged that Sermanoukian "would have worked as a nurse" if the government permitted it.[43]

Détente Destabilized

Sermanoukian's presence and Dr. Farrar's plans weakened the détente between prohospital and noninstitutional missionaries—a détente characterized in part by an unwritten agreement of mutual noninterference.[44] As a result, in 1961 missionary conflict flowed back into the US when Leslie Diestelkamp penned an open letter to West End COC (W-COC) objecting to their intended sponsorship of Dr. Farrar; Diestelkamp sent copies to missionaries in Nigeria and to three US congregations on differing sides of the controversy. While stating his desire to be transparent and nonthreatening, Diestelkamp argued that 1) sending a physician supported from church treasury funds would introduce doctrinal conflict into Nigerian COCs; 2) the supply of medical professionals in Nigeria met demand; and 3) Nigerian church unity was possible only if missionaries limited their work to evangelism. W-COC must avoid funding "secular schools, hospitals, nurses and doctors," he insisted, in order to maintain COC unity in Nigeria and to reach "every lost soul possible with the pure gospel."[45]

From Onicha Ngwa, Rees Bryant responded immediately. The advent of licensed professionals, Rees argued, constituted a practical improvement not an innovation because lay missionaries already delivered care. Church-salaried health professionals, too, were not innovative because

---

[41]R. Bryant to Proctor Street, July 1, 1961; Bryant and Bryant, Interview; Lawyer to Summerlin and Proctor Street, May 1, 1961; Taylor to R. Bryant, May 14, 1961.

[42]P. Bryant to Mattoxes, June 4, 1961; Lawyer, "Narrative," 37.

[43]Bryant and Bryant, Interview.

[44]H. Farrar to McInteer, February 24, 1967.

[45]Diestelkamp to West End, May 31, 1961.

COC funds already supported Sermanoukian—a tautological argument that perhaps redeemed her presence for Bryant while confirming Diestelkamp's fears. Moreover, Bryant noted that Nigeria's Federal Ministry of Health statistics recorded "1,079 registered medical practitioners" for its "35 million" citizens, with 189 of those providers in Lagos, and he further insisted that COC unity must arise from biblical teaching not human agreement. Finally, Bryant affirmed the primacy of evangelism and rejoiced that W-COC would send Dr. Farrar as a "gospel preacher" in 1963 in order to evaluate Nigeria's medical mission prospects.[46]

Both sides argued from the US Restoration Movement ideal that Christians should enact God's will as revealed in the Bible, that the Bible's message is clear, and that an honest reading of Scripture brings unity. Nonetheless, their disagreement about how Christians should care for the sick laid bare that theology's fault lines. Although in the 1950s, untaught Nigerians committed to following the Bible while not being sure what it said,[47] in the 1960s, Bryant and Diestelkamp committed to following the Bible while each was quite sure what it said. Even so, their letters reflected a tone of personal responsibility for each other, and despite intense rhetoric they continued as intra-COC missionaries to one another.[48]

Unplanned Leaving

While these events swirled around what Rees Bryant named "Project Letty,"[49] a pregnant Patti Bryant was admitted with severe amoebic dysentery to QEH in July 1961, and subsequently the concerned family abruptly left Nigeria to seek US care. Nigerians sent them off with customarily effusive well wishes, gifts, and pleas to return when strength allowed, while Bryants concentrated on the need to get home and healthy. In the US, the family temporarily lived in Lubbock with Patti's parents, F.W. and Mildred Mattox, while Rees Bryant preached for the Green Lawn COC. "Perfect" infant daughter Rebecca arrived safely in December.[50]

---

[46]Diestelkamp to Bryant, Massey, and Lawyer, January 18, 1961; Bryant to Elders, August 3, 1961. More on Bryants sentiments in R. Bryant to Lawyers and Masseys, August 2, 1961. The 1960 population of Nigeria was over 45 million.

[47]Reese and Echols, *Report*, 9.

[48]Diestelkamp to R. Bryant, Massey, and Lawyer, January 18, 1961; Bryant to Diestelkamp, January 24, 1961.

[49]Rees Bryant, appointment calendar/diary, January 5, 1961.

[50]Bryant, *Divine*, 144–48; Chronicle News, "Bryants Leave;" Church of Christ, Aba to Bryants, July 17, 1961; Church of Christ, Ibo-Land to Bryants, July 17, 1961; Student body of Bible Training College, Onicha Ngwa to Bryants, July 17, 1961; Farewell to Bryants (program), July 17, 1961.

Despite this geographical separation from Onicha Ngwa, Rees Bryant remained emotionally connected. His inability to stay until the Sermanoukian-related challenges were resolved generated a sense of personal frailty and lifelong regret,[51] but he did what he could from the US. Bryant followed up with Lubbock's Broadway COC about their $800 contribution for Sermanoukian's support that was still in Nigeria. After learning that Sermanoukian could not register as a nurse, the Broadway elders released those funds to Onicha Ngwa missionaries to use at their discretion, and Bryant encouraged the Lawyers and Masseys to use some for Sermanoukian and some to prepare the Bryants' vacated house for their Proctor Street COC-funded replacements: Bill and Mary Lou Johnson Curry with young children, Bart, Clifford, and Patty Nell.[52] Bryant may also have recouped his substantial expenditure of £125 for Sermanoukian's immigration and £300 for her early salary and expenses.[53]

Legal Action

In Nigeria, the Masseys and Lawyers terminated Sermanoukian, and she took legal action. Rejecting Bryants' advice to return either to Libya or the middle east,[54] she filed a breach of contract suit against the Registered Trustees of the Churches of Christ in Nigeria. Although the Trustees never employed anyone, she asserted that the missionaries violated promises of "support and American citizenship."[55] Jim Massey and Doug Lawyer reassured Rees Bryant that they did not fault him for the situation, and in typical good humor Lawyer framed the situation in biblical terms. "The matter is one of those unfortunate problems," he wrote, "which, if accepted in their place, makes us more noble Christians. The trying of our faith works patience. Believe me—it's worked some patience in me."[56]

The court case consumed substantial missionary time. Doug Lawyer hired a PH attorney, and the suit required missionary presence over many months in Lagos, Calabar, and Umuahia courtrooms. By December 1963, two high court judges concluded that while no contract existed, the mis-

---

[51]R. Bryant to Taylor, April 28, 1961; Bryant and Bryant, Interview.
[52]Proctor Street, "Bill Currys;" R. Bryant to Lawyers and Masseys, August 2, 1961; R. Bryant to Nicks, September 5, 1961.
[53]R. Bryant to Masseys, June 3, 1965.
[54]Bryant, *Divine*, 160–61; Bryant, *Gently*, bk. 3, 25; P. Bryant to Mattoxes, June 4, 1961; Lawyer, "Narrative," 37.
[55]Bryant and Bryant, Interview; Lawyer, "Narrative," 37.
[56]Lawyer, quoted in Bryant, in *Gently*, bk. 3, 5.

sionaries owed Sermanoukian two months of salary. The COC team paid the court-ordered funds, but Sermanoukian rebuffed Massey and Lawyer's attempted reconciliation, blaming them for the difficulties.[57] The unplanned experiment of in-the-field oversight of a missionary nurse had failed, and in 1964 Sermanoukian moved to Lagos and from there to the US. Lawyer later wrote that she was "ordered" to leave Nigeria.[58] Her departure reopened a COC quota position, likely refunded any of Bryant's remaining repatriation deposit on her behalf, and brought closure. There are no records or memories indicating that Sermanoukian met Henry Farrar when he came to Nigeria in 1963 and 1964, and nothing further is known of her life and work.[59]

Rees Bryant retrospectively described "Project Letty"[60] as his attempt "to do what I thought was Christian and wise," but bluntly called his decision to bring Sermanoukian from Lagos to Onicha Ngwa "the worst mistake I ever made in Nigeria." Fairly or unfairly, no one was more critical of Bryant than he, but his actions to immigrate Sermanoukian never undermined the long-term harmony either among prohospital missionaries or with sponsoring COCs.[61] Perhaps most remarkable was that the "long, unfortunate ordeal"[62] did not derail missionaries' healthcare dreams.

Moving Forward

The second Bryant furlough was spent in Lubbock and Searcy and lasted three years (1961–1964) because of health crises for Patti and then Rees.[63] During much of that time, Rees Bryant continued to raise money and recruit health professionals for Nigeria in numerous congregations; he would preach a Sunday morning "mission sermon" and then show scripted Nigerian slides with a donated state-of-the-art projector in the evening. Bryant was an excellent fundraiser, and hearers opened "their

---

[57]Joyce Massey, quoted in Bryant, *Divine*, 161.

[58]R. Bryant to Martins, January 1, 1965; Lawyer to R. Bryant, May 7, 1964, RPB:N; Lawyer, "Narrative," 37.

[59]Bryant, *Divine*, 161; Bryant and Bryant, Interview; P. Bryant and Joyce Massey, email to author, April 27, 2018; Farrar, "Chronology."

[60]R. Bryant, personal diary, January 5, 1961.

[61]Bryant, "Reflections;" R. Bryant to Masseys, June 3, 1965; Bryant and Bryant, Interview.

[62]Lawyer, "Narrative," 37.

[63]Bryant, *Divine*, 144–70; R. Bryant to Proctor Street, July 1, 1961; R. Bryant to Summerlin, November 5, 1963; R. Bryant to Underwood, December 28, 1961.

hearts and...pocketbooks."[64] Concurrently, Rees Bryant and Bill Nicks corresponded with Henry Farrar and W-COC elders, who committed to "complete support"[65] for Dr. Farrar as a preacher who would practice medicine "on the side."[66]

The Bryants longed for a third Nigerian tour, and when they felt ready, a soon-to-furlough Jim Massey persuaded his sponsor, South Park COC in Beaumont, Texas, to hire Rees Bryant as his replacement.[67] Meanwhile, missionaries continued to move to and from Nigeria in what Patti Bryant called "divine choreography." Among them, the Currys and Masseys were furloughing, and the Farrar family would arrive for the first time in 1964. The Currys planned to return to Nigeria at a new mission point in Enugu alongside COC novice missionaries Dayton and Ruth Keesee with young daughters, Dita and Tonya; Keesees were sponsored by Creswell Street COC in Shreveport, Louisiana.[68]

Conclusion

Missionary ideas of what a COC missionary nurse should be and do clashed with the reality of who one particular nurse was and what she did. The missionaries' primary goal was for a nurse to practice Christian service, while Sermanoukian focused on employment and immigrating to the US. Further complicating her integration into the Onicha Ngwa team were multiple interpersonal, professional, and communication issues, including unspoken missionary assumptions.

The context of her work also was problematic. In their eagerness, missionaries facilitated Sermanoukian's side-stepping of ordinary COC congregational vetting and oversight. Evangelists were expected to have church sponsors, but Sermanoukian's gender, occupation, and indirect communications may be what led missionaries down a different path. In yielding to the blur of her fast-moving travel plans, Rees Bryant became a *de facto* sponsoring employer—finding funds, prescribing work, evaluating outcomes, and dispensing salary. His sponsoring COC elders gave him this leeway post hoc in a sign of extraordinary trust.

---

[64]Bryant, *Divine*, 163–64; Bryant and Bryant, Interview.
[65]Summerlin to Bryants and Masseys, May 25, 1960.
[66]Bryant and Bryant, Interview.
[67]Bryant, *Divine*, 160–62; Summerlin to Bryants, November 3, 1963; Summerlin to R. Bryant, May 31, 1961 and January 20, 1964.
[68]Bryant, *Divine*, 161–62, 173–74; *Star Reporter*, "Keesee."

The combined result of these variables was Sermanoukian's conflict-infused transition from a paid government position into a not-yet-salaried-and-poorly-defined missionary role. Unfortunately, we have no record of what Sermanoukian thought or expected, but in a self-critical analysis, Rees Bryant reflected on his own motives in bringing her to Onicha Ngwa, and he labelled them as a combined "desire to help the suffering" and personal arrogance. He expressed gratitude that colleagues forgave him for the difficulties and that God continued to use "less than perfect [...] human beings to accomplish His will," for "there are no other kind."[69] Yet even the Bryants themselves found it remarkable that their hospital vision survived.[70]

---

[69]Bryant, "Reflections," 24.
[70]Bryant and Bryant, Interview.

8

The Evolution of Nancy Petty

(1940–1964)

All these seeds had been planted, so I was ready.
—Nancy Petty

Before Essien's letters, before Glenna Peden's work, and even longer before the idea of an Onicha Ngwa hospital, future missionary Nancy
Corinne Petty was born to Albert and Kitty Foster Petty. A physician attended her June 24, 1940 birth in her parents' two-story, log cabin home
in tiny Bear Creek, Tennessee, on the outskirts of the diminutive town of
Vanleer. Nancy was the firstborn in her family, and in southern US tradition, her parents named her after a family member: her Aunt Corinne.
The next year, sister Dianne was also born at home, and ten years later
brother Dale arrived at the Jackson Clinic in nearby Dickson.[1]

Nancy Petty recalled that roughly half her elementary teachers attended the Vanleer COC with the Pettys in their small close-knit community.
The other half went to the Methodist congregation, the only other
church in town. Townspeople attended each other's "gospel meetings,"
shared a conservative morality, loved Jesus, and believed he was "the
Way." Young Petty experienced the congregations as more alike than different, although the COC sang a capella and the Methodists used a piano.
She didn't remember "anybody ever changing" churches.[2]

Vocation Nursing

At age four, Petty was "called" to be a nurse and "never wavered." After
her father was wounded in WWII, Nancy became captivated by the
starched, white-capped professionals caring for her father at the Veterans

---

[1]Farrar and Petty-Kraus, Interview; Petty-Kraus, Interview 1; *Dickson County Herald*,
"Volunteer nurse arrives in Nigeria," ca. 1965.
[2]Farrar and Petty-Kraus, Interview.

Administration (VA) Hospital in Memphis. She announced to her family that she was going to be a nurse, and her mother lent whole-hearted support. Years later when high-schooler Nancy came home weeping over an aptitude test that classified her as secretarial material, Kitty Petty told her daughter in no uncertain terms to forget the test and pursue her nursing dreams. Only later did Nancy learn that Kitty had wanted to be a nurse like her own lay nurse mother, who delivered babies, cared for the sick, laid out the dead, and "just had a healing kind of nature." When Kitty secretly applied and was admitted to nursing school, her controlling father forbade her to go. "Nurses do things ladies should not do, and you're not going to do that," he told her.[3] Kitty refused to let Nancy suffer the same disappointment.

Thus, after her 1958 Charlotte High School graduation, Nancy Petty began nursing studies about fifty miles from home at Mid-State Baptist School of Nursing in Nashville—the same program that had accepted her mother. She remembered the school as "faith-oriented" and supplemented by a few classes from nearby Belmont College. Its three-year nursing diploma curriculum was intense, and she recalled only one two-week break.[4]

Petty graduated in 1961 with self-assessed strong clinical, triage, and decision-making skills. She felt well-prepared for her first job as staff nurse in the recovery room at Mid-State Baptist Hospital (now St. Thomas West) in Nashville.[5] Intensive care units did not exist then, and the recovery room admitted all high acuity patients. There Petty discovered what it meant to have a professional attitude toward self, work, and colleagues—something she appreciated later as good preparation for the mission field. She learned to rest and to respect everyone on the team. The head nurse enforced fifteen-minute breaks every ninety minutes for all staff regardless of workload, and she taught Petty not to underestimate colleagues. When new graduate Petty complained that an older Licensed Practical Nurse colleague, Mrs. Vanderpool, didn't do her share of the work, the head nurse disagreed, telling her that Mrs. Vanderpool "just reserves her strength" for what needs to be done. Petty never forgot a later hectic Saturday when Mrs. Vanderpool "saved" her "over and over and over."[6]

---

[3]Ibid.
[4]"Former CHS Student;" Ibid.
[5]Petty-Kraus, personal communication, April 10, 2017.
[6]Farrar and Petty-Kraus, Interview.

Location Nigeria

Nancy Petty entered nursing for its own sake, not as a pathway to missions, although her mission interests began in childhood. Whenever missionaries from Korea, Africa, and Germany visited the Vanleer COC, her parents would host them, exposing her to people and stories from around the world. Nancy's lifetime favorite hymns became missional ones: "Send the Light" and "Let the Lower Lights Be Burning."[7]

Petty's mission interests were further piqued during her nursing school years when Baptist peer Linda Porter returned from a three-month mission trip during their junior year.[8] Linda talked incessantly about how Nigerians would travel long distances for healthcare and classes, describing them as smart people who loved learning and worshipped enthusiastically.[9] Petty wondered if the COC sent missionaries to Nigeria,[10] and soon she began to hear reports of Glenna Peden's work from the LA-COC pulpit.[11] "I had a lot of teaching, and it fell on me," she reflected years later.[12]

These influences came together for her in 1962:

> One day...I was off duty and was standing in my little kitchen...sorting through white beans and picking out the rocks and stuff and washing them to cook. And I'm thinking and I'm thinking. And that's when I got the call to Nigeria, for sure. I knew it was Nigeria. [...] Now, I didn't hear an audible voice...but it was a clear message. I'm just going about my duties. But...all these seeds had been planted, so I was ready.[13]

Immediately Petty stopped sorting beans and phoned minister Clyde Hale (1901-1979) at Nashville's University COC, where she regularly attended. Telling Hale about her Nigerian call, Petty said that she didn't know anyone in Nigeria but didn't want to go alone. Hale told her of Dr. Farrar's plans and wrote Farrar asking if he would like "a trained regis-

---

[7]Petty-Kraus, Presentation to Keen-Agers.

[8]Farrar and Petty-Kraus, Interview; Hays-Savio and Petty-Kraus, Interview; Petty-Kraus, Presentation to Keen-Agers. Nancy misspoke name of classmate Linda Porter as Anna Mae Roberts in Farrar and Petty-Kraus, Interview.

[9]Farrar and Petty-Kraus, Interview.

[10]Petty-Kraus, Interview 1.

[11]Hays-Savio and Petty-Kraus, Interview; Petty-Kraus, Interview 1.

[12]Farrar and Petty-Kraus, Interview.

[13]Ibid.

tered nurse to work for" him on the mission field. Hale described Petty as "thoroughly qualified...in perfect health, and one of the finest Christian young ladies it has been my privilege to know." As Hale explained, Petty intended to go to Nigeria whether Farrar was interested in her coming or not, adding that he and Eugene Peden, then in Nashville, supported her plans and the University COC would help her financially.[14] Thus, whatever Hale meant by her working "for" Dr. Farrar, Petty and Farrar's relationship would be a functional, not an employer-employee one.

Petty's theological explanation for why she was called, while others were not, was simple: "God calls who He calls." She saw herself acting in response to God's will for her that was revealed to her through thoughts and ordinary life experiences. Petty admitted later that she was "really young...pretty arrogant," and overconfident, but she considered those flaws balanced by God's provision of what she needed—even when she forgot to ask for his help.[15]

Easy Choice

Petty earlier thought she "would die" when she couldn't go home for two weeks from nursing school, and friends were skeptical that she would leave her beloved Bear Creek for West Africa. They did not understand the relative weight of her missionary motivation, which now made the prospect of two years in Nigeria seem easy. As with her decision to be a nurse, Petty never wavered from responding to her missionary call. Jesus came "a far piece" for her, Petty explained colloquially, and she wanted to tell Nigerians about him as the way to be saved by God.[16] Besides, as Petty joked about heaven, the missionary "retirement plan is so good."[17]

Even her Christian, premedical studies boyfriend could not dissuade her. Petty recalled that his plan was "to work and...send money to missions," while her plan was, "I'm going." She promptly informed her family of her Nigeria commitment, which both parents took seriously.[18] Albert Petty later admitted that his twenty-two-year-old daughter's plans to move to sub-Saharan Africa caused him stomach distress;[19] and Kitty Petty vigorously defended Nancy's intentions against at least one

---

[14]Ibid.; Hale to H. Farrar, March 2, 1962; Harp, "Henry Clyde Hale;" Peden, "Chronology."

[15]Petty-Kraus, Interview 1.

[16]Ibid.; Farrar and Petty-Kraus, Interview.

[17]G. Farrar, Interview.

[18]Farrar and Petty-Kraus, Interview.

[19]H. Farrar, Interview 1; Farrars, personal communication, n.d.

woman's concerns that Nancy "was going to be so friendly with black people"—concerns that Kitty rejected as not Christian.[20] Whatever preschooler Nancy Petty thought nursing would be, she was not later disappointed. The vocation proved engaging and interesting. And whatever young Nurse Petty thought it meant to be a missionary, she saw it as God's personal call to her.

Childhood Preparation

From Petty's perspective, God readied her for missions from childhood. Her father modeled virtue and determination, her mother encouraged Nancy's vocational aspirations,[21] and her grandmother Jesse Foster taught her how to live without utilities, take a bath in a pan of water, and use a kerosene refrigerator and wick lamp.[22] Petty viewed even a positive childhood tuberculosis skin test and childhood illnesses as valuable.[23]

Nancy Petty credited her dad with teaching her how to act "when you're called." She saw him as a quiet, courageous man who finished what he started, and she never forgot his determination to recover from osteomyelitis caused by a WWII gunshot wound. Penicillin saved him, but VA providers told Albert Petty that he would never walk again. Not true, he bluntly informed them, because he was a farmer with a family to support. He designed a brace, called on Kitty to cut him out of traction, visited the VA prosthetic shop daily "until they made his brace," and then signed himself out of the VA against medical advice. Once home he went from brace to crutches, to walking cane, to farming, and then to driving big equipment as a forest ranger. Ruefully, Nancy admitted, she didn't learn enough from him about when to be silent; her reactions were more like her mother's: "the tea kettle, here it comes."[24]

From her father, Nancy learned to rely on Christian faith as a guide for life,[25] and from her mother she acquired a stubbornness to stick with decisions. By now she knew well the story of Kitty Foster's refusal to marry high school classmate Albert Petty during four years of dating because he was unbaptized. Albert would not change just to please Kitty but decided

[20]Ibid.; G. Farrar, Interview.
[21]Farrar and Petty-Kraus, Interview.
[22]Petty-Kraus, Presentation to Keen-Agers.
[23]Petty-Kraus, Interview 1.
[24]Ibid.
[25]Kraus, "On Daddy's Knee."

that "if the Bible was the word of God" he should read it. Reading led him to baptism, and Kitty and Albert married soon after.[26]

Being raised by those "godly parents" on a farm taught Petty other lessons that she used on the mission field, including the value of hard work and unearned benefits, as well as how little control a person has over life. As she reflected, sometimes "you reap what you don't sow" like blackberries and edible wild greens, and other times you sow and don't reap, as when you plant and rain doesn't come. Life was "adventuresome…fun…never dull," she discovered, and the one day she grumbled about boredom, her mother assigned enough work that she never complained again. Thus, by the time Nancy Petty decided to go to Nigeria, she had taken to heart these lessons of faith, hard work, perseverance, and reliance on God. Albert and Kitty Petty believed in her, and Nancy was thoroughly self-assured.[27]

Mission Preparations

During Nurse Petty's 1962–1965 preparation years for Nigeria, it quickly became apparent that she was not the only future missionary with abundant self-confidence. Shortly after Hale's letter, Dr. Farrar began sending what Nancy portrayed as "a long string of letters…with instructions on how you get to the mission field. Very specific instructions!"[28] Farrar's first missive, she laughed, "detailed what I should do for the next five years of my life."[29] Dr. Farrar did not let his inexperience stand in the way of advice-giving. He had never been to a mission field, except for a few weeks in late 1963, but was twelve years older than Petty and a surgeon who extended his authoritarian, captain-of-the-ship, operating room role to other relationships. While his sources of information were sound —the Nickses, Bryants, and other mission mentors from Harding College days—his early counsel was based almost entirely on second-hand reports.[30] Petty read, but rarely replied to Dr. Farrar's letters, perhaps because of her self-confidence, busy schedule, and self-assessed status as a poor writer.[31] Grace Farrar recalled Petty's postal silence as a source of

---

[26]Petty-Kraus, Interview 1.
[27]Ibid.; Farrar and Petty-Kraus, Interview.
[28]Farrar and Petty-Kraus, Interview.
[29]Petty-Kraus, Presentation to Keen-Agers.
[30]G. Farrar to Folks, September 15 and October 26, 1963; Farrar, *Stand*, ix–x.
[31]Farrar and Petty-Kraus, Interview.

endless frustration to Henry, who vowed "to meet her at the airport with a fountain pen and ask her if she knows how to use it."[32]

Dr. Farrar wrote to Petty that the field could be dangerous and recommended that she learn about missionary work. He suggested that former missionaries in Nashville were excellent resources and advised Petty to take courses at a COC-affiliated college.[33] Given the rarity of COC academic missions courses in the early 1960s, he may have assumed that enrollment would provide access to extracurricular mission-related activities; he thought of his own 1940s experiences in Harding College's China Club as helpful. Perhaps he reasoned further that Petty needed COC training because of her Baptist nursing education and that enrollment might reassure potential financial supporters that she was a faithful COC member, "fitted for" international missions.[34] Petty was young, Farrar had not met her, and his possible knowledge of Sermanoukian-related issues may have heightened his awareness that well-intended plans could go wrong. In turn, Petty believed that Dr. Farrar did not appreciate what she already knew from missionaries visiting her childhood home, her roommate's stories, her faith-based nursing program, and the Pedens at LA-COC.[35] And she did little to inform him.

Her Own Path

Petty came closest to following Farrar's advice when her friend Janice Keasling, RN, came through Nashville on her way to Abilene. Keasling planned to work as a school nurse at Abilene Christian College (ACC) while completing a bachelor's degree, and she invited Petty to come along. Petty went, and the two shared living quarters in Abilene for over a year, but Petty never enrolled in ACC. Instead, she added almost a year of nursing work experience at the local Baptist Hospital.[36] Participating in mission-related college offerings may have been Farrar's priority, but it wasn't hers, and she had no obligation to follow his recommendations. Petty modeled her dad, who "didn't do things just because people thought he ought to."[37]

---

[32]G. Farrar, Interview.

[33]H. Farrar, Interview 1; Farrar and Petty-Kraus, Interview.

[34]H. Farrar, Interview 1.

[35]Farrar and Petty-Kraus, Interview; Hale to H. Farrar, March 2, 1962.

[36]Farrar and Petty-Kraus, Interview; *Dickson County*, "Miss Nancy Petty."

[37]Petty-Kraus, Interview 1.

In 1964, when Petty heard that the Farrars were making final arrangements to leave for Nigeria, she quit her Abilene job and moved home to Bear Creek in hopes of traveling with them. Her failure to enroll in ACC freed her from academic obligations that might have held her back, and as she mused later, "The Lord is working when you're not helping too much."[38] Petty wrote Farrar about her plans on May 1, 1964, and he again welcomed her interest, reveling in her endorsement by Clyde Hale and others. He gave an overview of the current mission status in Onicha Ngwa, confirmed the need for her nursing expertise, invited her to move to Nigeria with his family in July, and offered to help raise financial support. While repeating that Africa could be dangerous, he affirmed that so could America. After all, he penned, John Glenn was injured in a home bathroom fall after safely orbiting the Earth.[39]

Reaffirmed Intentions

Nancy Petty reaffirmed her missionary intentions to Farrar in a telephone call during the Farrars' predeparture visit with Henry's mother in Nashville, and soon the Farrars became the latest in a string of missionaries visiting her home. Eager to recruit a COC nurse, Farrar and family drove the roughly hundred miles round trip over paved and dirt roads to Bear Creek for their only face-to-face meeting before moving to Nigeria. Undeterred by Petty's decision not to enroll in a COC-affiliated college, he discussed fundraising and practical matters with her and her parents and allayed their apprehension about safety despite his previous hints at danger.[40] The encounter established a lifetime, personal bond between the families that was grounded in their shared religious faith and support of Nancy.[41]

One week later, on July 15, 1964, Henry and Grace Farrar and their five children flew from Nashville to New York for a week's vacation at the World's Fair and a visit with Christians in the Bay Shore COC Exodus movement. From there, they flew to England, where Henry Farrar studied for five days at the London School of Tropical Medicine and Hygiene and the Hospital for Tropical Diseases. From London, the family board-

---

[38]Farrar and Petty-Kraus, Interview.
[39]H. Farrar to Petty, May 4, 1964.
[40]G. Farrar to Johnsons, July 15, 1964; H. Farrar, Interview 1.
[41]Farrar and Petty-Kraus, Interview.

ed a BOAC plane to Lagos and a Nigerian Airways one on to Port Harcourt (PH).[42]

Meanwhile, Petty waited on a visa and funding and worked at Goodlark Hospital in Dickson, Tennessee.[43] As she promised during the Petty-Farrar meeting, Petty asked the Vanleer COC for financial help, and its elders and seventy to eighty members agreed. In a letter possibly written for Nigerian immigration authorities, the congregation's three elders, including her father, committed to "full responsibility" for Petty's missionary costs.[44] Thus, just as LA-COC took on a larger Ikot Usen work than they initially thought possible, the Vanleer congregation acted beyond its size, making Petty their "first, and probably only, full-time missionary."[45] Petty benefited from her decades-long family membership at Vanleer COC in the same way that the Farrars benefited from W-COC connections. The personal relationships with their financial backers would have been impossible with a distant mission society.

Petty's funding situation, however, differed from Dr. Farrar's in at least two ways. First, a single congregation, the wealthy W-COC, underwrote almost the entire budget of Farrar as their "first 'preaching physician,'"[46] while the smaller Vanleer COC could cover only part of Petty's costs. Thus, fundraising became a Petty family project with money coming from Nashville's University COC, Walnut Street COC in Dickson, and other Tennessee churches.[47] Albert Petty spoke before congregations about his daughter's planned work, while Kitty Petty, as official reporter of Vanleer news for the *Dickson County Herald*, built community goodwill.[48] Henry Farrar raised some funds, and Nancy Petty cultivated local relationships by speaking to the Future Homemakers of America at her high school alma mater—an event reported with photo in unknown local newspaper.[49]

---

[42]Author's recollection; Farrar, *Stand*, 5–6; H. Farrar to McInteer, Cayce, and Sinclair, August 24, 1964, W-COC file.

[43]*Dickson County*, "Miss Nancy Petty."

[44]G. Farrar, Interview; Petty-Kraus, Interview 1; A.H. Petty, Bone, and Powell to "Whom It May Concern," April 4, 1965. Some sponsorship details in Minutes, Mission Study Committee, W-COC, May 21, 1967.

[45]Farrar and Petty-Kraus, Interview.

[46]R. Bryant to Lawyers and Masseys, August 2, 1961; McInteer, quoted in Farrar, *Stand*, ix; Summerlin to Bryants and Masseys, May 25, 1960. Per H. Farrar to Benson, ca. May/June 1965, Nicks raised funds for the Farrars' car.

[47]G. Farrar to Kee, Buice, and Tarbet, September 29, 1967; Farrar and Petty-Kraus, Interview; Green Lawn, *Nigerian Evangelism*; Minutes, Mission Study Committee, May 21, 1967, W-COC file; Petty to Gibbs, April 12, 1966.

[48]Farrar and Petty-Kraus, Interview; Petty-Kraus, Interview 1.

[49]H. Farrar, Interview 1; "Former CHS Student."

Second, Petty's financial support may have been more ecumenical than Farrar's.[50] Albert Petty often helped the elderly Vanleer Methodist minister with repairs and firewood "just as a neighbor," and now the Methodists donated to Petty's travel expenses. "She is one of us," the minister asserted, confirming for Petty the "special," "unique," "loving" and "real" character of her community that prepared her well for interdenominational relationships in Nigeria.[51] Similar ecumenical support for a missionary man might have raised concerns about COC orthodoxy, but no one questioned Nancy Petty's doctrinal purity. Perhaps she received less scrutiny because she was a woman and nurse, not a preacher, and the Petty family's lifetime membership in the COC spoke to her faith pedigree. Too, it is possible that few outside Vanleer knew of the Methodist funding that likely was received and disbursed through Vanleer COC. For Petty, funding from diverse supporters affirmed both her calling and God's providence. "I didn't do everything right at all," she acknowledged decades later, "But He helped us through the whole thing."[52]

Petty prepared professionally, personally, spiritually, and materially. Following Farrar's instructions, she registered with Nigeria's Council of Nursing, sending her diploma and other documents before leaving the US. Petty recalled that she "prayed a lot" and at her mother's suggestion bought $5,000 in life insurance to cover any debts should she not return. Although disinterested in driving, she also took Farrar's advice to earn a US driver's license, which would make it easier to obtain a Nigerian one. "You do not want to take the Nigerian driving test," he warned.[53]

Conclusion

By the end of 1964, Nancy Petty, RN, was ready to go, and from this she drew a single conclusion: God prepared the way for her. With help from parents, Farrar, Vanleer Methodists, and COC congregations, Petty gathered what she thought was needed. Then she waited impatiently for a visa on one side of the Atlantic Ocean, while COC missionaries waited impatiently for her coming on the other.

---

[50]H. Farrar, Interview 1. Per G. Farrar to Johnson, February 4 and February 27, 1964 letters, Henry Farrar presented slides to several non-COC, charitable, religious and secular groups after his 1963 exploratory visit. No contributions from those are documented.

[51]Farrar and Petty-Kraus, Interview.

[52]Petty-Kraus, Interview 1.

[53]Ibid.

9
The Revolution of Iris Hays
(1941–1964)

I'm going to be a missionary to Africa.
—Iris Hays, age 10

While Nancy Petty was being shaped by family and church in Tennessee, Iris Fay Hays was being molded in Texas.[1] Both women grew up in the COC, where they were inspired to be missionaries, but their paths, personalities, physiques, and sibling positions were strikingly different. Notably, Petty initially chose a career in nursing; Hays, a career in African missions.

Iris Hays's heritage was Irish, Cherokee, and Arkansas/Texas pioneer. When her widowed maternal grandmother, lay nurse Bonnie Ramsey, remarried and moved to west Texas, she became "the nearest thing to a doctor in their area." Bonnie's daughter Dove "Dovie" married Ruey "R.D." Hays, and Iris Hays was born to them in Monahans, Texas, on August 7, 1941. Iris was the youngest of four: Wanda was born in 1936 in Turkey, Texas; James Ernest was born in 1937 and Earl David in 1939, both in Snyder, Texas. [2] Iris and Wanda were especially close when they were growing up, and preteen Wanda used her newspaper route money to buy coveted, store-bought clothing items for Iris and herself.[3]

Iris's father was a sharecropper who "followed the harvest" from Turkey to Snyder and peddled fruit. He built a family house in Monahans, but walked away from his marriage, leaving his family in poverty. When Dovie's brother Elmer realized their situation around 1948, he moved her

---

[1]"Iris Fay Hays Savio," September 13, 2012, findagrave.com no. 97014106.
[2]Talley, "Bonnie Elizabeth Ramsey," 48930–vm; Wanda Hays Talley, phone call to author, August 1, 2013. During phone call, Talley explained that August 6 is sometimes listed as Iris Hays's birthdate because the attending physician filled out paperwork when he arrived at the hospital on August 6, then delivered Iris after midnight on August 7.
[3]Iris Hays-Savio, personal communication, May 16, 2012.

and the children into his own home in Andrews, Texas, until he could rent a separate place for them. In Andrews, Iris and her siblings found the COC a "strong and a wonderful place to grow."[4]

Vocation Missionary

Iris Hays chose her career at age ten during a service at the Andrews COC. Impressed by the slideshow of a visiting missionary from South Africa, she decided at once to "be a missionary to Africa." She "was determined; that was it." After her 1959 graduation from Andrews High School, she entered Lubbock Christian College (LCC), then a junior college in West Texas. LCC mandated Bible courses but did not prepare women for nursing, ministry, or missions, and she enrolled as a secretarial science major because she enjoyed typing.[5]

Nevertheless, she persisted with her mission dreams, despite having no plan, no missionary friends, and no connection to Africa. Hays was also sure about one other thing: She would never be a nurse. She was not persuaded by stories of Grandmother Bonnie caring for her community or by her many friends who "wanted to be nurses…[and] read those nursing novels that everybody reads." In truth, hospital smells made Hays so sick that she held her nose when visiting them, and the only career she deemed worse than nursing was teaching.[6] She did not know that her future held both.

During her freshman year at LCC, Hays abruptly changed—or as she saw it *was* changed—when she heard Rees Bryant speak during chapel about the desperate healthcare situation in rural Onicha Ngwa.[7] The Bryants were on their first furlough, and Rees was seeking COC physicians and nurses from "everywhere," who could follow "Christ's example" of healing.[8] Touched by his slides of devastating physical problems like swollen arms and legs from elephantiasis, Hays was convicted. Knowing that her gender and marital status might be barriers to her dream of mission work in Africa, a shy, but determined Hays approached Bryant: How could she prepare herself to go to Africa in case she never

---

[4]Talley, phone call to author, August 1, 2013. G. Farrar in undated personal communication told the story of RD dropping off a sack of potatoes at the house, and the family was so hungry that they ate them raw immediately; Talley said they moved to Andrews when she was in 7th grade.

[5]Andrews, *Mustang*; Hays-Savio, Interview.

[6]Hays-Savio, Interview.

[7]Ibid.

[8]Bryant and Bryant, Interview; Bryant, "Reflections," 22.

married? His answer was swift: "You can be a nurse because we're going to build a hospital;" too, Dr. Farrar is coming to Nigeria.[9]

Bryant's assertion that nursing would get her to Africa was persuasive enough for Hays. She changed her major to prenursing the next day. From among typical mid-century women's careers, nursing satisfied both Bryant's desire to recruit health professionals and Hays's desire to be a missionary. Nursing at least held more appeal for Hays than did teaching because she felt "petrified like a stick" in her LCC speech classes. Nonetheless, decades later Hays still marveled at her dramatic career reversal and never fully understood "why, when he said, 'We need nurses,' I said, 'Okay.'" Only God could have worked such a change in her, she affirmed, speculating that without Bryant she would neither have become a nurse nor made it to Africa.[10]

To her surprise, Hays enjoyed not only the difficult-for-her chemistry classes, but also the once-dreaded nursing. She paid her own way through a three-year diploma program at Lubbock's Methodist Hospital School of Nursing, which included some courses at Texas Tech University, and she discovered that nursing education added specialty knowledge to her compassion. Nursing empowered her to help people deal with illness as part of life, it suited her, and she loved it. "It was good," she remembered. Completing nursing studies in Lubbock also kept her within a comfortable network of friends and church family but created one enduring regret. Years later, while asserting that Methodist Hospital prepared her well for missionary nursing, she lamented that she never earned a baccalaureate—a pursuit that would have required her to move elsewhere.[11]

During nursing school, Hays lost contact with Bryant, and as she neared a 1964 graduation, her next step toward Africa was undefined. So, when medical missionary Dr. Ronald Huddleston spoke in her Lubbock church, College Avenue COC, Hays approached him about going with him to Chimala Mission and Hospital in Tanganyika (now Tanzania). His response was disappointing. Huddleston lacked Bryant's enthusiasm for her plans and offered no help with COC fundraising challenges. Instead, he suggested that she ask the US Peace Corps to place her at Chimala— an option Hays had already rejected, perhaps because she wanted to be a missionary, not a government employee. Huddleston "missed his oppor-

---

[9]Hays-Savio, Interview.
[10]Ibid.
[11]Ibid.

tunity…[and] that was the end of my conversation with him," Hays declared. And she turned her sights away from Tanganyika.[12]

Way Forward

The end of that conversation led to the beginning of another. One evening during her Methodist Hospital shift, Hays encountered anesthesiologist Dr. Jesse Paul, an elder at Green Lawn COC in Lubbock. He knew of her mission interests and suggested that she contact Rees Bryant, who was back in Lubbock. Hays was thrilled. The Bryants were preparing to return to Nigeria for a third tour, and Hays's missionary interest was again fanned into flame. Hays had not spoken to Bryant since her life-changing meeting with him at LCC, but the Bryants embraced her dreams and quickly became friendly, reliable advisors on all things Onicha Ngwa.[13] Probably alerted by the Bryants, Dr. Farrar began corresponding with Hays, and she delighted in sharing those mostly one-way, Farrar-to-Hays letters with fascinated classmates.[14]

A self-effacing Hays found Farrar's missives confidence-inspiring, in contrast to a self-assured Petty, who felt his detailed instructions discounted what she knew. When Hays informed Farrar that she knew almost nothing about tropical medicine, he reassured her that he could teach her "anything" she needed, and that satisfied her.[15] Soon, Hays would possess a nursing degree, professional license, and a few months of work experience. She anticipated that those credentials—coupled with personal determination—would finally take her where she had wanted to go for over half of her life: Africa.

Nascent Cause

Hays knew it would take more than desire to get to Nigeria; she needed a sponsoring church to cover travel, living, and work expenses. COC rules for missionary fundraising were unwritten but clear: A potential mission-

---

[12]Ibid.

[13]Ibid; P. Bryant, emails to author, June 18 and 19, 2012. Hays-Savio misspoke about Dr. Jesse Paul's name and details; P. Bryant emailed that her paternal uncle was Paul Mattox.

[14]Bryant and Bryant, Interview; Hays-Savio, Interview; Hays-Savio and Petty-Kraus, Interview. Some chronology during this time connecting Iris Hays, H. Farrar, Bryants, and Nancy Petty is unclear.

[15]Hays-Savio, Interview.

ary needed to convince elders in a local congregation to be the sponsoring church. For accountability and tax purposes, that sponsor would collect donations, disburse funds, provide legal and spiritual missionary oversight, and guarantee missionary salary and expenses. Noninstitutional COCs followed different, also unwritten protocols. Missionary men asked for salary from their sponsors based on the needs and size of their particular families, and married missionary women relied on their husbands' funding. Because wives were not paid directly, each missionary woman was free for intensive household management and to choose when, where, and how much direct ministry work she would do outside the home.

As a single woman, however, Hays's pursuit of church funding differed.[16] In the COC men were welcome to speak from pulpits to the full church and thereby could attract broad membership support of their mission plans. Moreover, congregants could easily identify men's foreign preaching and Bible teaching as fulfillment of Jesus's command to "go and make disciples of all nations" (Matthew 28:19) and thus worthy of their financial support. In contrast, Hays's professional nursing work was not as easily identified with evangelism, and her public church speech was limited to addressing women and children.

Hays met these fundraising challenges through interpersonal relationships, her own persuasive speech where possible, and the speech of others when needed. How single June Hobbs garnered support in the 1950s is not recorded. Nancy Petty did so with the help of parents and a lifetime of Vanleer COC membership.[17] Hays's family support and participation in a single congregation were less robust than Petty's, but her years of attending LCC and Lubbock's College Avenue COC nonetheless yielded the necessary financial, theological, and moral support for her work.

By the time Hays asked College Avenue to sponsor her, its elders had already accepted the doctrinal legitimacy of medical missions as a pragmatic means to evangelistic ends. They already partially funded Dr. Huddleston at the COC Chimala Clinic to enable evangelists to stay in Tanganyika,[18] even though the Clinic heightened conflicts with noninstitutional COCs.[19] Unlike the Tanganyika government, however, Nigeria's did not require missionaries to provide social services, and so the primary argument for an Onicha Ngwa hospital was theological: Christians have a

---

[16]Ibid.

[17]Farrar and Petty-Kraus, Interview; Petty-Kraus, Interview 1.

[18]Echols, *Beyond,* 31–34; Hays-Savio, Interview.

[19]Liggin, "Is Preaching," 7–10.

religious duty to care for the whole person.[20] College Avenue COC accepted this new moral reasoning and agreed to sponsor Hays, who found their endorsement "unusual" given the nascent state of COC healthcare. She was touched when the elders filed a (possibly Nigerian-required) letter at the bank that guaranteed coverage of any overdraft she might incur.[21]

With salary promised, Hays relied on other relationships for travel costs. Three men with whom she had existing rapport were especially helpful: a preacher, a professor, and a brother. Don Killough, College Avenue's fulltime minister, and Gerald Kendrick, Hays's former LCC teacher and a College Avenue part-time minister, accompanied her to local COCs and made financial appeals on her behalf.[22] An unidentified man presented her planned work to her brother's Albuquerque congregation, and Hays conquered her terror of public speaking long enough to represent herself before women's groups. Her courage was bolstered by her quiet passion, a copy of Rees Bryant's Nigeria slide set, and the universally positive reception from audiences. Onicha Ngwa missionaries briefed Hays on the people and places in the slides, so Hays could use them to illustrate her opportunities, and Hays expressed surprised that no one opposed her plans.[23] Jim Massey living in Texas may have helped with fundraising as well.[24]

COCs were still getting "used to the idea" of medical missions, and she and professor Kendrick emphasized that she was going to Africa not merely to remedy social ills, but "to present Jesus." Hays would heal in Jesus's name, teach Bible classes for women and children, and work in a "Christ-centered" hospital with regular devotionals. "We weren't going there just to give out Band-Aids and things," she insisted, "but we were there for a purpose and that purpose was Jesus." Hays remembered her gratitude, uncertainty, and relief during "precarious" fundraising, "but God made it come about" through many $1 and $5 donations.[25]

Perhaps (unintentionally) aiding her efforts was a September 1964, three-column, Lubbock newspaper story about Hays's history, her plans, and the health situation in Nigeria. A woman journalist touted Hays's successes: her 1961 LCC graduation as an "A" student in challenging subjects like New Testament Greek, her receipt of the LCC President's

---

[20]Bryant and Bryant, Interview.
[21]Hays-Savio, Interview.
[22]Ibid.; Dixon, "Graduate."
[23]Hays-Savio, Interview.
[24]Bryant and Bryant, Interview.
[25]Hays-Savio, Interview.

Award for Outstanding Religious Growth and Service, and her graduation from Methodist Hospital School of Nursing where classmates selected her for the Best All-Around Nurse Award. The article included
praise from Don Killough, Gerald Kendrick, F.W. Mattox, and Irene Wilson, the nursing school director, who described Hays as "a good bedside
nurse."[26]

Hays's fundraising for travel also coincided with an emerging COC
consciousness of Nigerians' health needs. For years Rees Bryant, who
transitioned back to Nigeria in August 1964 during Hays's fundraising,
had argued the case for sending nurses and physicians to Onicha Ngwa,[27]
and Hays's appeals overlapped with both his pleas and those of his influential father-in-law, F.W. Mattox. In late 1964 Mattox was reporting widely in Lubbock about his November visit to Onicha Ngwa, where he saw
the sick constantly seeking Dr. Farrar's help.[28] Donating to Hays now
presented a tangible way for Bryant's and Mattox's audiences to help
Nigerians. Much of her one-time travel funding came from individual
College Avenue members, who contributed above and beyond the congregation's commitment, and Hays felt spiritually supported as she saw
College Avenue's excitement about her work and heard their public
prayers for her.[29] Nigerian village women, too, later recognized the significance of this financial support when they expressed gratitude to the
Americans who sent Nurse Hays to them.[30] Thus, through fundraising,
Hays bridged the distance between strangers an ocean and a world apart.

Unlike missionary men, neither Hays nor Petty raised a separate,
monthly, business-expense, "working fund." Instead, they each gathered
exactly what Dr. Farrar recommended: a monthly salary of $250 plus
travel.[31] Perhaps the idea of working funds was considered but rejected
for several reasons. It would have been one more fiscal hurdle, the nurses
had no preaching-associated costs, and they were ineligible for tax-de-
ductible allowances for ministerial housing and offices because the COC
did not ordain women. Thus, while missionary men paid for cars, petrol,
materials, supplies, and housing expenses from their working funds, Hays
and Petty bought these things from their salaries. Nonetheless, they benefited from male colleagues' working funds that covered shared team ex-

---

[26]Dixon, "Graduate."

[27]Bryant and Bryant, Interview.

[28]P. Bryant to M. Mattox, November 12, 1964; Mattox to Bryants, December 3,
1964. More in "F.W. Mattox to Visit."

[29]Hays to Bryants and Farrars, October 7, 1964.

[30]Umuogbala and Ekwereazu Women to Nursing Sisters, May 5, 1965.

[31]Farrar and Petty-Kraus, Interview.

penses, such as compound electricity and grounds maintenance,[32] as well as some nurse-specific costs. Dr. Farrar's working fund paid for construction upgrades and furnishing of the nurses' house,[33] and College Avenue COC sent money through his business account to pay for shipping Hays's belongings.[34] Additionally, the nurses' salaries were proportionately large, with each one receiving fifty percent of the salary given to the Farrar family of seven and to the Bryant family of six.[35] The missionary team also advised Hays and Petty to raise separate funds for a car.[36]

Conclusion

Hays longed to be a missionary to Africa, and her desire enabled her to choose the "almost anyhow"[37] of despised nursing and to tackle her fear of public speaking. When Rees Bryant unhesitatingly recruited her as a future missionary nurse, there was no clinic, no hospital, and no COC immigration quota for nurses. His confidence betrayed an exuberant enthusiasm that all things necessary to a mission hospital would happen. Hays uncritically accepted Bryant's confidence and Farrar's reassurances, and their shared religious faith in the future exemplified "the substance of things hoped for, the evidence of things not seen" (Hebrews. 11:1; KJV).

Hays relied heavily on personal relationships to raise funds, and those efforts brought known US supporters and unknown Nigerians together. The most sustaining relationship for Iris Hays, however, was an ever-present sense that God was always with her. God, she said, fulfilled to her the promise that Jesus made to his earliest disciples when he sent them out to preach to the nations: "Go ye into all the world, and I'll be with you."[38]

---

[32]Farrar to Mission Committee, May 2, 1965, *WEV* (attached budget in W-COC file); Hays-Savio, Interview.

[33]Farrar to Mission Committee, March 1, 1965, *WEV*.

[34]Farrar to Mission Committee, September 1, 1965, *WEV*.

[35]Bryant and Bryant, Interview; Hays-Savio, Interview.

[36]P. Bryant to Hays, October 23, 1964.

[37]Nietzsche, quoted in Frankl, *Man's Search*, 101.

[38]Hays-Savio, Interview. Hays paraphrased Matt. 28:19–20 and Mark 16:15 (KJV).

10
Advice: Strife, Snakes, and Sheets
(1964)

Do you think I can survive over there with all the snakes?
—Iris Hays

Graduate nurse Iris Hays worked in Lubbock's Methodist Hospital emergency room while fundraising and waiting for her Registered Nursing (RN) Board exam results. "Everyone" told her that the busy evening shift would be "good experience," she confided to Bryants. At the same time, Hays minimized expectations, confessing to only "two months in surgery...two years ago" that made her little more proficient than "a bright new student nurse."[1] An unperturbed Henry Farrar continued to reassure her.[2] The missionaries' hospital plans required a COC nurse, and Hays fit that need.

Political Advice

Hays was so determined to get to Africa that she downplayed global racial conflicts. She later recounted how she dismissed warnings from her Methodist Hospital nursing supervisor, who had been evacuated from the Congo during its post-independence violence. The supervisor's experiences did not fit with COC or other Western narratives about Nigeria's stability, so Hays "didn't listen very well" and "spouted off" what she had been told. She remembered the supervisor looking at her as if she didn't know what she was talking about, and "I didn't," a later wiser Hays acknowledged.[3]

COC missionaries emphasized differences especially between the decolonization journeys of the Congo and Nigeria and spoke glowingly of

---

[1]Hays to Bryants and H. Farrar, October 7, 1964.
[2]Hays-Savio, Interview.
[3]Ibid.

93

Nigeria's government and political future.[4] A slide presentation script about the COC work in Nigeria—perhaps the same one that Hays used in fundraising—attributed to the March 1963 *Reader's Digest* this optimistic assessment of the newly independent, oil-rich Federation of Nigeria:

> Nigeria is one of the most democratic and stable countries in the entire under-developed world. The rule of law and the liberties of its citizens are scrupulously observed. Its press is the freest and liveliest in Africa. Its economy is based on free enterprise. Foreign investment…is pouring into the country at the rate of $70,000,000 a year. Population growth (estimated at 2½% a year) has been comfortably offset by a 4% annual rise in gross national product.[5]

Reports like this[6] reassured the West in general and missionaries in particular, while conveniently ignoring a colonial pattern of undermining Nigerian unity. Since Nigeria's earliest days, British colonizers politically favored northern Hausa-Fulanis and western Yorubas because their centralized governance structures were a better fit with the British system of indirect rule. In contrast, the decentralized governance structures of southeastern Igbos (among others) led some colonial officials to view Igbos as more primitive and inferior—intellectually, economically, and politically.[7] Such unfortunate tribal partisanship institutionalized mistrust between Nigeria's amalgamated people groups and reinforced a history of ethnic conflict.[8] Nevertheless, most international observers foresaw a bright future for the country.

Hays also viewed 1960s US racial tensions as irrelevant to her plans. Domestic conflicts neither delayed nor accelerated her intentions to move to black, sub-Saharan Africa, and she remembered no one discouraging her out of racial bias. Rees Bryant had told her she was needed in Nigeria, and she took his statements to heart and prepared to move as soon as she obtained education, license, funding, and a visa.[9] "The time seems to drag," penned an eager-to-go Hays.[10]

---

[4]Martin to McInteer, September 5, 1960; *Lubbock Avalanche*, "Peace."
[5]"Evangelist fund."
[6]Goff, *Great*; Snyder, "Western Africa;" Summerlin, "Elder's Evaluation."
[7]Korieh, *The Land*, 59–76.
[8]Achebe, *There Was*, 74–78; Madiebo, *Nigerian Revolution*, 3–14.
[9]Hays-Savio, Interview.
[10]Hays to Bryants and H. Farrar, October 7, 1964.

Snakes and Sheets

Although Hays remained unconcerned about racism and political conflict, she did worry about snakes, the subjects of her childhood nightmares. She feared they might "be dropping out of every tree" in Africa, and in her first meeting with Patti Bryant, she demanded answers: "What about snakes?...Do you see many snakes?...Do you think I can survive over there with all the snakes?" Bryant reassured her that snakes were no more common in Nigeria than in West Texas, and Hays decided she could "live with that."[11] Perhaps Hays did not hear about Joyce Massey's encounter with a snake hiding behind a crooked picture frame, another that fell out of a missionary woman's closet during Farrar's 1963 visit, or about the Pedens' memories of "lots of snakes" and massive rock pythons.[12]

By August the Bryants' face-to-face counsel to Hays shifted to written advice from the field after they returned to Onicha Ngwa for a third tour.[13] Those letters contrasted starkly with Bryant-Sermanoukian ones: Bryant-Hays correspondence was direct and woman-to-woman. Patti Bryant filled a September letter to Hays with humor, faith, friendship, news, and practical information.

"We just can't tell you how happy we are! ...You are an answer to prayer.[...] A day rarely goes by that we don't think about you," she penned. Patti wrote that Hays should ship three sets of bed linens and all kitchen linens, silverware, "everything necessary for housekeeping, [...] the works! [...] Prices are sky-high here for *everything*." Lightweight clothing would be best, Patti wrote, because rains that last two to three days would keep any cloth from drying quickly. Bring makeup, Bryant advised, but "don't bring soap or sanitary napkins...Bring one light weight blanket. A few small pictures and vases, etc. would make your place more homey." Bryant also recommended that Hays contact Nancy Petty to "decide who's going to bring what" for the house. She continued: Your own things will probably fill one shipping barrel; an iron is available; buy appliances in Nigeria because electricity is direct current from an evening-only generator.[14]

---

[11]Hays-Savio, Interview. On May 15, 2012 in personal communication Hays-Savio retold a story recounted by her brother of her terrifying encounter with a non-poisonous snake when she was about two years old.

[12]Carol Massey Dennison, in Beth Sheldon, "Nigeria Missionary Kids" Facebook group page, March 10, 2016; G. Farrar to Johnson, November 1, 1963; Peden, Interview.

[13]Bryant, *Divine*, 167–71.

[14]P. Bryant to Hays, September 18, 1964.

Then Bryant turned to personal and hospital matters:

> Everyone on the compound is well...Things get hectic at
> times what with untangling the [missionary] children (there
> are 12 of them), reminding the [US evangelist] college boys
> to bring their laundry down, getting the car tuned-up a sec-
> ond time (they tuned it down the first), trying to figure out
> what's wrong with a perfectly new kerosene iron (I suspect
> the trouble is in the washerman—but how to repair him?),
> dodging the cyclists on the road to P.H., etc., etc. Things are
> looking bright for the establishment of the hospital...Twen-
> ty-five villages are working together to raise money...Things
> seem to move slowly, but we know the providence of God is
> working in it all.[15]

Hays responded immediately, questions spilling from her pen. "Don Killough wants some information about my mode of transportation after I
arrive...What kind of beds will we have?" What about mosquito nets,
camera, contact lenses, and work shoes? Would donated surgical supplies,
syringes, and needles be useful? What is Nancy Petty's mailing address
and might the two travel together? Finally, in closing, an always unassum-
ing and affectionate Hays apologized for her "incoherent" letter, expressing happiness at receiving Bryant's note, asking her to "give my love to
the children" and reminiscing about their last devotional together in
Lubbock when they all "sang 'This Little Light of Mine.'"[16]

Patti Bryant circulated Hays's letter among Onicha Ngwa missionaries,
and Farrar scrawled input on its margins and back. Bryant combined Farrar's input with her own answers to Hays, consistently calling him "Dr.
Farrar" while using first names for others—something that became a pattern for the nurses themselves. Yes, the nurses should fly together, she
wrote. Bring mosquito nets from Sears, ship "any and all" medical supplies in your barrels, and bring comfortable shoes in which you can stand
all day. Tennis shoes would "not be good for your feet." The nurses
would have twin beds, and "*must* have a car." Perhaps they could jointly
purchase a new, economical "little VW" that could get them "*back* from
wherever" they went. She sent Petty's address and suggested that Hays

---

[15]Ibid. See Bryant, *Divine*, 164, 178–79, 196 for details on "the college boys" as
Conquest for Christ participants.

[16]Hays to Bryants and H. Farrar, October 7, 1964. P. Bryant's email to author, June
18, 2012, identified the likely donor of medical supplies as Dr. Iridell Adams, a
Lubbock pediatrician and member of Broadway COC.

hand carry her camera to avoid customs charges because if brought in its box, customs might think the camera new. Hays could bring contact lenses and was advised that "there is an eye surgeon in Aba." A pressure cooker and orange juicer would be useful. Because shipped goods could take two to four months to arrive, Bryant suggested that she send belongings as soon as possible and mail the paperwork so that the missionaries could pick up the barrels if they arrived before Hays did. Then, with a twinge of anxious uncertainty about Hays's professional status, Bryant penned: "By now you probably know how you did on state board examinations. I hope it was good! Let us know."[17]

Conclusion

The Bryants and Henry Farrar became the equivalent of a how-to missionary manual for Iris Hays, and she accepted their positive view of Nigeria—a view that fit with her plans. Missionaries gave honest advice in good conscience, and Hays always remained glad that she moved to Onicha Ngwa. Nevertheless, she later attested that missionaries were wrong about at least two things: Frequent "snake experiences…[proved] a test of faith," and Nigeria was less stable than they thought.[18]

---

[17]P. Bryant to Hays, October 23, 1964.
[18]Hays-Savio, Interview.

11

Active Waiting

(July 1964–March 1965)

It's Africa….not America.

—Grace Farrar

In July 1964, the seven-member Farrar family arrived in Onicha Ngwa and moved into the largest, newest house on the compound. The five-member Lawyer family had graciously departed it for the smaller mission house next door,[1] and Dr. Farrar's preacher status perhaps justified his family's occupying a house built for evangelists on a Bible Training College (BTC) compound; a single congregation, Proctor Street COC, oversaw that compound.[2] Wasting no time, Farrar dove into immigration work on behalf of Nancy Petty and Iris Hays, despite his jet lag, car shopping, and oldest son's emergency appendectomy at the American-style, Shell Oil Hospital in Port Harcourt (PH). Within days of arrival, Dr. Farrar flew to Lagos in order to rectify government confusion blocking visas for Hays and Petty.[3] Two weeks later Rees Bryant made the same trip regarding similar issues,[4] but neither man was successful. Immigration claimed the COC quota was full, while missionaries insisted that officials were counting expatriates already back in the US.[5]

As newly elected Secretary of the Trustees of COC, Rees Bryant pivoted. To circumvent the stalemate, he filed September paperwork to raise their quota from eleven to thirty-three positions, requesting an increase in nurses from zero to four, physicians from one to four, laboratory technologists from zero to two, medical students from zero to four, and other educational and evangelist positions by nine. With his typical optimism,

---

[1]Farrar, *Stand*, 6–10.

[2]R. Bryant to Summerlin, August 18, 1960; G. Farrar, Interview; Goff, *Great*, 33.

[3]R. Bryant to Massey, October 8, 1964; G. Farrar to Johnson, August 3, 1964; Farrar to Mission Committee, August 15, 1964, W-COC file.

[4]G. Farrar to Mrs. H.C. Farrar, August 16, 1964.

[5]G. Farrar to Johnson, August 3, 1964.

Bryant then wrote to Jim Massey that Hays and Petty would arrive in January 1965.[6]

Unfortunately, Bryant's confidence in government speed was misplaced, and Nigeria continued to deny visas for the nurses,[7] maintaining that Nigeria had enough nurses, and American nurses would take jobs from Nigerians. Not so, Farrar told regional immigration officials in Enugu; instead, US nurses would work only temporarily in the country in order to "train more Nigerian nurses."[8] This line of argument succeeded, and by December, Eastern Region immigration officials approved the COC quota increase, raising missionary hopes of final federal approval in Lagos after upcoming national elections.[9] In the meantime, Henry Farrar and the senior medical officer in Aba wrote to Lagos immigration authorities requesting swift authorization of US nurse visas, further bolstering positive expectations.[10] The country needed nurses who were educated to more up-to-date American standards, asserted Grace Farrar.[11]

Not America

Despite a January 1965 report from Henry Farrar that Nigeria's first, post-independence elections showed "political maturity," all was not well. Rigged parliamentary appointments, jailing of political opponents, and boycotting of elections suggested to some Western journalists that "Nigeria's unity…hung by a thread." Still, undaunted Farrar called for COC spending in Nigeria. Pointing to investments in the country by Gulf Oil, the Peace Corps, and the US government, he wrote to W-COC that Nigeria is "vibrantly and dynamically alive with potential. Now is the time to step in with the gospel."[12]

In Onicha Ngwa missionaries moved forward. The Lawyers, Farrars, and Bryants focused on practical housing arrangements for nurses Hays and Petty. They agreed that the two should have their own home and be responsible for their own cooking and housekeeping. The quickest, least expensive option was to improve the house earlier upgraded for Ser-

---

[6]R. Bryant to Massey, October 8, 1964.

[7]Hays-Savio, Interview; Mattox to Bryants, December 3, 1964.

[8]G. Farrar to Mrs. H.C. Farrar, December 6, 1964.

[9]R. Bryant to Martins, January 1, 1965.

[10]G. Farrar to Johnson, January 31, 1965; H. Farrar to Permanent Secretary, Ministry of Health, February 15, 1965.

[11]G. Farrar to Mrs. H.C. Farrar, December 6, 1964.

[12]Farrar to Mission Committee, January 9, 1965, in W-COC file; *Time*, "Nigeria: Model Breaks."

manoukian and currently occupied by three, soon-to-depart, college-age evangelists.[13] Proposed renovations included painting and adding a bathroom, a second bedroom, and electrical wiring. With help from a "rare" Nigerian subcontractor, Farrar assumed contractor responsibilities, buying materials and paying workers.[14]

The inexperienced Farrar, however, soon ran into trouble with the remodel. Other missionaries hired construction workers, but when trusted Nigerian electrician Luke was temporarily unavailable, Farrar "became impatient" and hired a "bush" (lay) electrician. When that electrician finished wiring and "turned on the power, there was an explosion." Across the compound, houses smoked, crackled, and popped. Then, despite his unfortunate connection of hot and ground wires, the electrician insisted on full payment for his month's work, "which was customary." Dr. Farrar, who was more interested in results than in time spent, was furious, claiming he would rather go to court; but US teammates persuaded him to yield and then hired Luke to repair the damage. "Everybody had to get their feet wet," reflected Doug Lawyer.[15]

Farrar financed the $1,000 remodel with five months of his working fund, and W-COC granted post hoc approval.[16] The congregation published a picture of the completed house in its church bulletin, and Dr. Farrar used the opportunity to point supporters to the future: "This concrete block construction with simple metal roof is what is planned for the hospital."[17] Inside Grace Farrar hung curtains, and the Bryants installed Formica-like countertops.[18]

Knowing that Hays and Petty would need help with labor-intensive housework, the missionaries next addressed the question of household staff for the nurses. Charla Lawyer proposed that the nurses hire Mark Apollos Ugwunna from Onicha Ngwa. Mark, who first worked for the Nickses, was apprenticing under Lawyers' cook-steward Friday Onukafor (also Onukafur). Bilingual Mark couldn't read or write, but he remembered any recipe explained to him, and Charla was rightly confident in his ability to function independently. Tennessean Henry Farrar expressed concern about how Southern US supporters might view a young, single,

---

[13]Bryant, *Divine* 196, 200; P. Bryant to Hays, September 18, 1964.

[14]G. Farrar to Johnsons, November 19, 1964; Farrar to Mission Committee, December 31, 1964, *WEV*; Lawyer, "Narrative," 39.

[15]Lawyer, "Narrative," 39; Author's recollection. "Bush lawyers," "bush electricians," and other "bush" professionals were those with lay preparation of variable quality.

[16]Farrar to Mission Committee, December 31, 1964, *WEV*; H. Farrar to Benson, February 20, 1965.

[17]Farrar to Mission Committee, March 1, 1965, *WEV*.

[18]P. Bryant to Mattoxes, March 8, 1965; G. Farrar to Johnson, March 7, 1965.

black man working for young, single, white women, but Grace Farrar's no-nonsense answer was simple: "They have to remember, that it's Africa….not America." Indeed, Dr. Farrar's worries were unfounded, and Mark proved "a jewel."[19]

Competing Interests

The team also moved ahead with outpatient dispensary plans. That work coupled with an upcoming Lawyer furlough, however, heightened Rees Bryant's concern that missionary numbers would soon be too thin to sustain both evangelistic and healthcare efforts. Not only was the nurses' coming still uncertain, but the Lawyers' imminent departure would vacate the BTC principal position and leave only two families in Onicha Ngwa. Doug Lawyer's sponsoring Proctor Street COC was obligated to support only him and could not afford a replacement.[20]

Relying on his past relationship with Proctor Street, Bryant handwrote an impassioned, four-page plea. Without a Lawyer replacement, medical work would crowd out evangelism, he explained. Dr. Farrar kept a rigorous surgical schedule three times a week at non-COC mission hospitals, preached on Sundays, and taught in the BTC. As COC hospital work increased, however, Farrar's BTC teaching would decrease, and Bryant already carried a full workload of teaching, preaching, and planning of the "Ndiakata-Owo-Joint Christian Hospital." Without a third mission family, Bill Curry might be compelled to leave his new, Enugu mission point and return to Onicha Ngwa, Bryant noted, and he called on Proctor Street to continue their status as "the sustaining force, with God's grace, which has backed one of the most fruitful mission efforts in the Lord's church in the 20th century." If they absolutely could not help, he asked them to assist in finding a COC that could. Then, not waiting for their response, Bryant began his own US search for a new BTC principal.[21] Nowhere did Bryant suggest that Farrar might have to curtail medical mission efforts in order to support evangelism.

Bryant's boldness was rewarded. Proctor Street reversed itself, agreeing to partial funding of Lawyer's replacement,[22] and an elated Bryant lauded

---

[19]G. Farrar, Interview; Nicks, "Why?," 67–69. See also Wilson, "Biography."

[20]Bryant, *Divine*, 204–5, 210–11; Mattox to Bryant, December 3, 1964; Bryant to Martins, January 1, 1965.

[21]R. Bryant to Elders, December 28, 1964; R. Bryant to Salmon, January 1, 1965. "Ndiakata-Owo-Joint Christian Hospital" was a descriptor, never a formal name.

[22]Bryant, *Divine*, 211.

their solidarity in evangelism's cause, expressing confidence in heaven's rejoicing that they had "again launched out in faith on behalf of those who sit in deepest darkness...who will (together with their children and their children's children) rise up in the day of judgement and call you blessed."[23] Side-by-side evangelism and healthcare could continue unimpeded.

Visa Approved

Meanwhile, Iris Hays raised money, shipped belongings,[24] and, in January 1965, quit her job. She assumed quick Nigerian visa approval but instead found herself without employment, income, or visa. College Avenue COC stepped into the breach, beginning her salary as if she were already in Nigeria, and an appreciative Hays recalled "sitting on pins and needles" not knowing if or when a visa might come.[25]

Fortunately, she did not wait long. In a land of bargaining, the COC's request for thirty-three positions allowed no-bribe negotiating space for twenty-two, and on February 18, 1965, the Nigerian federal government added to the COC quota "3 Doctors, 2 Nursing Sisters, 2 Laboratory Technologists, 2 Bible Tutors, 2 School Supervisors."[26] Rees Bryant's "many trips to Lagos...many hours sitting in offices,"[27] six consecutive February days with "the top man for a desperate effort,"[28] and assistance from well-positioned Nigerian supporters succeeded.[29] Likely the Honorable Ibanga Udo "Daniel" Akpabio, who was the Eastern Minister of Internal Affairs,[30] helped, as did Sunday Ezerie, a former BTC student who worked for the Permanent Secretary of Internal Affairs. Ezerie cut through red tape in a way that prompted Patti Bryant to compare him to Queen Esther of the Bible: "called for such a time as this."[31] Missionaries

---

[23]R. Bryant to Elders, February 28, 1965.

[24]G. Farrar to Johnsons, January 10, 1965.

[25]Hays-Savio, Interview.

[26]Federal Ministry of Internal Affairs, Immigration Division to Secretary, Church of Christ Mission, March 8, 1965. According to R. Bryant to Derr, February 11, 1965, another driver for the increased quota was evangelist Derr family's anticipated move to Nigeria from Ghana because of political upheaval.

[27]Bryant and Bryant, Interview.

[28]G. Farrar to Johnson, February 14, 1965.

[29]Bryant to Massey, October 8, 1964.

[30]Akpabio, *He Dared*, 257–59; P. Bryant to Mattoxes, September 7, 1964. The Hon. Akpabio was older brother to Udofia Udo "Edward" Akpabio MD, who later worked at NCH.

[31]Bryant to Mattoxes, March 8, 1965.

delightedly relayed the news to US supporters. Farrar emphasized the new quota as an "unequaled opportunity to preach the gospel," and Bryant stressed its doubling as the first increase since 1958.[32] Neither mentioned the denial of eleven additional requested positions, including four evangelist slots.

While Patti Bryant privately mused that "we don't know how long it will take to get *that* many missionaries,"[33] the *Christian Chronicle,* a US COC newspaper, printed Rees Bryant's enthusiastic report (International Edition, May 7, 1965). Pointing to a trend in Nigerian policy that favored "expatriate social servants more than…'religious' workers," Bryant proclaimed Nigerian Christians' expectations "that American brethren will rise to the challenge" of sending more missionaries. "An immediate effect," Bryant wrote, "is the granting of visas for nurses Iris Hays and Nancy Petty, who will soon join Dr. Henry Farrar here as he pioneers the establishment of a Nigerian Christian Hospital." A photograph of Bryant and missionary colleague Phil Dunn shaking hands with H.O. Omenai, Permanent Secretary of the Federal Nigerian Ministry of Internal Affairs, graced the front-page article.

Conclusion

Recruiting and maintaining enough COC missionaries to support healthcare and evangelism presented multiple challenges: housing, furloughs, funding, and Nigerian immigration decisions. Missionaries overcame the difficulties within the context of remarkable missionary-missionary and missionary-supporter trust that empowered them to deal with each other's mistakes and to initiate problem resolution from the field. Such was the atmosphere into which Hays and Petty arrived.

---

[32]Farrar to Mission Committee, March 1, 1965, *WEV*; R. Bryant to Elders, March 4, 1965.

[33]Bryant to Mattoxes, March 8, 1965.

12

Course Corrections

(August 1964–April 1965)

Progress is being made.
—Henry Farrar

While Rees Bryant worked to increase the quota and the two nurses prepared to come, Henry Farrar and colleagues struggled for nine months with financing, land surveys, and government approvals as necessary prerequisites for a COC hospital. Plans stalled, and frustrations grew. Farrar originally understood that locals and the government would jointly fund a facility as suggested by Aba's senior medical officer. That plan met West End COC (W-COC) expectations,[1] limited the need for US fundraising, created local engagement, and circumvented some objections of noninstitutional COCs.

Unfortunately, Nigerian money turned out to be in short supply. Local Igbos greeted the Farrars in July with numerous personal gifts but no hospital cash.[2] Worse still was the death of the Eastern Ngwa chairman who had been sympathetic to the missionaries' cause. The new chairman, a member of the African Gospel Church, was hostile toward the COC.[3] Thus, despite past written promises to the contrary, the new chairman refused to give council funds unless he controlled the hospital. Missionaries promptly rejected his plan as both unacceptable governance and uncharitable to his people.[4] Farrar adamantly insisted that Nigerians fund the hospital, while Nigerians waited to see how much Americans would invest. "A cat and mouse game," Grace Farrar called it.[5]

---

[1]G. Farrar to G.B. Farrars, January 31, 1965.
[2]G. Farrar to Mrs. H.C. Farrar, August 3, 1964.
[3]Bryant to Martins on January 1, 1965.
[4]G. Farrar to Johnson, August 10 and 26, 1964; Farrar to Mission Committee, August 15, 1964, W-COC file.
[5]G. Farrar to Mrs. H.C. Farrar, August 3, 1964.

The frustrated Farrars considered moving to another location where money was reportedly available and villages pleaded for them to come.[6] Earlier Ogba/Ebema had offered to build a COC hospital near PH and turn it over to missionaries,[7] and the town of Owo claimed to have £3,000 ready,[8] but the Farrars ultimately decided to stay in Onicha Ngwa; they liked its living arrangements and didn't want the expense of building a house elsewhere.[9] Moreover, by October, they received reassuring new written promises from Ndiakata Group villages that they would contribute £3,000 by the end of 1964, and the regional government promised matching funds.[10] Villages also promised to donate hospital land for lease,[11] because expatriate outright ownership of land was prohibited by law.

Soon individual Nigerians and nearby COCs began to fulfill their commitments to raise the £3,000. Locals collectively circumvented their council president by taxing their own palm fruit harvest, and Grace Farrar was soon serving endless cups of tea to "dignitaries and delegations" that offered assistance or brought donations to be secured in a missionary safe.[12] The Farrars were especially touched when "one poor preacher in debt himself made a special trip…to bring 6 shillings (about 84¢)."[13] Meanwhile, Henry Farrar delayed drafting the government-required, five-to-ten-year hospital plan, hoping that sheer population density would overcome individual poverty in producing promised funds.[14]

In November 1964, however, financing plans took a new turn when F.W. Mattox, Patti Bryant's father, visited Onicha Ngwa. During nightly meetings with Mattox, missionaries decided to raise all needed $45,000 from US donors for construction of a thirty to thirty-eight-bed hospital, including a clinic, maternity unit, isolation unit, kitchen-laundry building, and a twenty-eight-bed ward. They also determined to charge fees for

[6]H. Farrar, Interview 1; G. Farrar to Mrs. H.C. Farrar, August 3, 1964; Farrar to Mission Committee, April 1, 1963, W-COC file.

[7]Farrar to Mission Committee, April 1, 1965.

[8]P. Bryant to Mattoxes on September 7, 1964.

[9]G. Farrar to Mrs. H.C. Farrar, August 3, 1964; Farrar to Mission Committee, November 7, 1964, HGF.

[10]P. Bryant to Mattoxes, September 7, 1964; G. Farrar to Johnson, August 26 and September 17, 1964; Farrar to Brethren, October 5, 1964, *WEV*; Farrar to Mission Committee, July 28, 1964, W-COC file.

[11]Farrar to Brethren, October 5, 1964, *WEV*.

[12]G. Farrar to Johnson, September 17 and November 1, 1964.

[13]G. Farrar to Johnson, November 8, 1964

[14]Ibid.; G. Farrar to Johnson, August 26, 1964.

services.[15] Perhaps they used physician Dr. Joanaa Maiden's 1963 budget structure at a southeastern Nigeria Baptist mission hospital and clinic as a model.[16]

Dr. Farrar was reluctant to ask US supporters for hospital funds,[17] yet he wrote persuasively to W-COC about the new team consensus to "raise our own money, build our own hospital, and control it completely." While acknowledging this was not "the original plan," Farrar outlined their threefold rationale for the change. First, more Nigerian money meant more Nigerian control, and Farrar feared that non-Christians or the ill-informed would gain too much voice in hospital governance—a problem that he observed in neighboring facilities. Second, he argued that a modest $45,000 raised over time was enough to build a "creditable hospital," and finally, he described the Onicha Ngwa location as "ideal" given its proximity to the Farrars' existing house, the Bible Training College (BTC), six hundred COCs, US missionary families, and many Nigerian preachers.[18]

W-COC's response was mixed. They authorized Farrar to proceed with establishing electric and water utilities at an estimated $5,000–$6,000, but "thought it unwise" for them to assume other expenses beyond his monthly support; they did not object to others giving money for the hospital.[19] Meanwhile, Igbo fundraising bore little fruit, with villages collecting only about £300 of the promised £3,000 by December's end. "Their zeal exceeds their ability," observed a sympathetic Grace Farrar.[20] Yet in the face of this "hopeless" situation, three influential leaders, including Francis J. Ellah, stepped forward to prompt more local giving by lobbying the regional Enugu government for hospital approval. They assured Dr. Farrar that regional approval would increase village contributions while cautioning him against depending on full local funding.[21]

---

[15]P. Bryant to M. Mattox, November 12, 1964; Bryant to Friends, April 20, 1965; G. Farrar to Johnson, November 8, 1964. See rationale in Mattox to Cayce, January 22 and April 29, 1965, W-COC file. Messrs. Farrar, Bryant, Lawyer, Massey, and Curry were former students of F.W. Mattox at Harding College.

[16]Farrar to Mission Committee, April 1, 1963.

[17]P. Bryant to Mattoxes, March 24, 1965.

[18]Farrar, *Stand*, 37–40; Farrar to Mission Committee, November 7, 1965. See Cayce to H. Farrar, December 7, 1964 in W-COC file for objections to funding a hospital.

[19]Elders to W-COC members, January 14, 1965, *WEV*; Farrar to Mission Committee, December 31, 1964, *WEV*.

[20]G. Farrar to Johnson, December 29, 1964.

[21]Farrar, *Stand*, 51; G. Farrar to G.B. Farrars, January 31, 1965. See details about Ellah in his *Nigeria and States*.

New supporters also stepped forward in the US. Dr. Adrian Formby, Patti Bryant's physician uncle in Searcy, Arkansas, and Dr. George S. Benson, outgoing President of Harding College, offered to raise money for the hospital. Benson was a prolific fundraiser for Harding, and the Farrars were "thrilled."[22] Well-known for his strong opinions and micromanagement style, however, Benson promptly asserted that missionaries did not need $45,000 and insisted that they instead "build a small bush hospital...patterned after Dr. Schweitzer's" 1913 one—a demand inconsistent with Nigerian standards.[23] As Patti Bryant wrote, the $45,000 estimate would finance only a single-story, "unadorned concrete building...with the barest minimum of equipment...no windows, only wooden shutters...concrete floor, a 'tin' roof...no partitions for rooms, only three big wards, one for men and one for women and one for maternity cases," all with water and power.[24] Farrar responded to Benson with details,[25] but Benson's name dropped from subsequent correspondence, and he switched his fundraising support permanently to Zambian COC schools.[26] Still, Patti Bryant later recognized Benson and Formby as NCH fund-raisers.[27]

Interim Work

In the meantime, Nigerian officials continued to deny Farrar either permission or place to practice in Onicha Ngwa. They delayed approving nearby, abandoned buildings for a clinic and prohibited him from practicing outside a clinic—a rule that did not apply to native doctors. A stymied Farrar thus limited his surgical practice to secular and "denomi-

---

[22]G. Farrar to G.B. Farrar, January 31, 1965. See also McInteer to Mission Committee, January 14, 1965, W-COC file.

[23]P. Bryant to Mattoxes, March 24, 1965; R. Bryant to Mattoxes, April 1, 1965. G. Farrar in undated personal communication said that as Harding's school nurse, she was forbidden to hang clinic shelving until President Benson personally visited the clinic to approve shelf location; H. Farrar Jr. in undated personal communication remembered that during a Harding China Club meeting, Benson verbally paired men and women members into future marital partners who could go as missionaries.

[24]P. Bryant to Mattoxes, March 24, 1965.

[25]H. Farrar to Benson, February 20, 1965; H. Farrar to Benson, ca. May or June 1965.

[26]"George Stuart Benson," June 3, 2006, findagrave.com no. 14484814.

[27]Bryant, Divine, 242.

national hospitals"[28] and to treating ill missionaries.[29] Still, his frustration and pangs of conscience compelled him to care for a few ill and injured locals begging for help at his backdoor, and there he performed his first surgical operation in Nigeria: removal of his night watchman's abscessed teeth.[30] He also dispensed "a few pills,"[31] gave chloroquine injections to critically ill children,[32] visited a suffering family at home,[33] and drove one man, whose hand was "blown to bits by an old muzzle-loading gun," to a government hospital;[34] missionary neighbors transported others.[35] Farrar constrained his own practice not only because of government prohibitions but also from his own concerns that providing backdoor care or even establishing a clinic might demotivate locals to work toward a hospital.[36]

While Grace Farrar appreciated her husband's surgical work at Queen Elizabeth Hospital (QEH) and elsewhere, she was dismayed that other churches, not the COC, received credit for his work. Six months into their stay, she began to wonder if the nurses would ever arrive or a COC hospital ever materialize,[37] while Henry Farrar explained his practice at other hospitals to US supporters as the "first phase" of his medical mission efforts: He was learning tropical medicine. He worked not only in QEH, but also the Leprosarium in Itu, the Qua Iboe Hospital in Etinan, and the British Shell Oil Company Hospital in PH.[38] For reasons probably related both to church politics and his love of preaching,[39] Farrar listed his multihospital practice as the last of his "four-fold" responsibilities behind parenting, teaching in the BTC, and preaching in multiple church-

---

[28]P. Bryant to Mattoxes, September 7, 1964; G. Farrar to Johnson, November 1, 1964; G. Farrar to Folks, March 30, 1965; Farrar to Brethren, October 5, 1964, *WEV*.

[29]P. Bryant to Mattoxes, April 19, August 12, September 7, and September 22; R. Bryant to Friends, December 23, 1964; G. Farrar to Johnson, January 24, 1965; Farrar to Mission Committee, March 1, 1965, *WEV*.

[30]Farrar to Mission Committee, August 15, 1964, W-COC file.

[31]G. Farrar to Johnson, September 17, 1964.

[32]Farrar to Brethren, October 5, 1964, *WEV*.

[33]Farrar to Mission Committee, December 31, 1964, *WEV*.

[34]P. Bryant to Mattoxes, September 7, 1964.

[35]P. Bryant to Joe Mattoxes, April 11, 1965.

[36]H. Farrar to Brethren, October 5, 1964, *WEV*; H. Farrar to Mission Committee, August 15, 1964, W-COC file.

[37]G. Farrar to Johnsons, January 10, 1965; G. Farrar, Interview.

[38]P. Bryant to Mattoxes, August 18, 1965; R. Bryant in P. Bryant to Mattoxes, September 7, 1964; Farrar to Mission Committee, August 15, 1964, W-COC file; H. Farrar, Interview 1; Farrar, "Heroes" Interview.

[39]Hays-Savio and Petty-Kraus, Interview; Farrar, "Heroes" Interview.

es each Sunday.[40] "Henry Farrar is ideal for this work," scrawled Rees Bryant in the margin of a letter to F.W. Mattox.[41]

Farrar invested energy in other jobs as well. In his December 1964 report to W-COC's Mission Committee, he enumerated twelve accomplishments, ranging from establishing new COCs to hauling cement for the nurses' house.[42] His days included various combinations of teaching in the BTC, performing surgery, treating BTC students, meeting officials, preaching in open-air markets, conducting correspondence, preparing Sunday sermons, "meeting with many backdoor visitors, and [completing] odd jobs." An eager, cost-conscious Farrar also purchased drafting tools and put his precollege vocational-technical training to use in creating customized hospital blueprints for an American-style hospital that he thought an improvement on the British-style QEH.[43]

Concurrently, Grace Farrar served briefly as unofficial BTC school nurse, a task she added to her already full schedule of managing a Nigerian household, homeschooling, and treating her own children, particularly eight-year-old David, who was dangerously ill from stingray envenomization during a family Eket Beach trip. Care for BTC students consisted mostly of distributing aspirin and antimalarials that she thought wouldn't "hurt and might possibly help,"[44] and aided by experienced Charla Lawyer, she diagnosed most students' complaints as a desire for attention.[45] One day, Nurse Farrar absent-mindedly used her left hand to pass medication to a student, a forbidden and disrespectful act among Igbos. He paled and trembled before a dismayed Farrar. "I forgive you because you don't know our customs," he said.[46]

Grace Farrar also worked as a reluctant nurse to locals, who came to the family's back door every morning after her husband left for the day.[47] There, she attended to a bleeding circumcised female infant, a dog-bite victim whose family already "chopped" (ate) head and all of the potentially rabid animal, and others complaining of "waist pain" (low back

[40]Farrar to Missions Committee, November 7, 1964.
[41]R. Bryant in P. Bryant to Mattoxes, September 7, 1964
[42]Farrar to Mission Committee, December 31, 1964, *WEV.*
[43]Farrar, *Stand*, 45; G. Farrar to Johnson, November 19, 1964.
[44]G. Farrar to Johnson, January 24, 1965.
[45]Farrar, *Stand*, 77.
[46]Ibid., 116.
[47]G. Farrar, Interview.

pain), "internal heat" (anxiety), or impotence.[48] A few wanted lifesaving advice, including a woman desperate to save her acutely anemic infant after the loss of her previous twelve children, and a destitute couple wanting Farrar to tell them whether their measles-infected infant would live or die, so they could decide between paying for the infant's medical care or buying food for her siblings. The couple's request so overwhelmed Farrar that she "retreated into the house to think and pray," but when she re-emerged they were gone, leaving her with only a "haunting memory."[49] Later none were more relieved than she when Hays and Petty arrived and relieved her of backdoor caregiving, although the process of transition was unremembered.[50]

Tension

Dr. Farrar's multifaceted work, especially his practice in other hospitals, interfered with progress toward a COC hospital. At least that was the Bryant perspective.[51] From the Farrar perspective, Henry was spending months on related paperwork from the regional Enugu Ministry of Health by "again and again—revising, visiting, and waiting—revising, visiting, and waiting."[52] Despite his efforts, progress stalled, and in early April 1965, missionaries were still waiting on both government approval of their land survey and a well-drilling cost estimate requested in October from Balakhany, Ltd.[53] Power company officials in Aba and Lagos were arguing over which was responsible to electrify the clinic,[54] and regional Health Ministry officials rejected two sets of clinic blueprints, including Farrar's, because they were "not done by a 'professional' architect." Moreover, civil servants stashed the COC hospital application "in a

---

[48]Farrar, *Stand*, 77–79. Dr. Chi Ekwenye-Hendricks in email to author on July 22, 2019, wrote regarding the complaint of internal heat: "In the US, one would say it is some kind of anxiety disorder; but that is not a diagnosis here. So it won't work. Internal heat and chest pain are common and [may be]…acid indigestion…. But the psychology of ill health here needs to be understood! The 'bigger' and more mysterious your illness is,…[the better]! So internal heat can be anything—known and unknown!"

[49]Farrar, *Stand*, 117.

[50]G. Farrar, Interview.

[51]P. Bryant to Mattoxes, March 24, 1965.

[52]Farrar, *Stand*, 65.

[53]P. Bryant to Mattoxes, April 6, 1965; R. Bryant to Mattoxes, April 1, 1965; Farrar to Mission Committee, February 8 and April 19, 1965, *WEV*.

[54]Farrar to Mission Committee, February 8, 1965, *WEV*.

bottom drawer," unearthing it only during a face-to-face meeting with Farrar.[55]

Rees Bryant's distress grew as hospital dreams bogged down in bureaucratic processes. Whereas he earlier wrote home that Dr. Farrar "does a lot of good, and he keeps his surgical skill sharp,"[56] now Bryant was frustrated by Farrar's keeping a schedule that allowed only intermittent work in tackling delays. Rees entrusted hospital plans to "the will of God," but he also expected Farrar to do his part. Messrs. Bryant and Lawyer called a team meeting; its purpose was to convince Farrar to pursue government approvals aggressively at the cost of all other work. Nonetheless, a kindhearted Rees Bryant euphemized Farrar's waiting on officials to act without prodding as patience, a trait that even Farrar himself denied having.[57]

The March 25 Lawyer-Bryant-Farrar meeting to "thrash out" disagreements over Farrar's use of time[58] happily coincided with other driving forces. A vacation renewed Farrar's energy, Hays and Petty arrived by early April, and officials accepted a second land survey that allowed missionaries to begin lease negotiations for hospital acreage.[59] Farrar's more assertive pursuit of government authorizations re-established "very good rapport" among the missionary men. Too, hopes for final approval of new, professionally drawn clinic blueprints were bolstered after Farrar met with the original architect of the buildings that they planned to renovate into a clinic. That architect worked in the regional approving office, leading to Patti Bryant's optimistic assessment that "this time should really do it."[60]

Meanwhile, Farrar and Bryant sought financing for construction and equipment,[61] and hundreds of dollars poured in from individuals and churches.[62] Among them the BTC campus congregation donated £500, the Keesee missionary family in Enugu gave $450 that they had saved for a car, and Dr. Farrar's in-laws sent another $450.[63] In the end, all these

---

[55]P. Bryant to Mattoxes, March 24, 1965.

[56]R. Bryant in P. Bryant to Mattoxes, September 7, 1964.

[57]P. Bryant to Mattoxes, March 24, 1965 (orig.); R. Bryant to Mattoxes, April 1, 1965; Farrar, *Stand*, 16.

[58]P. Bryant to Mattoxes, March 24, 1965 (orig.).

[59]P. Bryant to Mattoxes, April 6 and April 19, 1965; R. Bryant to Mattoxes, April 1, 1965; Farrar, *Stand*, 64–65.

[60]P. Bryant to Mattoxes, April 19, 1965; R. Bryant to Currys, June 1, 1965.

[61]P. Bryant to Joe Mattoxes, April 11, 1965; Farrar to Mission Committee, December 31, 1964, *WEV*.

[62]Farrar to Benson, ca. May/June 1965.

[63]P. Bryant to Joe Mattoxes, April 11, 1965; R. Bryant to Mattoxes, April 1, 1965; Keesees to H. Farrar, n.d., in February 8, 1965, *WEV*.

events led the Bryants to conclude later that Farrar's long hours in other mission hospitals had facilitated the success of their own and that "the Lord was working through it all."[64]

A Clinic Advances

Finally, on April 23, 1965, the regional Enugu government authorized COC missionaries to proceed with renovating nearby buildings for a clinic.[65] Henry Farrar, however, was not the one who gained this approval. Instead, it was the Aba television station manager, a Nigerian who "understood what could and should be done for his people." The manager voluntarily made the 300-mile roundtrip to Enugu and hand-carried papers from official to official, waiting at each desk until approvals were complete. "It takes a Nigerian to understand how Nigeria moves," Grace Farrar concluded gratefully;[66] yet while missionaries celebrated him none recorded his name.

As with this station manager, individual identities sometimes receded behind professional and Christian roles. Missionaries writing to family, friends, and supporters perhaps reasonably assumed that titles and roles would be more meaningful to US audiences than would the names of strangers. Thus, Grace Farrar wrote only of the station manager and his wife, although she interacted with them as friends.[67] And though the Bryants came to love and respect Hays and Petty, Rees Bryant lauded them to his sponsoring COC on one occasion simply as two "American nurses," who were "young and capable." His use of the title "Dr." before Farrar's name suggested a similar pattern.[68] Likewise, to W-COC in May, Henry Farrar described the persons in one photograph as "two of our best" senior, BTC preaching students whom he was treating for tuberculosis, lauding them as "outstanding preachers of the gospel...faithful," sincere, and knowledgeable. He personally knew them well as Benedict Ibara and Victor Johnny Opidiwowu.[69]

In these accounts to supporters, both Bryant and Farrar emphasized evangelistic efforts more than medical work. Bryant dedicated only a single sentence to clinic approval in the middle of a two-page preaching and

---

[64]Bryant and Bryant, Interview.

[65]R. Bryant to Elders, April 24, 1965.

[66]Farrar, *Stand*, 66.

[67]Ibid, 105; Author's recollection.

[68]R. Bryant to Elders, April 24, 1965.

[69]Farrar to Mission Committee, March 1 and May 28, 1965, *WEV*; "Benedict Ibara and Victor Johnny Opidiwowu," photograph, 1965, HGF.

teaching report, and Farrar relegated it to the last paragraph of his report that was accompanied by four evangelism-related photographs. Aware that W-COC expected Nigerians to contribute to hospital costs, Farrar announced that local donations totaled $1,402, as evidence that "progress is being made."[70]

Meanwhile, at the clinic site, Farrar "swung into high gear," hiring carpenters, plumbers, and Anthony Agali, a trusted contractor, master mason, and COC member, to repurpose three vacant, formerly British buildings.[71] Colonialists had originally erected the structures as intermittent housing and courthouse for the British District Officer and his "entourage"[72] when they traveled into rural Nigeria to settle disputes. In 1957, they became the first Igboland home for the Nicks family, and in 1961, a proposed site for Sermanoukian's never-to-be clinic.[73] Now they would be a dispensary and outpatient clinic. Everything, except the water well, will be finished within a week, declared an overly optimistic Dr. Farrar.[74]

Located on Ndiakata village land, the structures were separated from the BTC compound by roughly a quarter mile of dusty footpaths through bush and farmland or about a half mile over paved and dirt roads.[75] The site was easily accessible at Mile 11 on the main Aba-Ikot Ekpene road, a coal-tar highway that ran east from PH through Aba and along the southern side of the clinic and proposed hospital land. The pavement then dipped down a steep hill past the dirt road turnoff to Onicha Ngwa and stretched across the little, wooden Nwaigwe Bridge that spanned a stream dividing Igbos from Annangs (also Anaangs/Ibibios), and that in present day, separates Abia and Akwa Ibom States. Continuing east from the bridge, the Aba-Ikot Ekpene road rose again on the Annang side where the Nwaigwe police station capped the opposite hill and bush roads branched off into villages. About nine miles beyond, across the Qua Ibo River, the coal-tar continued through the town of Ikot Ekpene and then split east toward the municipality of Itu and southeast toward Uyo. Smaller dirt roads from Ikot Ekpene led east to

---

[70]R. Bryant to Elders, April 24, 1965; Farrar to Mission Committee, May 28, 1965, *WEV*.

[71]"Biographical Sketches" (Agali), 190; Farrar, *Stand*, 66.

[72]H. Farrar, Interview 1.

[73]P. Bryant to Mattoxes, March 3, 1961; R. Bryant to Brooms, May 6, 1961; Nicks, "Okorobeke," 22.

[74]Farrar, *Stand*, 66.

[75]Author's recollection.

rural Ikot Usen and south to Ukpom. The British had unknowingly positioned the future COC clinic buildings well.

Conclusion

Farrar struggled much of his first year with local politics, regional and federal government processes, and numerous other details necessary to prepare a clinic as precursor to a hospital. For nine months, he labored without missionary nurses. The work was shaped by his own readiness to change within a context of locals willing to circumvent their council president, a college president who understood organizational financing, teammates willing to challenge him, and a television station manager unwilling to take "no" for an answer.

13
Making a Start: The Nurses Arrive
(March–April 1965)

I was supposed to help…But the Lord helped us both.
—Nancy Petty

Like those of mice and men, the best laid plans of nurses and missionaries went awry. Although Iris Hays and Nancy Petty intended to fly to Nigeria together, Hays decided to go alone when her visa arrived before Petty's. Hays was already on the College Avenue COC payroll, eager to realize her dreams, and convicted of her critical importance to Dr. Farrar's work. She "couldn't wait any longer;" no one knew when—or even if—Petty's visa would come.[1]

Not Alone

Hays had never flown before, and events immediately prior to the trip left her physically exhausted and emotionally drained. When her grandmother died only three days before Hays's scheduled departure, she stopped preparations for Nigeria, traveled to be with family, and "didn't sleep at all." After the funeral services, a weary Hays drove back to Lubbock, got into bed at 3:00 a.m. and rose two hours later to get to the airport. She recalled her fatigue during the Lubbock-to-New York flight and the six-to-eight-hour layover in New York, followed by an eighteen-hour, multi-stop trip from New York to Lagos, where she boarded Nigerian Airways for Port Harcourt (PH).[2]

Decades later, she described how Dr. Farrar's care ameliorated her fears. "Shy" and "scared to death," Hays fretted that she might end up in the wrong destination, so she clung to Farrar's minutely detailed travel

---

[1] Hays-Savio, Interview.
[2] Ibid.

instructions that included "every imaginable situation," even taxi fares. During the interminable "Pan-American puddle jumper flight [that] stopped in every African country on the way down," Hays read and reread Farrar's written guidance, holding it like a security, "fuzzy blanket."[3] His take-charge attitude that had created a kerfuffle regarding electricians now provided a much-needed confidence booster for the inexperienced traveler.

Comforting supporters on both sides of the Atlantic bookended Hays's trip, which proceeded without a hitch. Roughly seventy-five to one hundred members of College Avenue COC gathered at 7:00 a.m. (probably March 22) in Lubbock to see Hays off with a prayer. And all the southeastern Nigeria COC missionary families greeted her at 7:30 p.m. on March 24 when she stepped off the plane in PH. Missionaries met her as they met others, waiting to gather her and her luggage into their arms.[4] Entire families drove hours to PH to welcome every new or returning missionary and to see off every departing one. The adults used these occasions to do their PH shopping, and the children enjoyed a day off from school and a swim in the Olympic size pool on the Shell Oil Company compound. Most brought picnic lunches from home and purchased warm, glass-bottled "Fantas," a moniker applied to most carbonated beverages. A bottled drink was safe if the drinker wiped off the tropical-humidity-created rust deposited by its metal cap and then positioned lips inside the opening.[5]

Missionary families would make these trips even though they never knew whether the expected traveler would appear, given transportation vagaries and communication hurdles. Phone service was unavailable on COC compounds, and the fastest US to Nigeria messages were telegrams that took two to three days and were delivered to the Aba post office, eleven miles from Onicha Ngwa. Sometimes more travelers arrived than expected, sometimes fewer, and sometimes none at all. When no one got off the plane, the families would go home, but a few missionaries would return to PH to greet the next plane arriving from the US via Lagos, repeating the trip until either the person arrived or they learned no one was coming.[6]

Thus, when Iris Hays disembarked down the steep, mobile airplane stairs, she was greeted by a large, waving, enthusiastic crowd of missionary children and adults. They hoped Nancy Petty might be with her, but

---

[3]Ibid.
[4]Ibid.
[5]Author's recollection.
[6]Ibid. Example in G. Farrar to Mrs. H.C. Farrar, June 26, 1966.

their delight in Hays's arrival[7] was exceeded only by her reaction. Hays recalled seeing her welcoming party from the airplane door as "the most joyous sight in my life...because I thought...'I don't have to think any more about what I have to do or where I have to go...They can take care of me.'" They did, and for Hays "it was wonderful."[8]

At last, she was in Africa.

Like missionaries before her, Hays translated her gratitude for the waiting, waving COC crowd into a commitment to "meet every missionary that ever set their foot down on that African soil," and so she did for all her years in the continent.[9] Hays understood at once what all knew. It was not merely the necessity of shopping or the pleasure of a holiday that brought entire US families together from Ukpom, Ikot Usen, and Onicha Ngwa to the PH airport. One missionary could have greeted planes. But the coming of every worker was cause for community celebration. "Lucky us!" wrote nine-year-old Sara Bryant when her family's car "was chosen to bring Hays home."[10]

First Impressions

The car caravan ferrying Hays to Onicha Ngwa traversed the narrow, two-way coal-tar road through the large town of Aba after dark. Along unlit roads, Hays's first impression was the people. She had "never seen so many" walking along the road, and she wondered where they were all going. A second impression was the beauty of missionary homes in the headlights as the cars bumped up the compound's semicircular drive. She reacted to that view the same way she did to many things in her new life: "Wow! This is good."[11] Her twin bed in the Bryants' home, where she would live until Petty arrived, was draped with a mosquito net and looked like a curtained, royal couch to Hays. Later those nets became a "nuisance having to get in and out from under them," she conceded, but in that exhilarating moment she felt like "queen of the world."[12]

Missionaries also savored this time. Her coming marked another step toward the hospital in which they had invested so much time and energy, and the Bryants described Hays as "a wonderful, wonderful woman...tall,

---

[7]P. Bryant to Mattoxes, March 24 and April 6, 1965.
[8]Hays-Savio, Interview.
[9]Ibid.
[10]Sara Jo Bryant to Mattoxes, April 14, 1965; Bryant, *Divine*, 209.
[11]Hays-Savio, Interview
[12]R. Bryant to Mattoxes, April 1, 1965; P. Bryant to Mattoxes, April 6, 1965; Hays-Savio, Interview.

energetic!"[13] Unlike Sermanoukian, Hays followed advice, held professional documents, came as planned, and fit in well. To their further delight, Hays brought gifts, news, pictures, and a reel-to-reel audiotape from family and friends. Patti Bryant's delight in these presents reminded her how she had once wondered whether her family would become like other missionaries in so "longing for home...[that they] grasped at any news from America." They had.[14]

During the next two weeks, Hays rested, learned about tropical nursing, and set up housekeeping. She did little the first two days beyond recovering from the strain of her grandmother's death and her transatlantic trip, falling asleep every few minutes in chairs. But she did walk around the compound and meet Nigerian BTC teacher Josiah O. Akandu and family.[15] On day three, Hays accompanied Farrar to the miles-away Queen Elizabeth Hospital (QEH), where he performed surgery regularly in order to maintain and build skills.[16] There Hays assisted in surgery and on the wards, while observing QEH practices, methods, and terminology, which were British with a Nigerian flair.[17]

In the coming non-QEH days, Hays and Farrar bought her needed household goods in the market during what she called "quite a shopping experience," and it seemed to Hays that "Dr. Farrar reached in his pocket and pulled out money to pay for just about everything" to furnish their house and later the hospital.[18] Her house purchases included mosquito nets and a twenty-four by thirty by eighteen-inch refrigerator with copper tone door. The £80, gas refrigerator could be converted to run on electricity,[19] but when they got it home, "it didn't work!" As they bemoaned this expensive failure, a Wycliffe Bible translator dropped by; he learned of the problem, turned the refrigerator upside down for a bit, set it right side up, and then successfully turned it on. How glad they were to meet him, laughed Hays.[20] The working refrigerator joined the Nickses' refurbished gas stove in her kitchen, alongside her purchased kerosene-powered iron and Tilley lamps.[21]

---

[13]R. Bryant to Mattoxes, April 1, 1965; Bryant and Bryant, Interview.

[14]Bryant, *Divine*, 9; R. Bryant to Mattoxes, April 1, 1965; P. Bryant to Mattoxes, April 6, 1965.

[15]Hays-Savio, Interview.

[16]Farrar, "Heroes" Interview; H. Farrar to Morgan, September 5, 1964; Hays-Savio, Interview.

[17]Bryant to Mattoxes, April 6, 1965; Hays-Savio, Interview."

[18]Hays-Savio, Interview.

[19]Ibid.;. Bryant to Mattoxes, April 6, 1965; Petty to Corlew, April 12, 1965.

[20]Hays-Savio, Interview.

[21]Ibid.; P. Bryant to Mattoxes, April 6, 1965.

Household preparations were a learning experience, and in Hays's first solo attempt to prepare drinking water, she boiled stream water for twenty minutes as instructed and then poured it into the large filter container. When she returned minutes later, however, her floor was "flooded with good boiled water" because she forgot to turn off the filter spigot. Housekeeping alone was a fulltime job, and Hays was doubtless relieved when Mark Apollos ably took over these tasks after the Lawyers departed on May 18.[22]

Petty's Earliest Days

While Hays traveled, Petty waited. Nigerian officials insisted that her visa had been approved, but they couldn't find it, so an exasperated Rees Bryant traveled to Lagos to investigate. There his frustration turned to amusement when he discovered an official both figuratively and literally sitting on Petty's visa. A rather diminutive immigration clerk was perched on several files, including Petty's, in order to boost his height in a too-short chair.[23]

With visa found and sent, Petty cabled missionaries that she would arrive in Nigeria on April 7,[24] two weeks to the day after Hays's entry. She, too, departed the US surrounded by church members, and arrived in PH to an enthusiastic, multifamily, missionary greeting party.[25] It was then, beside the airport tarmac on a hot, humid evening that Hays and Petty met for the first time. For Hays, greeting Petty's plane was a first chance to fulfill her pledge of meeting every incoming missionary. For short, stocky Petty, a first glimpse of Hays generated good-humored dismay: "Oh Lord! Not tall *and* thin!"[26]

---

[22]Hays-Savio, Interview.

[23]P. Bryant, email to author, April 7, 2012; Bryant and Bryant, Interview.

[24]P. Bryant to Mattoxes, April 6, 1965.

[25]Farrar and Petty-Kraus, Interview.

[26]Petty-Kraus, unrecorded reading from her journal, Memorial Service for Iris Hays Savio, Church of Christ, Rockwall, Texas, September 15, 2012, NPK.

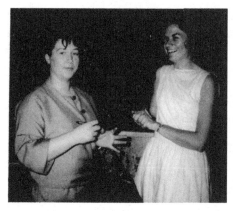

Photograph 13. First meeting of Nancy Petty and Iris Hays, Port Harcourt airport, April 7, 1965. (Author collection).

The two nurses spent that first night together in their petit, Onicha Ngwa house located on the highest back corner of the compound hill. Unprepared for the tropics, Petty arrived in heels, hose, corsage, and stifling suit to weather that was "hot, hot, hot, hot!" After changing into cooler sleepwear, Petty never donned that outfit again in Nigeria.[27]

A few hours later, Petty awoke to a surprise. In the heat she had left her curtains open overnight, and now looking in at each window were Nigerian men wearing "very little clothing" and carrying "huge knives." She "looked at them, and they looked at [her]...and they said, 'Good morning, Sister!' and off they went." Petty laughed about their cheerful curiosity but never left her bedtime curtains open again. Only later did she learn that men stripped down to loin cloths to climb oil palms and used large knives to harvest the kernels; her observers were simply on their way to "cut palm."[28]

Up and dressed, Nancy Petty met future friend and cook-steward, Mark Apollos, whom the Lawyers had assigned to the nurses during their first morning together. Then, making up for lost time, Petty plunged into practice. Hays suggested that she rest, but Petty insisted that she "came to work," and this suited hard-driving Farrar well.[29]

Her first-day adventure continued as she traveled with Hays and Farrar in Farrar's Peugeot 504 station wagon to QEH. Petty marveled that "Dr. Farrar did not slow down for anybody" over eight miles of bush paths with chickens flying in all directions, followed by twenty-eight miles of

---

[27]Farrar and Petty-Kraus, Interview.
[28]Ibid.
[29]Ibid.

narrow asphalt roads full of bicycles and lorries.[30] He drove like a Nigerian, weaving "in and out...so close to pedestrians you just knew they were going to get killed,"[31] and Petty felt certain that "at least three chickens" met their maker at his hand that day. Meanwhile, cyclists waved and called out *Ndewo* (hello) greetings.[32] Nor did Farrar slow his surgical schedule to accommodate Hays and Petty. If anything, he saw their presence as an opportunity to accelerate work, and Grace Farrar wrote that he felt "like a real doctor to have two nurses." Petty moved fast, too; once safely at QEH she worked all day on a surgical ward and began a close friendship with Canadian missionary nurse Dianne North.[33]

Petty crammed day two with activity as well. In the morning she attended BTC chapel, where she was deeply moved when students stood up "and sang 'Welcome Sister Petty.'" Missionaries would have no trouble raising money, she wrote to her sister Dianne Spann, if potential supporters could experience students' warm handshakes and hear them sing missional hymn "Send the Light." That afternoon, Petty shopped in the sprawling, open-air Aba market with Iris Hays and Henry and Grace Farrar. As they walked the narrow dirt paths between pole and thatch-roofed stalls, a man ran up to Dr. Farrar, holding up three fingers and respectfully observing, "3 wives." The missionary women laughed,[34] but similar stories emerged within days that Rees Bryant had one wife living in the house with him and two more wives in the house behind his—a polygamous arrangement mirroring Nigerian customs. COC missionaries, who preached monogamy, were amused.[35]

By the end of her second day, Petty, a self-confessed poor correspondent, had written eight pages of a now lost letter to her mother and over a page to her sister. Her love of home and family, combined with a desire to reassure them that she was doing well, overcame her usual reticence to put pen to paper. Nigeria, she announced, is "more wonderful than I ever dreamed it would be,"[36] but she did not report one swiftly uncovered flaw in her preparation. Her typical American clothing turned out to be miserable in the rainforest climate,[37] and Petty's only comfortable outfit was a sleeveless blue nightgown sewn by her mother. Petty wore it as a

[30]Ibid.; Morgan, "Report," 14.
[31]Bryant and Bryant, Interview.
[32]Farrar and Petty-Kraus, Interview.
[33]G. Farrar, Interview; Petty to Spann, April 9, 1965; Kotlarsky, "From Canada."
[34]Petty to Spann, April 9, 1965.
[35]Nau, *We Move*, 102–03; Bryant and Bryant, Interview.
[36]Petty to Spann, April 9, 1965; Petty-Kraus, phone call to author, July 6, 2015.
[37]Petty-Kraus, Presentation to Keen-Agers; Petty to Spann, June 20, 1966.

dress, and a US visitor captured Petty's photographic image in that night-gown. When the visitor later showed his slides at Vanleer COC, Kitty Petty "almost fell out of her pew."[38] No doubt to her mother's relief, Petty soon removed sleeves from her other clothes and bought Nigerian-made sleeveless dresses in breathable fabric.[39]

Conclusion

Decades later Petty asserted her belief that God cared for her and Hays in unexpected ways during their move to Nigeria. Moreover, differences between the two new friends were quickly apparent. For Petty, the nurses' separate intercontinental journeys were evidence that God had substituted his plans for theirs. "I was supposed to…help her…, but the Lord helped us both," she affirmed.[40] Then once in Onicha Ngwa, each nurse transitioned into missionary life in her own way; Hays gave herself time to rest, and Petty immersed herself in new religious, nursing, relational, and cultural activity.

---

[38]Farrar and Petty-Kraus, Interview.
[39]Petty-Kraus, Presentation to Keen-Agers.
[40]Farrar and Petty-Kraus, Interview.

14
Becoming "The Nurses"
(1965–1966)

Iris and I just fit so well. God did that.
—Nancy Petty

Living in Nigeria was not an intermission from life for Iris Hays and Nancy Petty. It *was* life, and they rapidly assimilated into the work and play of the missionary community. Dr. Henry Farrar wrote to West End Church of Christ (W-COC) that the nurses were "a great addition to the efforts here to preach and demonstrate the gospel…[and] their cheerful energy is an inspiration to all the missionaries."[1] Too, both promptly engaged in supporting missionaries' existing efforts. Hays typed for evangelists and taught Bible classes for missionary preschoolers, Petty visited churches on Sundays with evangelists, and both nurses practiced in nearby hospitals alongside Farrar.[2] They also participated in missionary men's Onicha Ngwa hospital planning meetings—meetings that Petty later described (over Hays's objections) as primarily venues for Farrar to hand down his decisions.[3]

Close Quarters

Friendship flourished in the nurses' tiny two-bedroom home, a building that matched Grace Farrar's description of her own house in character if not size:

Individually hand-molded, sun-dried blocks formed the walls [… with] galvanized ('zinc') roofing.[…] The floor was overlain with

---

[1] Farrar to Mission Committee, April 19, 1965, *WEV*.
[2] P. Bryant to Mattoxes, April 19, 1965; Farrar and Petty-Kraus, Interview; Farrar to Mission Committee, May 28, 1965, *WEV*; Hays-Savio, Interview.
[3] Hays-Savio and Petty-Kraus, Interview.

a red Colorcrete that took on a high gloss with an application of Red Mansion floor wax hand-rubbed with a halved coconut husk. Some of the windows were the casement type cranking outward [and opening like doors on side hinges] and others were of [horizontal] louvered glass.[4]

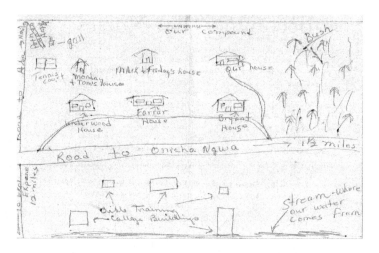

Map 2: Onicha Ngwa mission compound, artist Nancy Petty drawn in red ink on blue aerogram to Dianne Spann. September 27, 1965. To top left and outside of map would soon be NCH Clinic & Hospital. (NPK collection with permission).

According to Grace Farrar, the Colorcrete offered a cool sleeping surface on hot nights but was also like "living on a slick rock."[5]

The house where Hays and Petty lived was only the second missionary home built with an indoor kitchen after cooking shifted from open fires to gas stoves, and Petty found it comfortably furnished.[6] Like other missionary houses, theirs was fully paid for during its construction, so that the nurses had no rent or mortgage.[7] A compound generator supplied electricity from 6:00 p.m. to 10:00 p.m., water flowed by gravity feed from outdoor, elevated, fifty-gallon, steel shipping drums to interior faucets, and a teakettle on the stove could transform that cool water to hot as needed. In addition to roof runoff, the barrels were filled by a "water boy" who carried stream water on his head uphill for a quarter

---

[4]Farrar, *Stand*, 10–11.
[5]G. Farrar to Johnson, March 15 and May 22, 1965.
[6]Farrar, *Stand*, 11; Petty to Corlew, April 12, 1965.
[7]Farrar to Mission Committee, December 31, 1964, *WEV*; H. Farrar to Benson, February 20, 1965.

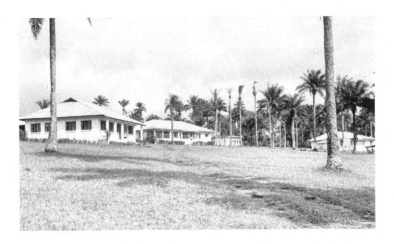

Photograph 14. Church of Christ mission compound, Onicha
Ngwa. (left to right) Lawyer/Morgan house, Farrar house, Petty and
Hays house, Bryant house. 1965. Photograph by J.R. Morgan. (JRM
collection with permission).

mile in a four-gallon square "tin"(can),[8] resulting in the occasional tad-
pole in the bathwater. Soon, Mark Apollos laundered their clothes,
cleaned, and cooked "for 6 or 7 shillings [~$1.00] a month…a very good
salary."[9]

Close living quarters provided ample opportunity for clashes between
the nurses, but as Hays observed, conflicts "fizzled away." The two easily
settled on who would get which bedroom, and after Hays confused their
toothbrushes for a few days, she laughingly observed that "if someone
can share your toothbrush you can share just about anything." Limited
evening electricity and equatorially consistent daylight hours partly syn-
chronized bedtime patterns of night owl Hays and morning lark Petty,[10]
and it would be hard to determine whether the remarkable peace between
them arose in spite of or because of their differences. Petty was an outspoken, take-charge extrovert; Hays, a shy and reserved introvert.[11] Petty
grew up as the oldest sibling in an intact nuclear, farm family; Hays, as
the youngest in a mostly city family with an absent father. Petty possessed
more nursing experience; Hays, more university education. Petty was
short and stocky; Hays, tall and slim. Petty always intended to be a nurse;

---

[8]Farrar, *Stand*, 11, 42, 84; Hays-Savio, Interview.
[9]Petty to Corlew, April 12, 1965.
[10]Hays-Savio, Interview.
[11]G. Farrar, Interview.

Hays chose nursing only when it matched her African ambitions.[12] Petty was bluntly straightforward, and Hays, keen to avoid conflict.[13]

What they did share, however, was significant: a strong personal faith, a COC history, and a commitment to missionary nursing. During their first US phone conversation before coming, Hays discovered "a meeting of spirit" between them, and missionary families agreed that the two were providentially well-matched for the unique demands of Nigeria. They never argued,[14] and so "fabulously"[15] did they live, work, and vacation together that Hays and Petty were soon identified as another family unit. As Hays put it, "We always went everywhere together…[and] everybody called us…'the Nurses.' Just like 'the Farrars.' Just 'the Nurses.'"[16]

Aba and Beyond

The two shared a tiny Ford Anglia that Hays described as "like a little toy car you could put…in your pocket." Petty's family facilitated a US car loan, and the two nurses split payments from their wages. Hays, who had driven since age fourteen,[17] took the Anglia wheel, an arrangement decided between them like most things: without discussion. Each simply assumed her more comfortable role. Although Hays did not like standing before groups to teach, she instructed Petty one-on-one in what was novel also to her: a steering wheel on the right, floor stick shift on the left, and motoring on the "wrong side" of the road.[18]

Soon Petty and Hays braved the main coal-tar road to the massive Aba market. This meant navigating a narrow highway lined with deep ruts and crowded with cyclists, pedestrians, and lorry drivers who hurtled down the road in seemingly full commitment to mottos emblazoned on their trucks, such as "I leave everything to God."[19] In the market where white faces were rare, the nurses garnered special attention, an advantage Hays and Petty embraced as they shopped separately among hundreds of rambling stalls. When it was time to leave, each simply asked, "Have you seen

---

[12]Farrar and Petty-Kraus, Interview; Hays-Savio, Interview.
[13]Author's recollection.
[14]Farrar and Petty-Kraus, Interview; Hays-Savio, Interview.
[15]G. Farrar, Interview.
[16]Ibid.; Farrar and Petty-Kraus, Interview; Hays-Savio, Interview.
[17]Hays-Savio, Interview.
[18]Ibid.; Farrar and Petty-Kraus, Interview; Petty to Spann, April 30, 1965.
[19]G. Farrar to Mrs. H.C. Farrar, October 4, 1964.

my sister?" Nigerians, who always knew the location of each, would direct them together.[20]

Hays and Petty also enjoyed opportunities to entertain, swim, cycle, explore the local area, play tennis on the COC compound's court,[21] and dress up for an occasional evening out.[22] Taking Mark Apollos along on one occasion, they enjoyed a ride down the nearby Qua Ibo River as a birthday gift to ten-year-old Sara Bryant and preteen Marty Farrar.[23] After packing a picnic dinner, they drove ten miles to the river and settled on a price of eight shillings with the owner of a dugout made from a single tree—a boat that held all five with room to spare. Peacefully floating down the river, they were surrounded by birds and tropical trees, wild flowers, and ferns of incredible size. After the trip ended, the nurses discovered they were short on change, forcing them to borrow three shillings from Mark to pay their bill, and Mark delighted in this opportunity to take "good care" of them.[24]

Hays and Petty also enjoyed social outings to Aba and beyond. For ten shillings a month, they joined a private Aba club, where they could swim and access a clean bathroom on shopping days. Missionary families were members, too, and a cool evening swim in the uncrowded pool provided a pleasant alternative to an antiseptic-infused, shallow bath at home.[25] Sometimes they drove west to PH for trips that Hays found refreshing to body and spirit with opportunities to shop "in a real store and ride the only escalator in [that part of] Nigeria, eat in an air-conditioned restaurant, and take a bath in more than one inch of water."[26] In PH each might don "heels and girdle" to see a movie in the luxurious Presidential Hotel, then spend the night with oil company friends from the US before returning to Onicha Ngwa for Sunday evening church services.[27]

Other times they drove in the opposite direction, east and deeper into rural Nigeria. There in Ukpom or Ikot Usen they dined and overnighted with COC missionaries, including Don and Joyce Huffard Harrison, the

---

[20]Hays-Savio, Interview.

[21]Petty to Spann, April 30, 1965; Petty to Spann, December 1, 1966. Per Farrar in *Stand*, no one appreciated missionaries' need for personal rejuvenation more than Douglas Lawyer, who constructed concrete tennis courts, barbeque pit, and picnic table, and kept BTC grounds groomed (186–87).

[22]G. Farrar, Interview; Petty to Spann, May 16, 1965.

[23]G. Farrar to Johnson, May 22, 1965; Hays-Savio, Interview.

[24]Petty to Spann, May 24, 1965.

[25]P. Bryant to Mattox, April 19, 1965; Farrar, *Stand*, 144; Petty to Spann, April 30, 1965.

[26]Savio, "Nigerian Christian Hospital," 48.

[27]Petty to Spann, May 31, 1965.

Eno and LaVera Otoyo family of three, the John and Dottie Beckloff family of six, or the Phil Dunn family of four.[28] Moreover, on rare occasions they vacationed further afield in Enugu or at the Obudu rest house and cattle ranch on the country's northeastern, cool plateau near the Cameroon border.[29]

Community as Family

Onicha Ngwa missionaries embraced the nurses as family, and the nurses felt "welcomed and honored and praised."[30] When any new missionary arrived, one experienced family would assume a primary role in orienting and helping the novice to settle in. The Lawyers volunteered to do this for the nurses, and Hays laughingly recounted how the nurses were so determined to honor the Lawyers with a thank-you dinner that she and Petty borrowed plates, silverware, pots, pans, and chairs from the Lawyers themselves to do so. Too, the Bryant or Lawyer families often invited Hays and Petty to spend evenings with them in those early days, creating space for relationship building, saving the nurses from labor-intensive dinner preparations, and laughing together at American television re-runs broadcast from the Aba station.[31] "You couldn't be in a better environment" socially, remembered Petty.[32]

Hays later attributed the team's close relationships to their shared faith and sense of purpose that eased the inevitable "bumps in the road" of life together.[33] Using words similar to those with which Petty praised her Vanleer community, Hays pronounced the team's love for each other as "special and unique...wonderful...really good." Missionaries' disagreements, she mused, never destroyed the bonds between them—a rarity even among "good, Christian people."[34]

Hays and Petty connected with the missionary children, too. Their tiny residence became a safe, fun place, and the nurses served as parent-trusted role models.[35] From their home, the nurses enjoyed a panoramic view

---

[28]G. Farrar, Interview; Don Harrison, emails to author, August 15, 2017 and October 6, 2019; Petty to Spann, July 18 and November 23, 1965. Joyce Huffard Harrison was the daughter of Elvis and Emily Huffard in Chapter 2.

[29]Farrar, *Stand*, 103; Petty to Spann, January 10, 1966.

[30]Farrar and Petty-Kraus, Interview.

[31]P. Bryant to Mattoxes, April 6, 1965; Hays-Savio, Interview.

[32]Farrar and Petty-Kraus, Interview.

[33]Savio, "Nigerian Christian Hospital," 48.

[34]Hays-Savio, Interview.

[35]Ibid.; G. Farrar, Interview.

of the four Bryant, five Farrar, and three Lawyer (later replaced by three Underwood) children at play in the sweeping, grassy space stretching behind family homes. Serendipitous surveillance taught the nurses a lot about children, and they learned how the children would calculate when and where to cry after getting hurt so that their mothers could hear.[36] The children reciprocated the nurses' affectionate attention, sometimes running en masse up to the little house to report on their adventures and misadventures and giving birthday gifts to Hays and Petty.[37] Sara Bryant and Marty Farrar also invited Hays to a favorite Onicha Ngwa space that they had christened the Garden of Eden. The three cycled to that atypically wide bush road canopied by the branches of ancient trees planted evenly along each side, and Hays savored the girls' welcoming her into their "secret, little worlds."[38] On a different day, Hays and Petty completed an all-day cycling jaunt with preteen and teen missionary girls in pursuit of Girl Scout badges, an activity of missionaries' Troop on Foreign Soil established by Grace Farrar.[39]

The two nurses also enjoyed the missionary children during their regular dinners with other families on Mark's days off.[40] One of Petty's long-remembered stories centered on Dr. Farrar's efforts to encourage his oldest son to good posture at the table. "Sit up there, Paul," his father said. "Who wants to marry a hunchback?" "Mama did," teenager Paul responded, and Petty said she almost choked on suppressed laughter.[41] Similar events prompted a later visitor's observation that the Farrars could sell tickets to their lively mealtimes.[42]

Nigerians also joined the nurses' extended family, and the nurses sometimes hosted them for meals.[43] Mark Apollos in particular became a protective, "close brother."[44] His wide smile and laugh were infectious, and his turns of phrase, adopted as part of in-house missionary language. When a village man unexpectedly called on the nurses one evening, Mark would not leave. After cleaning up the kitchen, Mark took the unprecedented step of getting himself a "Fanta" and sitting with them in the liv-

[36]Farrar and Petty-Kraus, Interview; Hays-Savio, Interview; Petty-Kraus, Presentation to Keen-Agers.

[37]Bryant, "Diary," August 7, 1965; Petty to Spann, April 16, 1965.

[38]Hays-Savio, Interview.

[39]Ibid.; G. Farrar, Interview; G. Farrar to Johnson, October 18, 1964.

[40]G. Farrar, Interview; Petty to Spann, August 6, 1965; Petty-Kraus, personal communication, May 16, 2012.

[41]G. Farrar, Interview.

[42]Rebecca Dorfmueller, personal communication, n.d.

[43]Petty to Spann, December 29, 1965; Petty-Kraus, Interview 1.

[44]Farrar and Petty-Kraus, Interview.

ing room until the man concluded his visit. "You never know what is in the mind of a man," Mark cautioned them[45]—a saying that mid-1960s Onicha Ngwa missionaries quote to this day when confronted with suspicious behavior. His phrase, "John Morgan bread," also entered missionary lore after Mark baked an outwardly beautiful loaf that fell in the middle. Hays and Petty discovered its hollow interior, put the loaf back together, and asked Mark to make sandwiches. When Mark sliced into the bread he was horrified, clucking his tongue and throwing away all his bowls and pans as potential culprits. After the nurses could no longer restrain their laughter, a chuckling Mark realized the joke and lightheartedly christened the loaf after that day's lunch guest.[46]

The nurses and families from the three COC compounds celebrated anniversaries and US holidays together, and Petty enjoyed the cake decorating opportunities.[47] Within days of their arrival, Hays and Petty delighted in Farrar children's birthday parties replete with Zebu cattle hamburgers and cocoyam fries that were eaten hot and bathed in ketchup to overcome their starchiness.[48] The nurses also enjoyed the compound's US-affiliated Boy Scout and Girl Scouts' July 4, 1965 ceremony, including "the pledge of allegiance... all the patriotic songs...[and] four firecrackers."[49] In fall, everyone decorated for Halloween, and Mark greeted trick-or-treating missionary children at the door with a sheet over his head;[50] special community meals and gifts marked US Thanksgivings and Christmases.[51]

Conclusion

Hays and Petty swiftly became an entity: "the Nurses." United in fun, faith, and purpose, they smoothly assumed complementary roles within a cohesive COC community of Americans and Nigerians. "Quite a wonderful addition to our little 'mission' family,"[52] Patti Bryant described the two nurses—"a breath of fresh air....[and] sunshine in our lives."[53]

---

[45]Author's recollections.

[46]H Hays-Savio, Interview; Petty-Kraus, Interview 1.

[47]Petty to Spann, July 18, 1965.

[48]Author's recollection; Petty to Spann, April 30, 1965; Petty to Corlew, May 13, 1965.

[49]Hays-Savio, Interview.

[50]Farrar, *Stand*, 144; Ibid.

[51]G. Farrar to Johnson, November 30, 1965; Petty to Spann, December 29, 1965.

[52]P. Bryant to Mattoxes, April 19, 1965.

[53]Bryant and Bryant, Interview.

15

Goodwill Ambassadors

(April–July 1965)

Remember our sons and daughters.
—Umuogbala and Ekwereazu women

Shortly after the nurses' arrival and while clinic buildings were still under renovation, Henry Farrar recommended that Iris Hays and Nancy Petty teach health classes for women in their own villages. This previously unconsidered activity would build relationships with clans who owned the contiguous land that missionaries wanted for the hospital, as well as acknowledge Igbo women's dignity and value.[1] Everyone welcomed the idea, and Hays and Petty made the rounds to nineteen villages from May to July 1965.[2] Attendance was excellent as Igbos embraced the educational and economic benefits offered by Westerners, and perhaps women lineage leaders mandated the women's presence.

In Their Spaces

Women-to-women health teaching by missionaries was not new. COC 1950s evangelists praised their wives' Bible and health classes as strengthening churches,[3] and in 1960 Rees Bryant pronounced similar classes as evidence of US wives' co-equal missionary status with their preacher husbands. Declaring a spiritual quota beyond the legal immigration one, Bryant asserted "that there are *four* missionaries now working at Onicha Ngwa, two preachers and their faithful wives...What a shame that they [the women] are often not...*counted*."[4]

---

[1]G. Farrar, Interview; H. Farrar, Interview 1; Hays-Savio, Interview; Savio, "Nigerian Christian Hospital."

[2]H. Farrar, Interview 1; Hays-Savio, Interview; Petty-Kraus, Interview 1.

[3]Goff, *Great*, 25.

[4]R. Bryant to Summerlin, August 18, 1960.

In the mid-1960s nurse Grace Farrar instructed Nigerian women about health, teaching children, and principles of Christian living. During the COC's annual women's Bible lectureships in Ukpom, she taught hygiene, basic anatomy/physiology, and health topics, such as "how a baby is formed and born."[5] Nurse Farrar discovered that "covering food from flies and not drinking the same water you bathe in was news to many... [and] their language had no word for germs."[6] Moreover, her content about antenatal care and menopause garnered such interest that she could hardly speak above attendees' excited conversations among themselves.[7] She also taught against female circumcision and superstitions related to ancestors and multiple births, while well aware that information alone was insufficient to overcome those traditional practices. Still, she hoped that "little by little" knowledge would win.[8]

Hays and Petty's 1965 classes, however, were different from those delivered by other missionary women. The nurses' gatherings included all village women, not just COC members, and were held in community spaces, not COC buildings. Their primary aim was to build relationships by giving special attention to the women and delivering health education in a Christian context but unaccompanied by biblical instruction. Hays and Petty's professional expertise and freedom from family responsibilities made them well-suited to this goodwill ambassadorship.[9]

Across the Divide

Igbo women seized the opportunity of these health classes to make their own voices heard, and two petitionary letters preserve their unique welcome to Petty and Hays.[10] Both typed documents were in a colonial-era style common among hired letter-writers, whose job it was to transform oral Igbo into written English. Letter-writers, often school children, village teachers, or government employees, frequently appealed in petitions to a Western understanding of fairness, democracy, and social obligation. Some represented their clients' sentiments precisely, while others used

---

[5]G. Farrar to Johnsons, August 23, 1966; G. Farrar to Johnsons, August 11, 1965.
[6]G. Farrar to Johnson, August 17, 1964.
[7]G. Farrar to Johnsons, August 23, 1966.
[8]G. Farrar to Johnsons, August 11, 1965.
[9]Hays-Savio, Interview.
[10]Jonnah, Joel, Achibiri, and Benson to Petty and Hays, May 2, 1965; Umuogbala and Ekwereazu Women to Nursing Sisters, May 5, 1965.

letters to display their language prowess, and it was impossible to know which was true in any given case.[11]

Like earlier Igbo-to-colonialist petitions, the two 1965 letters placed rural women as central actors in negotiating their own future. Each single-page message bore a "welcome address" heading, expressed greetings, articulated solidarity, called on a social contract, and then closed with supplication—a request for action from missionaries as benefactors. Letters were neither hostile nor passive.[12] Each was likely read aloud and presented to Hays and Petty at class time, and it seems improbable that the Americans either recognized the extent to which they represented white colonial power or understood the economic and social power of Igbo women.[13]

In the first letter, women from the village of Onicha Onicha Ngwa welcomed their "nursing sisters" and then asserted their primacy as original area landowners—a status according them special honors, rights, and privileges. As evidence of their preeminence, the women pointed to the nurses' coming to their village first before any other because God himself had so directed them.[14] More likely was that the nurses' interpreters as insiders made this critical scheduling decision, but their timing facilitated Onicha Onicha Ngwa women's appropriation of the white nurses' actions into their own narrative. The Igbo women further declared their positive expectation of teaching by "our nursing sisters"—an ambiguous phrase suggesting the nurses were from among them and belonged to them in ways that carried community obligations. Additionally, they confirmed their eager anticipation of "our new hospital" brought by the "American People...under the Church of Christ." The women listed specific ways the village had helped COC missionaries in the past that now obligated missionaries to them, and finally, they made a direct moral appeal on behalf of their families for health care and jobs for their children. The letter closed with four individual signatories' typed English (not Igbo) names as a final declaration of power.[15]

---

[11]Korieh, "May it please;" Korieh, "*Life*."

[12]Jonnah et al. to Petty and Hays, May 2, 1965; Umuogbala and Ekwereazu to Nursing Sisters, May 5, 1965.

[13]Chuku, *Igbo Women*.

[14]Chi Ekwenye-Hendricks email to author, August 23, 2019.

[15]Chi Ekwenye-Hendricks, Interview 1; Jonnah et al. to Petty and Hays, May 2, 1965. Nigerians used the British term "nursing sisters" for nurses. According to Ekwenye-Hendricks some Igbos adopted an Anglo name on their own and others may have been required to do so at Christian baptism—not a COC practice. Anglo names were regarded as prestigious and used selectively to gain influence.

The second letter was from the women of Umuogbala and Ekwereazu (or Ekwereeazu), and its composition suggested its writer was better educated.[16] Key sentences began in poetic parallelism: "We…welcome you… We are grateful…We are tired [of traveling to hospitals]…We have long expected [the missionary hospital]…We shall patronize [the hospital, and]…We shall give you every assistance."[17] In a nod to an Igbo sense of community and gender complementarity[18] and to the broader religious and ethnic context, the women thanked both American Christian men who sent the nurses to them and the nurses "who have taken up the pioneering work." Mixing Western idioms, biblical quotations, and religious language, the letter writer expressed shared values and solidarity with missionaries in the difficulties of transporting people to distant hospitals—actions that the women attributed to missionary "kindness to the poor." The women promised to reciprocate this past missionary aid to them by supporting the COC hospital. And finally, they made an oblique request on behalf of their children for employment and other benefits: "Remember our sons and daughters"[19]—a request akin to the biblical injunction to "remember the poor" (Galatians 2:10). They likely expected the nurses as women to understand the profound significance of this request in support of maternal-child relationships that comprised the "keystone" of Igbo society.[20] Their letter closed in religious solidarity with a typed group signature: "Yours in Christ, Umuogbala and Ekwereazu women."[21]

In response, Hays and Petty reached back across the same Igbo-US divide with American voices filtered through trusted, Nigerian interpreters, Comfort Eguzo and Rhoda Udogwu.[22] The village women and the US nurses both lacked fluency in the language and culture of the other and so were dependent on third parties to bridge the gap. All evidence suggests each party's desire for mutually beneficial relationships. Hays and Petty scattered bits of Igbo and Pidgin English in their speech, but neither learned Igbo, despite initially engaging a language teacher.[23] Reasons for this neglect probably included missionary precedent, other prior-

---

[16]Chi Ekwenye-Hendricks, email to author, July 23, 2019.

[17]Umuogbala and Ekwereazu to Nursing Sisters, May 5, 1965.

[18]Chuku, *Igbo Women*, esp. 6–9, 18–24, 244–45.

[19]Umuogbala and Ekwereazu Women to Nursing Sisters, May 5, 1965.

[20]Agbasiere, *Women*, 85.

[21]Umuogbala and Ekwereazu Women to Nursing Sisters, May 5, 1965.

[22]Monday John Akpakpan, email to author, June 24, 2019; G. Farrar, Interview; Hays-Savio, Interview; Annette Whitaker, undated personal communication.

[23]Petty to Spann, April 16, May 31, and August 19, 1965.

ities, the difficult-for-Americans tonal character of Igbo, English as Nigeria's national language, and the existence of over 500 Nigerian languages and dialects. Igbos sometimes required Igbo interpreters themselves.[24]

Men usually served as missionaries' interpreters, but Doug Lawyer or Jim Massey likely identified Rhoda and Comfort[25] as persons familiar with medical terminology; Henry Farrar may have paid them from his work expense fund. A Nigerian physician had earlier taught Comfort about nursing in his private practice,[26] and both unlicensed women possessed "practical nurse experience," according to Grace Farrar.[27] She later described them as "our first two Nigerian nurses."[28] Hays thought Rhoda and Comfort "wonderful" and quite young, and so was surprised to learn that Comfort was thirty-one years old with seven children.[29] Comfort's motherhood status probably facilitated respect from village women, who undoubtedly wondered how Petty and Hays were still unmarried.[30]

The Routine

Two to four days a week, Hays drove the two nurses and two interpreters down the narrow paths that passed for roads to one or more villages. The nurses' gray Ford Anglia with red upholstery was so small and the potholes so big that the car would disappear briefly into them before reemerging on the other side.[31] Greetings, devotionals, and etiquette were similar in each village, beginning with one woman summoning others from their work with a drum, a routine that avoided unnecessary work interruptions in a less than predictable West African world where a speaker might be delayed. Women then assembled over thirty to sixty minutes, although by June audiences sometimes gathered before the nurses arrived.[32] Perhaps this change was because the nurses consistently came on prompt American time rather than on the more leisurely African

---

[24]Chuku, *Igbo Women*, 12.

[25]Bryant and Bryant, Interview.

[26]G. Farrar, Interview; G. Farrar notation in member check of H. Farrar's Interview transcript, July 2, 2010.

[27]Farrar, *Stand*, 101.

[28]G. Farrar, Interview.

[29]Petty to Spann, May 31, 1965; Hays-Savio, Interview.

[30]Petty to Corlew, May 13, 1965.

[31]P. Bryant to Joe Mattoxes, May 24, 1965; G. Farrar to Johnson, May 11, 1965; Hays-Savio, Interview; Petty to Corlew, May 13, 1965.

[32]Hays-Savio, Interview; Petty to Spann, May 16, 1965.

time illustrated in the Igbo proverb, "Whenever a man wakes up is his own morning."

Petty remembered how "they all gathered up to look at us...There was me, the short, wide one and Hays the tall, thin one...Usually, the chief of the village would...greet us" because communities wanted hospital jobs.[33] Villages set up a speakers' table that faced audience chairs or benches either in a roofed, half-walled village council hall with doorless entry[34] or in a common space under a canopy of "huge tropical trees."[35] When outdoors, nurses and their audiences were subject to the vagaries of nature, such as the day that a downpour soaked the group[36] and another when a huge limb crashed down behind them from the massive tree overhead. That "scared us to death," Petty recalled, and if the tree was a sacred Iroko (*Ojii*) tree, then their audience's reaction may have been dramatic as well.[37]

Other incidents were more humorous. One day, Petty tried her hand at their talking drum, and locals erupted in laughter, making her wonder what she "said." On another occasion while women gathered, the village proudly placed their radio before the nurses on a table covered in "a beautiful white cloth."[38] Unexpectedly, Petula Clark's rendition of *Downtown* began playing, and the stark contrast between the surrounding tropical rainforest and song lyrics about neon lights and traffic jams threw Petty and Hays into uncontrolled giggling. Seeing their guests' happy laughter, local women joined in; the nurses were well-received, and the moment memorable.[39]

The gatherings followed a similar pattern. As women came from their work, Americans and Igbos smiled greetings to each other of "'Good morning' or 'Ndewo'"(hello).[40] Then when all were seated, the Igbos began fifteen to twenty minutes of call-and-response singing followed by the local chairwoman calling them to order. The US nurses then greeted the group and led a prayer, followed by Petty's singing a hymn of blessing in English to a pleased audience. Petty lectured first, followed by Hays.[41] They taught the same content in each village, then conducted a question-

---

[33]Farrar and Petty-Kraus, Interview.
[34]P. Bryant to Joe Mattoxes, May 24, 1965; Savio, "Nigerian Christian Hospital," 46.
[35]Savio, "Nigerian Christian Hospital," 46.
[36]Petty to Spann, May 12, 1965.
[37]Farrar and Petty-Kraus, Interview; Basden, *Niger Ibos*, 148.
[38]Petty to Spann, May 12, 1965.
[39]Ibid.; Farrar and Petty-Kraus, Interview; Savio, "Nigerian Christian Hospital," 46.
[40]Petty to Spann, June 7, 1965.
[41]Hays-Savio, Interview; Petty to Spann, June 7, 1965.

and-answer session intended to verify understanding, which in one case instead alerted Hays to her accidental omission of content. Petty covered health promotion and disease prevention, including infant care, nutrition, preparation of safe drinking water, and how to avoid parasites; Hays presented first aid for urgent or emergent situations like burns, machete cuts, or what to do "if a hernia pops out."[42] Marty Farrar's white, infant-size doll with eyes that opened and closed provided a model for demonstrating bathing to reduce fever, and the doll so enthralled audiences that women touched it to find out if it was alive.[43]

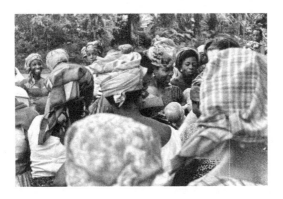

Photograph 15. Laughing women crowd around Petty to enjoy white doll teaching aid after village health class. Summer 1965. Photograph by J.R. Morgan. (JRM collection with permission).

Petty later laughed at the nurses' naïveté about what to teach. Hays's hand drawn pictures of a typhoid bacillus must have seemed like "some kind of juju," and when Petty instructed women how to soak an infected foot in warm salty water, she didn't realize that many owned only a single pan for cooking.[44] Yet despite the Americans' shortcomings, Hays found the Igbo women "very attentive"[45] and "so hospitable." They nodded and never contradicted the nurses, considering it more important to give answers they assumed US visitors wanted, than to correct speaker mistakes.[46]

A typical class, Petty wrote to her sister,

---

[42]Hays-Savio, Interview.

[43]Morgan, "Report," 12.

[44]Farrar and Petty-Kraus, Interview.

[45]Hays-Savio, Interview.

[46]Basden, *Niger Ibos*, 34; Farrar and Petty-Kraus, Interview.

...isn't anything like talking to a group of women at home...
1. Dogs, chickens, & goats come and go freely throughout
the meeting. 2. If a child needs to use the bathroom they do
so right in front of the mother. 3. If someone speaks out of
turn all the other women stand up, yell & shake their fist at
her. 4. Men come & stand around the Council Hall, but if
they dare open their mouths the women chase them off. 5.
They usually have our gifts or dashes behind us in a small
room and the chickens squawk out at the most crucial time
of our speeches.[47]

At the conclusion of each session, village women presented their guests
with customary dashes (gifts). Poor villages gave a few bananas, a chick-
en, or eggs that Petty thought the women needed for themselves;[48] rich
villages presented stalks of bananas, tropical fruits, or even a goat[49]—a
gift Petty equated with a beef cow in the US.[50] "Unusual dashes included
canned evaporated milk [and] bottled drinks."[51] Sometimes the nurses
made two trips in their diminutive car in order to get the four women and
considerable gifts back home.[52]

Hays and Petty's ambassadorship went well. Igbo women's letters, gifts,
and gracious reception strengthened missionary-Igbo relationships and
provoked Petty's deep affection for them. She felt welcomed, and she
valued their generosity. Dashes of food were prolific enough to share
with the other missionaries[53] and practical enough to reduce the nurses'
grocery bills to $5 per week for six weeks. Since our arrival, Petty wrote,
"we have not bought any eggs, pineapple, oranges, bananas, coconuts,
chickens (or goats, HA!)."[54] Still, Petty refused to eat the goat barbecued
by the Farrar's cook because "it was so cute."[55]

---

[47]Petty to Spann, June 7, 1965.

[48]Farrar and Petty-Kraus, Interview. Traditional Igbos believed that eating eggs
might make a child into a thief.

[49]Hays-Savio, Interview; Farrar and Petty-Kraus, Interview.

[50]Petty to Corlew, May 13, 1965.

[51]Morgan, "Report," 12.

[52]Hays-Savio, Interview; Petty to Corlew, May 13, 1965; Petty to Spann, April 16,
1965.

[53]G. Farrar to Johnson, May 11, 1965; Farrar and Petty-Kraus, Interview; Petty to
Corlew, May 13, 1965.

[54]Petty to Spann, June 14, 1965.

[55]Petty to Spann, May 31, 1965.

"Exciting Day"

Misadventures also occurred. One day, a cyclist collided with their car, and a frightened Hays followed missionaries' prior instructions to leave the scene as fast as possible in order to avoid mob justice of being dragged from the car and stoned. Hays took Rhoda and Comfort home, then headed to the Farrars' house. All the US men were away, and the missionary "women gathered around to give us advice." When angry locals descended on the group, the Nigerian compound staff sided with the missionaries. "About 30 Nigerians and 5 white women all talking at once. Total confusion!" Petty wrote.[56]

Fortunately, Henry Farrar arrived and escorted everyone to the police station, where the case was settled in the nurses' favor. Nonetheless, Hays and Petty felt sorry for the cyclist, and their gift of £2 for his bicycle repair may be why nothing further came of the matter; the bicycle was likely his only transport. Petty later summarized that "very exciting day" in a letter home:

> We have had a car accident, We were given a goat, two stalks of bananas, one chicken, five pineapples, about 3 pounds of groundnuts, We have been to the police station, We were caught out in a tropical rainstorm, The carpenters have been in our house, It was wash day and the clothes didn't get dry, I got word my [shipped] barrel will be here Friday, We had a spiritual song fest at the Bryants, We put too much butter in the candy, and late this afternoon I finished reading a very interesting book…[but it could not] hold a candle to Nigeria.[57]

Gender Perspectives

In her work, Petty observed the power and powerlessness of Igbo women, and like COC missionary men, she lamented husbands' near ownership of their wives.[58] Petty admired their physical stamina, grieved

---

[56]Petty to Spann, May 12, 1965.

[57]Ibid. Ground nuts are peanuts; the barrel contained her US personal belongings.

[58]Goff, *Great*, 25. In R. Bryant, "Newsletter No. 6," October 1, 1958, Bryant records the account of a BTC student who stopped beating his wife after becoming a COC member. Okorocha, quoted in Chuku, *Igbo Women*, 28, tells a judicial anecdote illustrating that bride dowry payment meant that the woman and all her property belonged to the husband.

the silencing of their voices, and decried polygamy as a problem in local congregations, where missionaries proclaimed marriage as between one man and one woman. "You cannot imagine how hard these women work," Petty wrote to her sister. "They carry heavy loads to work the farms," and owners with extensive acreage purchase more wives, instead of hiring employees. Educated women are more expensive, she added, and women marry the person paying the highest bride price, then have "one baby after the other."[59]

While true that marital abuses occurred and women's lives were hard, Petty's understanding at the time was incomplete. Childbearing was celebrated, she soon learned, and Igbo women valued high fertility as fulfillment of a woman's responsibility to her husband and confirmation of premarital chastity. Additionally, the local Igbo society and economy were grounded in agriculture with family members comprising most of the farm labor force; community owned land was divided patrilineally and usage rights were emphasized.[60] Igbo women often achieved economic stability and supported their families through "subsistence farming and sale of surpluses."[61] Too, they exercised considerable authority over marketplaces, and women's organizations were powerful.[62]

Polygamy was common, and marriages arranged, although intermediaries might obtain a woman's agreement before marriage, even in cases of infant betrothal.[63] Still, no evidence suggests that COC missionaries distinguished between women who of necessity acquiesced to polygamist marriages versus those who supported or even desired them. Nor is there evidence that they understood the host of traditional, familial, religious, and socio-economic difficulties arising from a Christian prohibition of polygamy. COC missionaries faulted the men for taking more wives, even though the first wife, who held seniority regardless of age, might advocate for more wives to share her work and add to her own prestige as well as to her husband's.[64] Moreover, some men, through no desire of their own, sometimes found themselves gaining multiple wives because of customs and parental plans.[65]

---

[59]Petty to Corlew, May 13, 1965.

[60]Agbasiere, *Women*, 12, 86–87, 103, 128; Chuku, *Igbo Women*, 37; Korieh, *The Land*, 36–40.

[61]Agbasiere, *Women*, 37.

[62]Ibid.; Chuku, *Igbo Women*; Farrar, *Stand*, 117.

[63]Agbasiere, *Women*, 101–02.

[64]Basden, *Niger Ibos*, 228–239; Nau, *We Move*, 133–36, 292–93, 296–303.

[65]Nau, *We Move*, 121–27.

Within this context, US and Igbo women engaged one another. Igbo women communicated their requests in religious, socio-economic, and gendered contexts—requests likely intertwined with Igbo men's agendas,[66] while US women reached out in ways intertwined with American men's agendas. Both Nigerian men and women sought to improve their families' lives, and both missionary men and women wanted to promote goodwill toward the planned hospital. Additionally, Henry Farrar delighted in the affirmation of Nigerian women's dignity provided by missionary nurses' classes. Perhaps like Howard Horton earlier, he saw women-to-women relationships as indispensable to Christian evangelism. Others agreed. "The woman missionary...alone" can intimately connect "native women" with the faith, wrote 1940s Lutheran missionary Nau in his discourse on Ibibio women, polygamy, and Christianity.[67]

Conclusion

Hays and Petty went out to Igbo women, and Igbo women welcomed them in. And through antiphonal song and speech, the women's back-and-forth gave birth to an emerging solidarity in pursuit of a better present and future. Each side wanted something from the other; each pursued those desires through relationship-building; each became part of the other's story. Greeting, solidarity, and reminders of mutual obligations reinforced Igbo spoken and American unspoken requests. Aided by letter-writers and gifts of food, village women competed and cooperated in seeking access to missionary economic and health resources. Aided by translators and gifts of education, missionary nurses sought access to future hospital land.

---

[66]Chi Ekwenye-Hendricks, email to author, September 5, 2019; Farrar and Petty-Kraus, Interview.

[67]H. Farrar, Interview 1; Horton, quoted in Goff, *Great*, 25; Nau, *We Move*, 295.

16
Watershed Moment: Decision to Stay
(Spring–Summer 1965)

We can do what we can do. The Lord will have to do the rest.
—Iris Hays

Iris Hays and Nancy Petty fully engaged from the start. Monday through Saturday, the nurses prepared and taught village lessons, shopped for the planned clinic, worked in nearby hospitals, and selected future staff. Their salaries covered most of their expenses, and Queen Elizabeth Hospital (QEH) contributed in-kind reimbursement to Petty, Hays, and Henry Farrar in the form of workday lunches[1] and medications for the future COC clinic. Dr. Farrar's working fund covered travel.[2]

Sundays were different, but involved no less effort. In the mornings, Petty accompanied missionaries on preaching appointments; in the afternoons, the nurses took turns helping missionary women teach a single Bible class for fifty to one hundred and fifty Nigerian children from infants to teens. All listened in rapt attention to stories illustrated with flannelgraph figures or enacted with puppets.[3] In the evenings, missionaries, staff, and US visitors from Port Harcourt (PH) oil companies worshipped together and sometimes shared a meal afterwards, complete with ice-cream from a hand-cranked freezer.[4]

---

[1]G. Farrar to Johnson, May 11, 1965; Hays-Savio, Interview.
[2]Farrar to Mission Committee, September 1, 1965, *WEV*.
[3]Bryant and Bryant, Interview; Hays-Savio, Interview.
[4]Author's recollection; Farrar, *Stand*, 33, 60, 97.

145

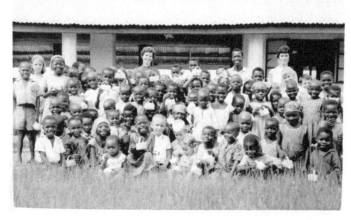

Photograph 16. Iris Hays and Patti Bryant's Sunday afternoon Bible Class for Nigerian and US missionary children with Friday Onukafor as interpreter. Onicha Ngwa BTC. ca. 1965. (Bryant collection with permission).

Mixed Blessing

Working at QEH proved a mixed blessing. Although Hays felt welcome, she was frustrated that British Matron Ann Bent relegated her and Petty primarily to observing for six months,[5] and the roughly forty-five-minute car rides home two to three times a week from QEH provided ample opportunity for the nurses to air their complaints. They had come to work, not watch.

Moreover, Hays was "shocked" by some QEH practices. Staff did not organize surgical instruments into case-specific packs, and she saw one student nurse's finger protruding through a hole in her glove during surgery, and no one stopped her. Hays observed that "even Dr. Farrar was always butting heads" with British doctors who insisted, "This is the way we do it here in the tropics." They were disinterested, for example, in Farrar's proposal to treat osteomyelitis in casted compound fractures by removing the cast, cleaning the wound, and replacing the cast. Hays called Farrar's ideas "just good medicine," and she remembered QEH as "a real eye-opener." Such QEH standards seemed "years behind American methods" to Hays and Grace Farrar,[6] and one American surgeon at

---

[5]P. Bryant to Mattoxes, April 19, 1965; Hays-Savio, Interview.
[6]Hays-Savio, Interview; G. Farrar to Johnson, December 6, 1964.

QEH, Dr. Preston Manning, was so exasperated that he returned to the US.[7]

Matron Bent allowed COC nurses to rotate through all inpatient and outpatient areas, where they learned about common illnesses, available medicines, and accessible resources. Petty especially enjoyed clinic work with Farrar, and both nurses used QEH experiences to plan for the COC hospital. A laughing Hays reported being particularly determined to avoid "Izal medicated toilet paper," a British restroom staple with the texture of tracing paper. Both US nurses agreed that individual patient cards would provide more efficient record keeping than did QEH ward books filled with repetitive documentation, and they also rejected the elaborate QEH process of starting intravenous (IV) fluids. Simpler US insertion technique employed preassembled needle, tubing, and bag, whereas starting an IV at QEH required Hays to use a syringe and a tray with "all these little individual dishes on it everywhere," including "a little bowl for the cotton wool and another…[for] the alcohol, and…forceps to pick up the things…and…so many extra pieces of things on the tray that…I probably didn't even use half of them."[8]

"The best" thing about QEH for Hays and Petty were newfound friendships with Irish nurse Rosemary Sweetham and Canadian nurse Dianne North.[9] The four enjoyed work and leisure together, including Hays and North's memorable bicycle ride to Onicha Ngwa at the end of one workday. The adventure was less fun in reality than imagination, and Hays laughed about bumping on and off the coal-tar highway on Paul Farrar's too-small bicycle as they dodged lorries and cars until they could reach safer dirt, bush roads. Additionally, North mentored Hays in COC clinic planning, and she was impressed with Hays's sketches of proposed curtained examination rooms with separate areas for wound care, injections, pharmacy, and laboratory that were based on her US emergency room experience.[10]

---

[7]Farrar, *Stand*, 53. He later donated to NCH per Manning to Farrar, November 11, 1967, W-COC file.

[8]Hays-Savio, Interview.

[9]Petty-Kraus, Interview 1.

[10]Hays-Savio, Interview.

Watershed Moment

The most defining QEH moment for Hays and Petty, however, was the day that "legendary"[11] Anglican missionary Matron Ann Bent told them flatly that they were incompetent to do the work for which they had come to Nigeria. As Petty recalled, "Miss Bent…told us that we…absolutely could not start a hospital. It was not going to work. We may as well go home.[12] [She] told us…there was no way we could train nurses, that we were not qualified whatsoever. 'You can't do it,' she said."[13]

Petty and Hays were stunned. Whatever Bent's intentions, her unexpected commentary devastated any quixotic notions they held. Bent was "highly trained and qualified, a midwife topnotch,"[14] while the relatively inexperienced COC nurses knew little about Nigeria and nothing about starting a hospital. As nursing "oddities," they also lacked the midwifery training of Nigerian Registered Nurses (NRNs), who were educated under British curricula.[15] When entering the country, Hays and Petty likely wrote "nursing tutor" or "nursing sister tutor" on their immigration papers at Dr. Farrar's suggestion in order to communicate that they would prepare—not displace—Nigerians.[16] Hays remembered writing whatever title was required to get into the country without knowing "exactly what that was going to entail,"[17] and Petty asserted that they registered as nurses, although Dr. Farrar retrospectively maintained that they came without license reciprocity because registration was not required for nursing teachers.[18] Evangelists had successfully submitted Farrar's credentials for Nigerian medical licensure before his coming.[19]

Whatever their precise legal status, Hays and Petty were unusually quiet on the long drive home. Then Hays broke the silence. "She's right," Hays announced, but "there is nobody else here…It's us. So…We can do what we can do. The Lord will have to do the rest." Hays and Petty weren't leaving. They knew that they lacked Bent's skills and knowledge, but they also knew they were the only nurses in Onicha Ngwa, where they were surrounded by people needing care. Their qualifications might be inade-

---

[11]Farrar and Petty-Kraus, Interview.
[12]Petty-Kraus, Interview 1.
[13]Farrar and Petty-Kraus, Interview.
[14]Ibid.
[15]Petty-Kraus, Interview 1.
[16]G. Farrar, Interview; *Dickson County*, "Miss Nancy Petty.
[17]Hays-Savio, Interview.
[18]Petty-Kraus, Interview 1; H. Farrar, Interview 1.
[19]Bryant to McInteer, September 5, 1960.

quate, but Hays and Petty shared a conviction that God could do whatever they could not.

They arrived back at Onicha Ngwa that day less naïve but more resolved. Bent's assessment, they decided, would not stop them from seeking "God's will," doing "the right thing," and staying their two years. If they left early because of homesickness, physical illness, or any reason, they believed it would be more difficult for future, young missionary women to garner support.[20] And so they stayed—for themselves and for those to come—a decision that sustained them through future challenges.[21]

Missionary colleagues were proud of the nurses' determination, and the team long told and retold the story of Hays's declaration of faith. No one recorded it, however, until decades later,[22] perhaps because they feared that Bent's assessment would threaten US support for the entire project, or maybe it was embarrassing. The team, including Petty and Hays, had no backup plan, and Bent's unmasking of the nurses' professional limitations must have highlighted every insecurity. At the same time, because QEH physicians rejected Dr. Farrar's practice suggestions, the missionaries were probably not surprised that the Matron questioned Hays and Petty's competence. As Grace Farrar summarized in retrospective triumph decades later, the British do things by the rules, but "the Americans just launch out [believing that] it'll work out. Kind of like the Africans. We can do it. We never started a hospital before, but why not? We can do it."[23]

Nevertheless, the nurses' decision to stay was not merely an assertion of American grit. Instead, it was grounded in personal humility and religious conviction. Hays and Petty recognized their weaknesses, gave up any burden of personal bravado, and fell back on their Christian faith. Perhaps they felt this was the only choice they had if they wanted to stay. Like others on the team,[24] they believed that the hospital would happen if God wanted it to happen. Their only obligation was to do what they could.[25]

---

[20]Farrar and Petty-Kraus, Interview.
[21]Hays-Savio and Petty-Kraus, Interview.
[22]"Biographical Sketches" (Savio), 208.
[23]G. Farrar, Interview.
[24]R. Bryant to Mattoxes, April 1, 1965.
[25]Farrar and Petty-Kraus, Interview.

Conclusion

In all this, Hays and Petty acted in continuity with past and present COC missionary colleagues. Others had already refused to let personal frailties, lack of resources, or limited knowledge stop them from pursuing the material and spiritual good that they saw to do. The two nurses, like their COC coworkers, understood their work, not as a mere physical enterprise, but as a divine vocation, and Matron Bent underestimated what such faith-based resolve would do.

17
Recruiting, Repercussions, and Redemption
(Summer 1965)

It was amazing. It really worked.
—Iris Hays

One physician and two nurses would not be enough to staff the COC clinic, let alone a future hospital, but the team had no money to hire professional providers. Consequently, they decided to educate their own personnel from the villages owning contiguous land proposed for the hospital. Missionaries reasoned that employing locals would help compensate for lost farmland,[1] provide interpreters, express gratitude to landowners, recognize historically reciprocal relationships, and fulfill a missionary pledge to educate—not displace—Nigerians.[2] The proposal was well-received by all and consistent with Igbo women's requests to "remember our sons and daughters."[3] Igbos wanted healthcare, education, and jobs. US missionaries wanted qualified workers and a hospital, and their plan to hire locals demonstrated the autonomy granted to them by supporting churches.

The team agreed that one US nurse should be in charge of preparing a workforce, while the other should be a nursing matron in charge of hospital operations. Iris Hays volunteered to be the educator, before Nancy Petty could speak, and in so doing, reversed herself about a teaching role as dramatically as she had earlier changed her mind about a nursing career. Petty's longer clinical experience favored her appointment as ma-

---

[1]Hays-Savio, Interview.
[2]G. Farrar to Mrs. H.C. Farrar, December 6, 1964; Savio, "Nigerian Christian Hospital."
[3]Umuogbala and Ekwereazu Women to Nursing Sisters, May 5, 1965.

tron, and both job allocations proved a fit.[4] On July 7, Hays wrote in her diary: "I am the Director of Nursing Education. What a title!"[5]

Technical Nurses

As a department of one, Hays planned a twelve-month curriculum similar to US Licensed Vocational Nurse (LVN) training. She would teach some skilled care, but unlike Nigerian Registered Nurses (NRNs), her graduates would have "no legal standing," title, or employment qualifications beyond COC facility walls.[6] QEH Matron Bent was right that Hays and Petty possessed neither hospital nor qualifications to prepare NRNs as grade one midwives (head nurses or directors of nursing) or grade two midwives (bedside nurses and midwives).[7]

Whether or not they obtained government approval for Hays's nursing education program is unremembered, but no one challenged it. At the time, private Nigerian physicians trained their own clinic workers, and perhaps Dr. Farrar's presence as chief medical officer met that role expectation. Moreover, a nursing shortage existed,[8] local support was strong, and licensed professionals would direct nursing auxiliaries' care.

Educating their own staff held several advantages. First, missionaries could set admission standards that allowed them to select "the brightest."[9] Applicants would be required to complete only Standard 6 (roughly equivalent to US eighth grade), instead of secondary school (roughly equivalent to US high school or community college) as required by NRN schools. Because few locals attended secondary school, this decision created a larger applicant pool and more village opportunity. Additionally, preparing their own staff honored the missionary-Igbo social contract as articulated by local women, and staff retention was likely to be strong given students' villages of origin and the lack of transferability of credentials. Finally, the US team could teach the specific skills they

---

[4]Farrar and Petty-Kraus, Interview; Hays-Savio, Interview; Hays-Savio and Petty-Kraus, Interview.
[5]Hays-Savio, Interview.
[6]Ibid.
[7]Ibid.; Petty-Kraus, Interview 1.
[8]G. Farrar, Interview; Farrar, *Stand*, 94; Hays-Savio, Interview.
[9]G. Farrar, Interview.

wanted, as opposed to hiring those educated to British preferences or in heterogeneous private physician clinics.[10]

Recruiting

In the summer of 1965, the team tackled student selection. Missionaries called for unmarried, Standard 6 graduates from land-owning villages.[11] COC membership was not required because the US team was specifically interested in landowner children, and they prized intellectual merit.[12] Hundreds responded, applying for "every job imaginable."[13] One applicant asked to be considered—meaning accepted—"in your office as a patient," and his petitionary letter modeled the diplomacy of less powerful supplicants and invoked missionaries' obligation to him as a member of the COC community.[14]

Approximately 400–435 men and women applied for the ten to fifteen class positions,[15] and the nurses accepted 325 as "legitimate" applicants based on English proficiency demonstrated in completed paperwork.[16] Accepted applicants then took a written examination in English that Hays and Petty created with guidance from LaVera Eugene Hamilton Otoyo (1927–2019), the US-born, master's-educated, dean of women at Ukpom's Nigerian Christian Secondary School (NCSS). LaVera and her Nigerian husband, Eno Otoyo (1930–), also at NCSS, were familiar with secondary school entrance examinations, as well as with US and Nigerian educational standards.[17] The nurses' resulting "simple" examination covered English, math, and general knowledge. Hays and Petty selected a few questions from the widely available Standard 6 reader and added original critical thinking questions, including a story completion item.[18]

---

[10]Ibid.; Farrar, *Stand*, 94; Hays-Savio, Interview; Jonnah et al. to Petty and Hays, May 2, 1965; Umuogbala and Ekwereazu Women to Nursing Sisters, May 5, 1965. Chi Ekwenye-Hendricks, email to the author, July 22, 2019, described mid-1960s Standard 6 as "closer to high school" and higher than 21st century Standard 6. To reach standard 6 might then take "8–10 years."

[11]G. Farrar to Johnson, June 16, 1965; Hays-Savio, Interview; Savio, "Nigerian Christian Hospital," 46.

[12]Bryant, *Divine*, 280; Chi Ekwenye-Hendricks, personal communication, November 15, 2016; H. Farrar, Interview 1; Hays-Savio, Interview.

[13]Morgan, "Report," 24.

[14]Korieh, "May it please;" Petty to Spann, July 18, 1965.

[15]G. Farrar to Folks, August 24, 1965; Farrar and Petty-Kraus, Interview; Hays-Savio, Interview; Petty-Kraus, Interview 1; Savio, "Nigerian Christian Hospital," 46.

[16]Savio, "Nigerian Christian Hospital," 46.

[17]Eno Otoyo, emails to author, May 19 and 21, 2018; *Christian Chronicle*, "Otoyos."

[18]Hays-Savio, Interview; Morgan, "John's Journal," July 17, 1965.

They kept tests under lock and key in order to protect their staff from pressure to share them with applicants, but those security measures did not stop potential students' families from bringing unsolicited gifts to the nurses.[19]

Hays and Petty administered four different versions of the examination to four separate groups of about eighty applicants each on three consecutive Mondays and a Saturday in July.[20] The testing process went well,[21] and outcomes not as well. Visiting US medical student, John Morgan, wrote that "grades were very poor, few good, & only one very good. Cheating was a problem" as evidenced in similar narrative answers.[22] For Hays, the entire process of writing, duplicating, securing, administering, and grading tests, as well as beginning interviews for the one hundred who passed was exhausting. "I really think I could sleep for fifteen hours without waking," she recorded in her diary.[23]

Moreover, Hays and Petty were daunted by the prospect of identifying only ten students from the hundred who passed the exam, and Dr. Farrar suggested that the nurses look in candidates' "eyes...[for] the light of intelligence." This they did during one-on-one, English-only interviews with candidates over many July and August days.[24] Farrar and Morgan sometimes participated, with each interviewer asking different questions in no particular order.[25] Happily, missionaries' independent ratings of each candidate as "yes or no or a maybe...were pretty much the same," and Hays was astonished that the process "really worked." Still, differences between missionaries' American-English and Nigerian-English created some amusingly awkward situations. In one instance, when "Dr. Morgan asked an interviewee what a pint was," she responded that it was a woman's undergarment. Missionaries were taken aback,[26] and the interviewee might have been equally surprised in hearing a question about "pants."

---

[19]Farrar and Petty-Kraus, Interview.

[20]P. Bryant to Mattoxes, July 11, 1965; Hays-Savio, Interview; Morgan, "John's Journal," July 17 and 31, 1965; Petty to Spann, July 18, 1965.

[21]Hays-Savio, Interview; Petty to Spann, July 18, 1965.

[22]Morgan, "John's Journal," July 17, 1965.

[23]Hays-Savio, Interview.

[24]Ibid.; G. Farrar to Folks, August 11, 1965.

[25]Morgan, "John's Journal," July 31, 1965.

[26]Hays-Savio, Interview.

A disappointed Hays and Petty accepted only seven candidates, but were pleased that each came from a different village;[27] they anticipated that this distribution would satisfy landowners and that each candidate would have a special commitment to her own people. Yet to hire even seven, the Americans were forced to set aside their own selection criteria twice in order to include Efik-speakers because Ibibio "patients from across the stream…wouldn't take their medicines" from an Igbo. Only later did they learn that several of those already selected also spoke Efik, making those exceptions unnecessary.[28] Their exceptions included Ihoma, who was Efik, and married Eunice Ukegbu, who predictably soon brought new baby, Chidi, to class with her.[29]

For Dr. Farrar, employing these women further demonstrated the merits of the medical mission. Writing enthusiastically to W-COC, he rejoiced that the team accepted "seven of the healthiest and most intelligent young women to train" as nursing assistants. Even so, he noted, they illustrated Nigeria's poor population health: Four had treatable parasitic infections, and four women were anemic with hemoglobin levels so low that they would not register on his hemoglobinometer that measured down to 7.5 grams per deciliter (normal 12–15 gm/dL). "Surely the Lord is pleased with your compassion for the sick in sending a doctor!" he concluded.[30] What Dr. Farrar did not write was that all were circumcised and planned to circumcise their own daughters. Female circumcision, observed Grace Farrar, "was passed down through the ages and you just didn't contradict it."[31]

Unfortunately, the number of auxiliary trainees soon dropped to five. Hays and Petty discovered that they had been "right the first time" in not hiring Ihoma; she failed every class exam and was dismissed early. Also, another student dropped out to go on to secondary school.[32] Thus, by

---

[27]Ibid. Primary sources differ on student numbers and names. The 1965 first cohort included seven per concurrent sources: color photograph "clinic staff1" by John Morgan; Farrar to Missions Committee, September 1, 1965; H. Farrar to Morgans, December 9, 1965.

[28]Petty-Kraus, Interview 1.

[29]Hays-Savio, Interview; Petty to Spann, November 23, 1965.

[30]Farrar to Mission Committee, September 1, 1965, *WEV*.

[31]G. Farrar, Interview.

[32]H. Farrar to Morgans, December 9, 1965; Hays-Savio, Interview.

year's end, only these remained: Lydia Agbara, Elizabeth Egbu, Esther Nwaghaghi Uzuogu, Eunice Ukegbu, and Comfort Amuta Nwosu.[33]

Gendered Employment

NRNs and nursing students at other hospitals where Hays and Petty worked were almost entirely women, and no men qualified for the COC nursing class. Hays was glad that gender issues would not complicate her class interactions, and she falsely assumed that her students were unmarried teens, based on the age at which US students would usually complete eighth grade.[34] Photographs of her students, however, suggested physical development typical of women in their twenties and thirties,[35] by which time they would have likely consummated traditional marriages, if not legal or church ones. If they were atypically single, the reason could have been their Standard 6 education that was considered advanced training in 1960s Nigeria and perhaps commanded a higher dowry.[36] Moreover, entering nursing auxiliary training might have affected marriageability because some Nigerian mothers discouraged their sons from marrying nurses.[37] Employment as a nurse or teacher could be seen either as an asset in generating a steady income or as a problem if husband and wife differed on whether or not earnings should be spent in traditional ways to support children and husband.[38]

In contrast to auxiliary positions, the COC team hired men for lay laboratory and pharmacy positions. Missionaries could not afford professionals for those jobs any more than they could afford NRNs, and Hays worked on applicant calls for laboratory, pharmacy, and auxiliary positions concurrently.[39] Interviews for a pharmacy dispenser focused on rea-

---

[33]Ngwakwe and Uzuegbu, quoted in Ekwenye-Hendricks, email to author, December 3, 2012. This retrospective list of class members in this citation was corrected using concurrent sources; naming conventions and spellings varied. According to Ekwenye-Hendricks, Interview 1: Women used English or Nigerian names depending on who was addressing them, and they sometimes took a husband's last name, first name, or both last and first name. Too, someone might be given a new English first name at baptism and another at confirmation—not a practice of COCs—and those working with whites selected English names pronounceable by whites. Farrar wrote in *Stand* that she received letters to Mrs. Grace Henry (30).

[34]Hays-Savio, Interview; Petty-Kraus, Interview 1.

[35]Chi Ekwenye-Hendricks, personal communication, May 4, 2012.

[36]Ekwenye-Hendricks, Interview 1; Petty to Corlew, May 13, 1965.

[37]Chi Ekwenye-Hendricks, personal communication, May 4, 2012,

[38]Agbasiere, *Women*, 37–38.

[39]Hays-Savio, Interview.

soning and dosage conversion math, and the team hired sixteen-year-old applicant Mark Peter, who hailed from one of the largest land-owning villages. He was "sharp...capable...honest," and accurate—all that was needed for a role that did not require mixing medications. Henry Farrar also hired Peter Uhiara and later Sylvanus Nwagbara as lay, laboratory staff-in-training.[40] Hays welcomed hiring men for those positions because the nursing students were all women,[41] and soon the team added an orderly class for men who could help with heavier physical work.[42] Men also filled clinic registrar as well as later hospital laundry, janitor, and cook positions.[43] John Nwogu joined staff as a second pharmacy dispenser by early 1967.[44]

Repercussions

The team's good deed of choosing locals for education and employment was punished by community displeasure. Not everyone in the villages liked missionaries' selections—or rather, missionaries' non-selections. Families of unsuccessful applicants were disappointed, a discontent perhaps heightened by the US nurses' accepting their gifts during the application process. "They were used to paying their way through school" whether or not they could do the work," Petty observed,[45] and she felt drained by efforts to satisfy unhappy locals. Despite her avowed love for them, she steeled herself against petitioners "in order to survive." A constant stream of family members appeared at the nurses' back door with requests that they "or their son or their daughter or their wife" should be hired. When turned away, the same people came again the next day "with an even bigger and better reason why" they should be offered a position. Meritocratic explanations were no match for families' "sad stories."[46] Hays escaped these encounters, perhaps because locals viewed Matron Petty and Chief Medical Officer Farrar as those with hiring power. "They went straight to the head man [Farrar]...in the palavering business," Hays

---

[40]Ibid.; Uhiara to Buice, October 2, 1967.

[41]Hays-Savio, Interview.

[42]Petty-Kraus, Interview 1.

[43]G. Farrar to Mrs. H.C. Farrar, September 25, 1966; G. Farrar to Johnsons, September 6, 1966; H. Farrar, Interview 1; Petty to Spann, January 21, 1966.

[44]Farrar, Nigerian Christian Hospital Payroll, April 1967, W-COC file.

[45]Farrar and Petty-Kraus, Interview.

[46]Petty to Spann, August 6, 1965.

noted,[47] and perhaps petitioners saw the Matron as a potential intermediary with him.

These unhappy families were not mere inconveniences. Missionaries feared that dissatisfied villages might refuse to lease their land for the hospital, and so Farrar promptly offered something new: first-aid classes for landowner children. The new classes would have no application, literacy, or language requirements and no examinations for entry, continuation, or graduation. The only admission criterion was that students be landowners' grown children; landowners without children could send someone of their choosing.[48] Rhoda Udogwu and Comfort Eguzo, who served as village class interpreters for Hays and Petty, also attended, and missionaries promised participants only a certificate of completion[49] "with the possibility"—but not a guarantee—that those who excelled might be hired.[50]

Dr. Farrar's plan restored goodwill with villages, and he conscripted nurses Nancy Petty and Grace Farrar to teach first-aid sessions with him.[51] Hays was spared because of her auxiliary classes,[52] and Petty's reaction to her assignment was blunt and angry: "Dr. Farrar, of all the things you've asked us to do, this is the craziest." She saw the classes as a waste of her valuable time that was already booked in organizing clinic operations, equipment, supplies, drug sources, and personnel.[53]

Nonetheless, Petty and the two Farrars began teaching afternoon first-aid classes by late August 1965 to about one hundred, mostly women students.[54] Learners sat for instruction at wooden desks under the metal, corrugated roof of the Bible Training College (BTC) classroom in the sweltering afternoon heat and humidity because BTC students occupied it during cooler mornings. Following lectures, nurses Petty and Farrar oversaw students' skills practice outside[55] in a move likely as much about comfort as space.

---

[47]Hays-Savio, Interview.

[48]Farrar, *Stand*, 95; G. Farrar, Interview; Farrar and Petty-Kraus, Interview; Hays-Savio, Interview.

[49]Hays-Savio, Interview.

[50]G. Farrar to Johnson, November 16, 1965; Petty-Kraus, Interview 1.

[51]G. Farrar, Interview.

[52]Hays-Savio, Interview.

[53]Farrar and Petty-Kraus, Interview.

[54]G. Farrar to Folks, August 24, 1965; G. Farrar to Johnson, November 16, 1965; Hays-Savio, Interview; Petty to Spann, November 17, 1965.

[55]Petty-Kraus, Interview 1. Morgan, "Nigeria: Summer" slides include BTC structures.

Grace Farrar registered students and taught anatomy, physiology, and "general health principles"[56] two to three afternoons a week after her mornings of homeschooling.[57] In anatomy, she covered what she thought was US high school level content while avoiding "fine muscles and everything like in medical school."[58] Her texts were local schoolbooks and a US Red Cross first-aid manual on resuscitation, wounds, splinting, hemorrhage, and more,[59] but after three months of first-aid classes she became frustrated. Of 104 registered students, many had simply paid a landowner to get into classes, and only about five passed each exam. One unashamed top student volunteered information that she and others cheated, and so she wondered how Farrar would grade exams. As Farrar observed, cheating was considered a strategy for success and not at all unethical.[60]

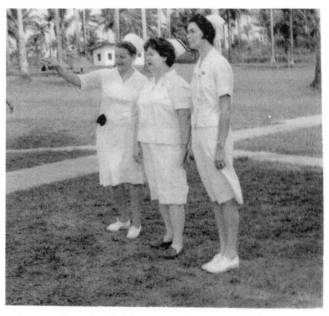

Photograph 17. Labelled "Founding Nurses:" Grace Farrar, RN, Nancy Petty, RN, and Iris Hays, RN; Hays and Petty's house in background, Onicha Ngwa mission compound. ca. 1965. (Author collection).

[56]G. Farrar, Interview.
[57]Author's recollection; G. Farrar to Folks, August 24 and November 16, 1965.
[58]G. Farrar, Interview.
[59]Ibid.; Farrar and Petty-Kraus, Interview.
[60]G. Farrar to Johnson, November 16, 1965; G. Farrar, Interview.

Grace Farrar now agreed with Petty that the first-aid classes were a waste of time, and her usual love of teaching devolved into exasperation at students' limited critical thinking and focus on test scores. In efforts to reduce cheating and improve reasoning, she wrote exams that required analysis instead of the rote memorization the students were accustomed to in school, but in the end she concluded that "this sort of thing was so new to them that they couldn't put it together." For example, students were unable to connect pallor, thirst, and weak rapid pulse with excessive bleeding.[61]

By November 30, Grace Farrar and Nancy Petty finished grading exams and dismissed students for the customary Nigerian school break that stretched from December to mid-January, a time that paralleled tradition-al, dry season holidays when food-production stopped.[62] Petty made passing references to her part-time teaching and to grading help from Nigerian staff friends, Friday Onukafor and Jacob Achinefu.[63] No one recorded first-aid course length and presentation of certificates.

Redemption

Three things transformed Petty and Grace Farrar's unhappiness about the first-aid classes into appreciation for them. The first redemptive event was immediate: Classes provided a ready pool from which missionaries could hire the brightest; one of these was a local chief's son.[64] The sec-ond redemptive event years later provided evidence to Petty that "when God is working, you may not appreciate it." After the 1967–1970 Nige-ria-Biafra War more than fifty first-aid class graduates came to see her; holding up their completion certificates, each told her, "When I present-ed this, I became a medic…You and Sister Farrar saved my life."[65] Grace Farrar's frustrations, too, were erased when she learned about the medic appointments and when she encountered other grateful graduates.[66] She felt particular pride in "good student" Ephraim, who years later told her, "Everything I know, you taught me." Not otherwise educated in health-

---

[61]G. Farrar, Interview.

[62]Basden, *Niger Ibos,* 195; G. Farrar to Johnson, November 16 and November 30, 1965.

[63]Petty to Spann, February 15, April 4, and April 19, 1966. Author's recollection of surnames.

[64]G. Farrar, Interview; G. Farrar, personal, communication, January 2, 2011; Petty-Kraus, Interview 1.

[65]Farrar and Petty-Kraus, Interview.

[66]Ibid.

care, Ephraim learned to assist Dr. Farrar in surgery, gaining skills that qualified him for a similar good job in Aba.[67]

Conclusion

Missionaries rejected the assumption that only an NRN-preparing nursing school could produce the staff they needed, and they invested their US-financed time into selecting local people as trainees. The team valued aptitude above religious qualifications, and they were pleased with their small, staff-in-training cadre who, according to Petty, could help them to do "everything that needed to be done that there was nobody to do."[68] And despite an unhappy mismatch between missionaries' meritocratic hiring and landowners' feelings of entitlement to jobs, goodwill was restored in a way that created unexpected long-term secondary benefits for all parties. These successes Petty credited to God.[69]

---

[67]G. Farrar, Interview.

[68]Petty-Kraus, Interview 1.

[69]Farrar and Petty-Kraus, Interview.

18
"Nigerian Christian Cracker-Box"
(April 1965–August 1965)

A great help and encouragement to me.
—Henry Farrar

During the summer of 1965, everyone on the Onicha Ngwa compound engaged in preparations to open the COC Clinic that they called "stage one" of the Nigerian Christian Hospital (NCH).[1] Dr. Henry Farrar served as general contractor for renovations that transformed empty formerly colonial buildings into an outpatient facility by reconfiguring internal walls, painting, applying asbestos roofing, wiring, and adding an electric generator. Floor plans were dictated by existing external walls, Iris Hays's sketches, and Farrar's preferences.[2] Some missionaries set up shelves and sorted US-donated equipment and supplies, while Iris Hays and Nancy Petty bought fabric for towels and exam room divider curtains and tasked a cloth seller with fetching auxiliary uniform fabric from Lagos.[3] Patti Bryant and Irondi, a local tailor, sewed all on their treadle machines.[4] Clinic progress begat fundraising success, and missionary hopes of adding inpatient units within two years rose.[5]

"Cracker-Box"

Hays laughingly christened the diminutive clinic as the NCC—"Nigerian Christian Cracker-Box."[6] The main, patient-care building and two side

---

[1] R. Bryant to Mattoxes, May 13, 1965.
[2] R. Bryant to Elders, August 9, 1965; Bryant and Bryant, Interview; H. Farrar, Interview 1; Hays-Savio, Interview.
[3] Hays-Savio and Petty-Kraus, Interview.
[4] P. Bryant to Mattoxes, August 18, 1965; G. Farrar in footnote to H. Farrar, Interview 1 transcript.
[5] R. Bryant to Elders, August 9, 1965.
[6] Petty to Spann, May 16, 1965.

buildings were concrete block construction with concrete flooring and corrugated roof. The largest structure was divided into two areas: a fully-walled patient examination area and an open, half-walled patient waiting area. The waiting area had open doorways, no windows or screens, and plain, wooden benches for roughly fifty patients and family members. A narrow wrap-around veranda surrounded three sides of the waiting area, and the fourth side, where the registrar sat, backed up to the exam area. A bamboo pole and thatched roof affair created a nearby parking lot for row upon row of patients' black bicycles, each with a handlebar bell for use in passing or in frightening chickens and children out of the way.[7]

Inside the main building, unbleached muslin curtains divided one large room into three or four smaller exam rooms,[8] each furnished with a simple wooden table covered in heavy "Macintosh" rubber sheeting, as well as a side table for minimal equipment. Tables were designed by Dr. Farrar and likely constructed by local furniture builder, John "Carpenter" Igwe. Natural light filtered through screened windows with security bars, half curtains for privacy, and wooden shutters that could be closed against tropical downpours or opened for ventilation.[9]

Other rooms were used as a "fully equipped" pharmacy "with a good supply of drugs,"[10] a laboratory with microscope, an office each for Dr. Farrar and Matron Petty,[11] and a patient injection and wound dressing area. The second building became Hays's classroom[12] and the third structure housed the government-required, flushing men's and women's latrines—a "hole in the floor European kind."[13] Nigerian health officials mandated these "modern toilet facilities," which required a reliable water supply.[14]

---

[7]R. Bryant to Elders, August 9, 1965; Farrar and Petty-Kraus, Interview; Morgan, "Nigeria: Summer."

[8]P. Bryant to Mattoxes, July 11, 1965; R. Bryant to Elders, August 9, 1965; Farrar, "Story;" Farrar and Petty-Kraus, Interview; H. Farrar, Interview 1.

[9]"Biographical Sketches" (Igwe), 200–01; Hays-Savio, Interview; Morgan, "Nigeria: Summer."

[10]R. Bryant to Elders, August 9, 1965.

[11]P. Bryant to Mattoxes, July 11, 1965; Hays-Savio and Petty-Kraus, Interview.

[12]G. Farrar, Interview; H. Farrar, Interview 1; Hays-Savio, Interview; Farrar and Petty-Kraus, Interview; Morgan, "Nigeria: Summer."

[13]Farrar and Petty-Kraus, Interview.

[14]R. Bryant to Elders, August 9, 1965.

Piecing It Together

Clinic renovations continued from April into August, and an eager Dr. Farrar constantly set and reset the grand opening date. In June, he set it for mid-July, then for late July, and then for early August. As each date approached, too many pieces of the Clinic puzzle were missing, and the timeline was pushed forward.[15] Meanwhile, Petty enjoyed as many daily BTC chapel services as possible, knowing that the Clinic would soon occupy all her time.[16]

Establishing a Clinic water supply proved particularly challenging. Unable to get a well-digger before August and facing a related $3,000 price tag, Dr. Farrar decided temporarily to pump water uphill to the Clinic from the same stream where missionaries got household water. His plan required laying pipe, installing a petrol-powered pump, constructing an elevated water storage tower, and fitting "filters at the taps;"[17] John Morgan, a visiting senior Vanderbilt University medical student, became invaluable to its implementation. Smith, Kline, and French (SKF) Laboratories had funded Morgan for a ten-week summer internship with Dr. Farrar, and all anticipated that after medical school John would replace Farrar during US furloughs.[18]

Arriving on June 9, John and Donna Morgan moved into the vacant house where the Lawyers had lived, integrated quickly into the team, and became close friends with the two other young adults on campus, Hays and Petty.[19] In Nashville, the Morgans were members of LA-COC, and in Nigeria, both helped in Clinic setup. Donna Morgan, a third-grade teacher, assisted with missionary homeschooling, taught local women, typed for Dr. Farrar,[20] and assisted missionary women in writing a Bible storybook for Nigerian children.[21] Meanwhile, John Morgan participated in evangelism, healthcare delivery, and missionary family life. He preached on Sundays, assisted in surgery at nearby hospitals, Interviewed

---

[15]R. Bryant to Currys, June 21, 1965; G. Farrar to Johnson, June 16 and July 6, 1965; H. Farrar to G.B. Farrars, July 16, 1965.

[16]Petty to Spann, August 6, 1965.

[17]G. Farrar to Johnson, July 6, 1965.

[18]*Christian Chronicle*, "1–35,000;" Farrar to Lafayette [sic] Church, September 21, 1965; Farrar to Mission Committee, March 1, 1965, *WEV*; Nigerian Christian Schools, "Two too late?"

[19]G. Farrar to Johnson, June 16, 1965; Hays-Savio, Interview; Petty-Kraus, Interview 1.

[20]G. Farrar to Johnson, June 16, 1965; G. Farrar to Folks, August 11, 1965; Morgan, Morgan, and Farrar, Interview.

[21]P. Bryant to Mattoxes, August 18, 1965.

auxiliary applicants, and enjoyed bicycling and working on Boy Scout badges with preteen Paul Farrar.[22] The four-member medical team of Hays, Petty, Farrar, and Morgan shopped together for medical supplies and equipment in Aba and Port Harcourt (PH).[23] "Morgans are a real joy," Dr. Farrar wrote. "He is a great help and encouragement to me."[24]

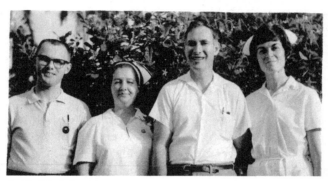

Photograph 18: COC Healthcare team, Onicha Ngwa, Summer 1965: John Morgan, Nancy Petty, RN, Henry Farrar, MD, and Iris Hays, RN. (Author collection).

Morgan proved "worth his weight in gold"[25] to NCH by supervising installation of Clinic water and electrical systems.[26] "I don't know how Henry could have gotten the clinic in operation without him!" marveled Grace Farrar.[27] Because Dr. Farrar feared heights, he asked Morgan to assemble the Clinic's 5,000-gallon water tank atop four, thirty-foot concrete-and-steel-reinforced columns constructed by Anthony Agali and crew. There, Morgan guided workers in fitting together the reservoir's steel plates,[28] astonishing Nigerians and missionaries alike "that one man" could do so many things so well. Farrar delightedly christened the tank, "John's erector set."[29]

On August 7, the senior medical officer in Aba approved missionaries' opening of the NCH Clinic at Dr. Farrar's discretion. Finally, after years

---

[22]Ibid.; G. Farrar to Folks, August 11 and 24, 1965; Hays-Savio, Interview; Morgan, "Report;" Morgans and Farrar, Interview.

[23]Hays-Savio, Interview.

[24]H. Farrar to G.B. Farrars, July 16, 1965.

[25]G. Farrar to Folks, August 11, 1965.

[26]Farrar to Lafayette [sic] Church, September 21, 1965.

[27]G. Farrar to Folks, August 24, 1965.

[28]P. Bryant to Mattoxes, August 18, 1965; G. Farrar to Folks, August 11, 1965; Farrar to Mission Committee, July 7, 1965, WEV.

[29]Farrar, Stand, 83; G. Farrar to Folks, August 11, 1965.

of stops and starts and investments of time, energy, and roughly $10,000,[30] the team now needed only cooperation from Nigeria's weather. Seasonal downpours delayed their laying the NCH stream-to-clinic pipeline, creating a water supply problem described by Farrar as "too much from above, and not enough below."[31]

Meanwhile, Rees Bryant communicated to his sponsoring South Park congregation that evangelism remained his top priority. He announced approval to open the Clinic at the end of his five-page report on preaching and teaching in which he described missionaries' "biggest project" in August as "a special gospel campaign" in Enugu. Bryant enjoyed his evangelistic work, and he wrote that he was also happy "to render some assistance to Dr. Farrar in this worthy work of medical benevolence among these suffering people." Never missing an opportunity to promote the hospital, Bryant reminded supporters of plans for NCH stage two: a "full-fledged hospital" that would require $36,000 for "an operating room building; a five bed maternity unit; a five bed isolation unit; a 30 bed male ward; a 30 bed female ward; a kitchen-laundry building; and a mortuary." As Bryant calculated for them, $1,500 per month for two years would cover those costs, and $175 per month had been pledged.[32]

That cost estimate omitted the roughly $5,000 for utilities promised by W-COC and remained close to the original quote of $45,000, but with an expansion in bed numbers from the original thirty to now seventy. This equaled roughly half the size of the Qua Iboe Hospital whose 140-bed capacity restricted its physician's church work.[33] Together, Americans and Nigerians, evangelists and healthcare providers, resident missionaries and visitors, brought a Christian clinic and dispensary into being as stage one of NCH.

[30]R. Bryant to Elders, August 9, 1965; G. Farrar to Folks, August 11, 1965.
[31]G. Farrar to Folks, August 11, 1965.
[32]R. Bryant to Elders, August 9, 1965.
[33]Bryant, "Reflections," 22.

19
Opening the "Cracker-Box"
(August 1965)

We laughed a lot.
—Nancy Petty

Better than crying.
—Henry Farrar

By late August 1965, the "Cracker-Box Clinic" buildings were ready, staff were hired, and water pipes and pump in place. But when the team turned on their stream-to-clinic water system, nothing happened. Several pump pieces were missing, and the entire setup was useless until the vendor could fly in the parts.[1] Undeterred, the team took a reservoir-half-full approach and decided to run the rainwater collected in the Agali-Morgan water tank to their flushing latrines and faucets by gravity feed. Where no sinks existed, hand-washing basins would have to do.[2] Only later did Henry Farrar find two of the needed pump pieces sitting in the vendor's warehouse,[3] and a few weeks afterwards a working pump could fill the water tank within four hours.[4]

Grand Opening

On Saturday, August 21, 1965, the Nigerian Christian Hospital (NCH) Out-Patient Clinic opened with great ceremony, followed by traditional refreshments of "rice with beef fried in palm oil and hot peppers,

---

[1]P. Bryant to Mattoxes, August 18, 1965; H. Farrar, Interview 1; Morgan, "John's Journal," August 23, 1965.
[2]G. Farrar to Johnson, June 16, 1965; H. Farrar, Interview 1.
[3]G. Farrar to Morgans, October 3, [1965]; H. Farrar to Morgans, September 21, 1965; H. Farrar, Interview 2.
[4]H. Farrar to Morgans, September 21, 1965.

169

ground nuts (peanuts) and Pepsis & Kola nuts" for everyone.[5] A torrential downpour forced missionaries and 400–500 attendees indoors at the Bible Training College (BTC) for the ribbon cutting. Present were local chiefs, council members, and two Eastern Ngwa dignitaries, and the entire program was presented in Igbo, Efik, and English. Not one for fanfare, Henry Farrar first belittled plans for a formal opening, but on the big day, he delighted the audience by quoting Bible verses in Igbo and Efik. Missionaries also took private satisfaction when Eastern Ngwa officials publicly recanted their past opposition to NCH. Chief Oguduro donated £20, and both he and Chief Ahukana appeared disappointed that the press was not present for this occasion.[6]

Many sick came to the celebration hoping for care and bringing empty pill bottles for medicine,[7] but NCH did not receive its first official patients until two days later on Monday, August 23.[8] John Morgan, who penned the most complete firsthand report of opening day, wrote that missionaries did not know what to expect but their "questions were soon answered."[9] Clinic doors were opened "to an overwhelming crowd" of over 200 patients and family members who filled the waiting area and spilled over into NCH's temporary seating shelter of bamboo poles with palm frond thatch roof.[10] Few in the stifling crush of patients and families, who crowded into the tiny Clinic, were curiosity seekers, and by 2:00 p.m. the team had registered 178 patients. They saw fewer than half of those,[11] sending the rest home with "paper slips to guarantee their being seen the next [clinic] day."[12] Patient numbers were similar on the second clinic day of Wednesday, and Iris Hays carefully recorded in her diary a daily census of patients treated: 79 patients on Monday (August 23), 78 on Wednesday, 101 on Friday, and 133 the next Monday (August 30).[13] No official Clinic records survived, but missionary estimates varied little

---

[5]G. Farrar to Folks, August 24, 1965.
[6]Ibid.; R. Bryant to Masseys and Lawyers, September 8, 1965; Hays-Savio, Interview.
[7]G. Farrar to Folks, August 24, 1965.
[8]Farrar "Letter;" Hays-Savio, Interview; Morgan, "Memories."
[9]Morgan, "Report," 22.
[10]Savio, "Nigerian Christian Hospital," 46.
[11]Farrar and Petty-Kraus, Interview; Hays-Savio, Interview; Morgan, "Report," 22–23.
[12]Savio, "Nigerian Christian Hospital,"47.
[13]Hays-Savio, Interview.

on the total number of patients enrolled in those first days.[14] Rising numbers suggested growing efficiency.

The dire physical plight of many patients on August 23 surprised the COC healthcare team. They referred for surgery a twelve-year-old who had been "unable to open her mouth for four years" yet had never seen a doctor, and they drained and prescribed penicillin for one woman's untreated "massive" abscess.[15] They likely also saw negative outcomes of native doctor practice, such as injection-related abscesses, loss of digits, infected skin slashes, and multiple small cuts in children intended to rid them of tuberculosis. Perhaps, too, as in later days, patients included those with vesico-vaginal fistulas, complete uterine prolapse, and parasitic filarial onchocerciasis (river blindness).[16] Many were malnourished; hookworm and malaria were prevalent. Others were so anemic that their hemoglobin levels were not measurable, and Dr. Farrar found himself teaching dietary practices to numerous feverish, nauseated, and vomiting patients.[17]

Hays's nursing auxiliary students began work that first day, but probably required as much time in instruction as they contributed in services. Hays worked with some in the wound and injection areas, while Matron Nancy Petty ran the pharmacy—both dispensing and teaching Mark Peter to do so. Meanwhile, some of Hays's students likely took vital signs, a skill they learned the previous week,[18] while Dr. Farrar rounded through examination rooms with translating auxiliaries,[19] whose medical vocabulary must have been little different from that of the patients. Additionally, registrar Joseph Nwaoguegbe (or Nwagwebe) signed patients in, called them to be seen, and typed a registration card for each patient that served as the person's medical record of history, diagnosis, prescription, treatment, and billing.[20] Peter Uhiara, the Igbo lay laboratory technician-in-

---

[14]G. Farrar to Johnson, September 13, 1965; H. Farrar to Mrs. H.C. Farrar, August 29, 1965; Farrar to Mission Committee, September 1, 1965, *WEV*; Hays-Savio, Interview; Morgan, "Report," 22.

[15]Morgan, "Report," 22–23. More case details in Farrar to Mission Committee, September 1, 1965, *WEV*.

[16]G. Farrar to Mrs. H.C. Farrar, June 26, 1966; Farrar to Lafayette [sic] Church, September 21, 1965; Farrar to Mission Committee, September 1 and October 4, 1965, *WEV*; Petty to Spann, July 13, 1966.

[17]G. Farrar to Johnson, September 13, 1965; H. Farrar, Interview 1.

[18]Hays-Savio, Interview.

[19]Farrar and Petty-Kraus, Interview.

[20]H. Farrar, Interview 1.

training, also began work, and Farrar probably used his own 1950s master's degree in parasitology and chemistry to teach Uhiara.[21]

Not everyone who helped in clinic that day saw patients. Knowing that the first week would be a test of systems, the Farrars suspended home-school for their two oldest children, preteens Paul and Marty, so that the two could serve as runners between Clinic and compound. One child was stationed at the Clinic and the other at Farrar's house, and Marty felt important delivering supplies, lunches, and messages across the roughly one quarter mile of dirt paths.[22] Because senior medical student Morgan could not independently see patients, he spent part of his time photographing the providers, crowd, and facilities, including Uhiara at his microscope, Petty with Mark Peter, NCH flushing latrines, and more. Where Uhiara obtained his white laboratory uniform is undocumented, and photographs of nursing auxiliaries show them out of uniform on day one and in NCH-provided uniforms on day two.[23]

Those early Clinic days generated both delight and moral distress for the missionaries. Rees Bryant rejoiced in seeing his 1950s healthcare vision coming to fruition with "Christian doctors and Christian nurses caring for the sick people in a Christian hospital."[24] In contrast, Farrar, Hays, and Petty felt the heartache of treating so many who were so ill, for whom they could do so little. They were now face-to-face with preventable death, disease, and an estimated ratio of one physician for every 35,000–50,000 patients.[25] Yet Hays wrote on many pages of her diary, "We had fun."[26]

As Petty recalled, "We were young…We laughed a lot."[27]

"Better than crying," replied Farrar.[28]

---

[21]H. Farrar, Unpublished, untitled biography, ca 1963. HGF.

[22]Author's recollection.

[23]Hays-Savio, Interview; John R. Morgan, email to author, August 17, 2012; Morgan, "Nigeria: Summer." In his email to author, Morgan denied taking the photo in his collection labeled "clinic patients" that showed a nursing auxiliary with cap and white pinafore; caps were awarded a year later.

[24]R. Bryant to Masseys and Lawyers, September 8, 1965.

[25]Farrar to Lafayette [sic] Church, September 21, 1965; Hays-Savio, Interview; Morgan, "Memories."

[26]Hays-Savio, Interview.

[27]Farrar and Petty-Kraus, Interview.

[28]Ibid.

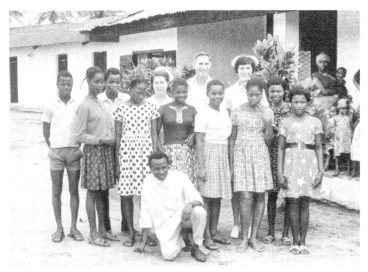

Photograph 19. NCH staff on opening day in front of main Clinic building. Front:
Peter Uhiara. Back, left to right: Mark Peter, Elizabeth Egbu, Joseph Nwaoguegbe,
possibly Esther Uzuogu, Nancy Petty, auxiliary student, Henry Farrar, Comfort Nwosu,
Iris Hays, Lydia Agbara, and two other auxiliary students. Photograph by J.R. Morgan.
August 23, 1965. (JRM collection with permission).

Clinic Routine

Patients started their days long before the missionaries did. Families traveled to the Clinic before sunrise, collecting numbers from the registrar or
the "day watch" (security) as they arrived. Men and women sat together
in the waiting room, in contrast to sitting separately in church,[29] and beginning at 7:00 a.m. NCH staff would hold two short devotionals. Registrar Nwaoguegbe would first teach "a short Bible class" to staff and construction workers. Then after the missionary team arrived at 7:30 a.m.,
either Farrar or a Nigerian preacher would read a Bible passage, com-
ment on it, and lead a prayer with staff, patients, and families. Missionaries pointed to these activities as a demonstration of the facility's Christian
emphasis.[30]

After the devotionals, staff would explain the two main Clinic rules to
waiting patients. The first was that patients would be called by number
unless Hays or Petty triaged them as too ill to wait; the second was that

---

[29]Ibid.; H. Farrar, Interview 1.
[30]Farrar to Mission Committee, October 4, 1965, *WEV*; Hays-Savio, Interview;
Savio, "Nigerian Christian Hospital," 47.

everyone was expected to use the indoor flushing latrines. The team then triaged and treated as many as possible until time ran out. The seriously ill were seen immediately and, when necessary, transported to a hospital probably by NCH driver and purchasing agent Friday Onukafor (formerly the Lawyer family's cook).[31]

Patients carried their registrar-typed cards with them from exam room to billing to pharmacy or treatment areas and finally returned the card for filing.[32] Petty found it extraordinary that Farrar allowed a five-minute tea and cookie break each morning at 10:30 a.m., after which the team resumed care until their two-hour lunch break. Afternoon hours ended between 4:00 and 5:00 p.m.[33] with what Farrar called "the hardest job of all:" Staff sent unseen patients home with registrar-issued numbers to be seen first on the next clinic day. We "rejoice at what little we can do. Pray for us," Farrar penned to W-COC.[34] Still, his energy and enthusiasm surged as he reveled in release from his pre-Clinic prison of medical inaction.

Petty chuckled that Farrar "thought it was his duty when we were having our tea break to give us some kind of little lecture,"[35] and sometimes these provided the opportunity for good-natured ribbing. One day Dr. Farrar pontificated that boils were caused by stress and refused to concede that the boils behind his own knees were promoted by skin moisture trapped by his long pants; other missionary men wore shorts in Nigeria's oppressive humidity; he refused. Immediately after that mini-lecture, a three-month-old infant presented with boils, and Matron Petty couldn't resist: "That poor little stressed out thing! What...do you do for a child...that stressed?" she teased Farrar.[36]

In the beginning, Dr. Farrar personally saw every patient because, according to Petty, "he didn't trust any of us."[37] Meanwhile, Hays rotated auxiliary students through examination rooms, teaching them how to record a chief complaint and brief history on the patient card and prepare the patient for examination. Farrar circled through rooms, spending about five minutes per patient reviewing complaints, doing cursory examinations, instructing patients, and writing prescriptions, lab work, needed

[31] Farrar and Petty-Kraus, Interview; Petty to Spann, July 14, 1965.

[32] H. Farrar, Interview 1.

[33] Farrar and Petty-Kraus, Interview; G. Farrar to Johnson, May 17, 1966; H. Farrar to Mrs. H.C. Farrar, August 29, 1965.

[34] Farrar to Mission Committee, October 4, 1965, *WEV*; Savio, "Memories," 47.

[35] Farrar and Petty-Kraus, Interview.

[36] Petty-Kraus, Interview 1.

[37] Farrar and Petty-Kraus, Interview.

treatments, charges, and any return appointment dates on the cards. Patients then paid their bills and went to the wound room, injection room, or pharmacy as needed. The US team hoped these routines would allow them to see roughly 200 patients per day,[38] and eight months later they were treating up to 180.[39]

Patients and families provided their own food during the long hours of waiting, and local entrepreneurs took notice. Petty christened the collection of food vendors who gathered under a nearby tree "the Nigerian Christian Hospital Snack Shop." One sold cooked beans, another rice and stew, and a third, groundnuts (peanuts). Hays suggested that Petty check out the other side of the clinic, where Petty discovered a woman was running "a drink fountain: palm wine in gourds, jugs and bottles with leaves rolled up and stuck in the top for lids. To make sure it was palm wine," Petty removed the stopper from one bottle and sniffed, an action that she said cleared her sinuses "for a long time." The woman never returned, and Petty speculated that she either sold out or feared the Matron's disapproval, although Petty did not rebuke her.[40]

"Cracker-Box" Cases

Onicha Ngwa missionaries' backdoor care mostly halted when the Clinic opened, and US nurses felt their efforts made a positive difference in people's lives. Petty recorded her sense of "great victory" in healing tropical ulcers up to three inches wide and down to the bone,[41] and she enjoyed lighter moments with patients. "I found a toy airplane in one of the packages of medicine and gave it to a little boy," Nancy wrote to her young nephew John, "But he didn't know what it was and…it scared him."[42]

Rabies was common, and Nigerian responses to suspect animals highlighted the differences between Western and Igbo knowledge. In one case, the team wanted to avoid giving rabies shots to a pregnant woman who had been bitten by a potentially ill dog. They "explained the dangers" and instructed the couple to monitor the animal. The family revealed that they already killed the dog, and so Dr. Farrar asked them to take its head to Aba government offices where it could be tested for ra-

[38]Ibid.; H. Farrar, Interview 1.
[39]Petty to Spann, April 19, 1966.
[40]Petty to Corlew, November 9, 1965.
[41]Petty to Spann, November 8, 1965.
[42]Petty to J. Spann, September 23, 1965.

bies. In response, the infuriated husband stormed out of the clinic, and the next morning, to her sickened dismay, Petty learned why. The family had eaten the dog—"head and all."[43] The team felt compelled to administer the injection series.[44]

Hays never forgot one small boy who also needed the prescribed two weeks of daily, large-volume rabies vaccinations. For three days the family held down their child on a narrow clinic bench, even sitting on him, while Hays struggled to give the shots using all new (instead of sharpened) needles that still seemed dull to her. The "screaming and fighting" child made a bad situation worse, and Hays dreaded the daily, traumatic routine. On the fourth miserable day, Hays asked what the child was saying. "He's saying to turn him loose, that he can do it by himself," the translator responded. "Turn him loose," Hays instructed, and the boy endured each following injection without complaint. He rewarded her with a "most handsome smile" in the end, and years later she remembered his "incredible" courage. "He was the strongest…determined little boy…He just didn't want to be held down."[45]

Abscesses created by native doctor injections were another common issue. In one case, the team saved the life and left arm of BTC student Lordson Egbutta (also Egbutu). His letter of gratitude to Petty contained no petition, but instead overflowed with profuse thanks to her, Hays, and the Farrars.[46] Years later, preacher Egbutta became an operating room technician at NCH, where missionary surgeon Maurice Hood called him "one of the most dependable, kind and gentle workers."[47]

In the Clinic, Hays and Petty experienced victory, joy, uncertainty, and discomfort. They savored small successes when they knew what to do and could do it, but felt doubt and shame when they imagined what could be done if not thwarted by the urgent and emergent. Although Petty resigned herself to triaging hundreds, she expressed retrospective chagrin that the team did so little preventive care and nutrition teaching. Patient needs were just "overwhelming if you thought about it too much," she sighed.[48]

---

[43]Petty to Corlew, November 9, 1965.

[44]Hays-Savio and Petty-Kraus, Interview.

[45]Hays-Savio, Interview; Savio, "Nigerian Christian Hospital," 47.

[46]Egbutta to Petty, November 17, 1965; Farrar to Mission Committee, October 4, 1965, *WEV*.

[47]"Biographical Sketches" (Egbutu), 196.

[48]Farrar and Petty-Kraus, Interview.

Conclusion

Bringing the NCH Outpatient Clinic to life took an international village. Dr. Farrar credited Hays and Petty with "pivotal" work that made it possible,[49] while Hays and Petty saw in the Clinic more work than they could do. The team coped by dividing responsibilities and uniting in laughter. "It took a lot of nerve," Grace Farrar observed later, for two single women to come "without any experience in Africa, without any orientation program," and they did such a "wonderful job…amazing…They just landed there fresh and raw and took over."[50]

---

[49]H. Farrar, Interview 1.
[50]G. Farrar, Interview.

20
"Many Colors Together"
(1965–1966)

I had forgotten that I was white.
—Iris Hays

Identities and interactions of Nigerians and Americans continued to evolve. As a new nursing graduate, Iris Hays immediately assumed a nurse educator role—perhaps because the idea of becoming NCH matron was even more terrifying. Still, standing in front of any group in her words "was terrible," and she remained forever mystified by how she overcame her dread of teaching. Nonetheless, overcome it she did, and her initial, cautious delight contrasted sharply with previously avowed fears. "Lectured to my first class of students," Hays recorded in her diary on August 18, 1965. "I really enjoyed it. We learned how to take temperatures. I am quite pleased with them. I only hope that I'm not disappointed later."[1]

Hays's ambitions for her 1965 cohort of nursing students were immense, and her teaching environment, tiny. The clinic outbuilding classroom held barely enough "little chairs" for them, and the only illustrations she had were the "little pictures…in books." She pecked out handouts and exams "one carbon copy at a time" on her miniature typewriter purchased when College Avenue COC sent her extra money to buy something personal. Only three inches tall, it was "the smallest little portable…[she'd] ever seen before or since" with a regular-size keyboard. The biggest chalkboard she could find in Aba was a twelve-by-eight-inch "slate," and she taught medication math by writing the first part of a problem on the front and the rest on the back. That restriction might be why in October Hays wrote in her diary, "I'm going out of my mind trying to teach these girls proportions." Moreover, frequent afternoon rains

---

[1]Hays-Savio, Interview.

pounding on the classroom's metal roof drowned out all sound and forced Hays to halt instruction until the downpour moved on.[2]

Hays modeled the auxiliary curriculum after her own, using standards grounded in US care expectations. No doubt this missionary-compatible education contributed to Dr. Farrar's later calling Hays's graduates "the best nurses he ever had,"[3] and perhaps also why nursing auxiliaries on occasion evaluated their own skills as better than those of NCH's British-educated Nigerian Registered Nurses (NRNs).[4] "We had a good nursing school," Grace Farrar recalled,[5] in first-person language that revealed her team member identity.

Nigerian oral traditions prepared students well for classes in which Hays talked and they listened. With no student books, no classroom supplies, and minimal handouts, Hays used "review and review and review, a bit of the rote memory stuff that they're good at." Lectures, tests, and simulated practice preceded application, and Hays drew content from US textbooks and a British text, "*Nursing Essentials for Tropical Nurses* or something like that," which she purchased in Aba. She was pleased with the way her students learned "all the basics:" anatomy, nursing fundamentals, pharmacology,[6] medical terminology, wound care, injection techniques, medication administration, ratio and proportions, vital signs, bed-making, history-taking, and nursing care of medical, surgical, pediatric, and obstetrical/gynecological patients. Her content was heavily skills-focused, and each auxiliary received a uniform and small salary.[7]

She taught no more than one or two days of classes before the Clinic opened to patients, creating a patient care immersion experience for students on Mondays, Wednesdays, and Fridays. On Tuesdays and Thursdays, Hays lectured, but she was confident that her students also learned a good deal while interpreting for Dr. Farrar, who loved to teach while seeing patients. As fast as Hays could teach and test her content, she moved students into skills acquisition, knowing that she and Matron Petty couldn't physically handle the patient load very long, given patient numbers, limited facilities, and their wider responsibilities. Yet Hays conscientiously avoided educational shortcuts, explaining principles and pro-

---

[2]Ibid.

[3]G. Farrar, Interview.

[4]Chi Ekwenye-Hendricks, Interview 2.

[5]G. Farrar, Interview.

[6]Hays-Savio, Interview.

[7]Ibid.; Petty-Kraus, Interview 1; Farrar, "Nigerian Christian Hospital Financial Report August 6–October 1, 1966;" Farrar, "Nigerian Christian Hospital Financial Report, Nov. 13–Dec. 15, 1966, Salaries," W-COC file.

cedures step by step. Wound care, for example, included a strict routine of cleaning, sulfa powder, and rebandaging, and Hays laughed that during return demonstrations auxiliaries bandaged each other "from head-to-toe!"[8]

While Hays tolerated a bit of imperfection in some tasks, she taught injection skills last because she required errorless injection technique from her students. Additionally, she instructed them how to sharpen, soak in solution, and weekly autoclave their reusable needles and syringes.[9] NCH avoided the hip muscle for injections because it was the preferred site for native doctors, who used nonsterile syringes containing "who-knows-what." The NCH team treated many resulting abscesses.[10] Nigerians preferred invasive over noninvasive treatments, and Hays may have feared that her students might try out their new injection knowledge in the community. Within eight months, top student Lydia Agbara administered shots, and within twelve, Hays would have trusted any student to inject Hays herself.[11]

Hays invited others to teach, too. Farrar and Petty lectured occasionally, Patti Bryant taught a Bible class,[12] and Rees Bryant focused on core values. The most important person at NCH, Rees Bryant emphasized, was not the doctor, not the nurses, and not the senior medical officer from Aba. The most important person in the hospital was the patient—an idea that became a team mantra and a nursing exam question.[13] Dr. Farrar acknowledged that Hays and Petty knew better than he "what nurses were supposed to do." Too, he expressed confidence that they would imbue students with missionaries' shared belief that they were all "working for Jesus" to meet spiritual as well as physical needs.[14] His noninterference with the nursing classes no doubt freed both him and the US nurses for their respective duties.

Iris Hays wrote auxiliary examinations, and Petty helped to monitor them.[15] Students' test scores were always positively related to their prior

---

[8]Hays-Savio, Interview.

[9]Ibid.

[10]Morgan, "Report," 10.

[11]Hays-Savio, Interview; Petty to Corlew, April 4, 1966.

[12]Bryant and Bryant, Interview; H. Farrar to Morgans, December 9, 1965; Hays-Savio, Interview; Hays-Savio and Petty-Kraus, Interview; Petty-Kraus, Interview 1.

[13]R. Bryant "Reflections," 26; Bryant and Bryant, Interview; "Onicha Ngwa Bible Training College Health Class Examination -1st Quarter," completed by Bernice Ugboyo, April 11, 1967. Per Bryants, the saying was Rees's adaptation of F. W. Mattox's statement that the most important person in a university is the student.

[14]Farrar to Mission Committee, July 7, 1965.

[15]Petty to Spann, November 23, 1965.

educational levels. The top students were always Lydia and Comfort who had completed the most secondary schooling, followed each time by Elizabeth, then Eunice, and then Esther in order of their years of formal education. Skill proficiencies paralleled exam grades.[16]

Additionally, as the Igbo women learned nursing, Hays and Petty learned teaching. If everyone did poorly on a test, Hays knew it had been too hard and added points. She was disappointed that her comprehensive, end-of-year exam "didn't go down too good," but otherwise thought her strategies worked well.[17] Meanwhile, Petty learned clinical coaching, and, with the notable exception of pharmacy dispenser Mark Peter,[18] she found Igbo students fearless in taking on new tasks. She quickly realized that she must ask students to demonstrate a skill rather than accepting their universal "yes-I-can-do-it" answers at face value. When Petty realized that students answered that way in order to please her, she began communicating differently. Still, the Matron found extracting the truth from eager-to-please Nigerians to be one of the hardest parts of missionary nursing.[19]

The US nurses taught to American standards, but Igbo staff-in-training sometimes insisted on Nigerian ones. Mid-1960s Western scientists maintained that infants must sleep on their stomachs in order to prevent Sudden Infant Death Syndrome (SIDS); Igbos disagreed. They had not heard of SIDS, but "they had seen it." As they explained to Petty, if you put babies face down, "spirits can come in...through their nose and take their life." Thus, as soon as Petty or Hays weren't looking, the auxiliaries flipped babies onto their backs.[20] Decades later, after scientific Western observations caught up with traditional Nigerian ones, Petty reflected on their knowledge. "God is good," she mused, and "I was living with a very gracious people. So, whatever I tried to push on them, if it wasn't going to work, they didn't tell me. They just went away and didn't do it."[21]

Differing assumptions led also to other treatment disagreements and to communication improvements. Petty was interested in relieving pain, but Nigerians thought pain should be endured and were reluctant to give pain medicines. They complied only after Matron Petty learned to rebuke them in writing and require their written response on what she had in-

---

[16]Hays-Savio, Interview.
[17]Ibid.
[18]H. Farrar to Morgans, October 27, 1965.
[19]Farrar and Petty-Kraus, Interview; Petty-Kraus, Interview 1.
[20]Petty-Kraus, Interview 1.
[21]Farrar and Petty-Kraus, Interview.

structed them to do. Oral correction did not produce behavioral change.[22]

Friendship

Student-teacher relationships between the Igbo and US women grew into friendships, and group differences between them in age, role, "or anything" faded. The US nurses sometimes hosted the auxiliaries in their home for games and traditional food prepared by cook-steward Mark Apollos,[23] and student Lydia Agbara documented her perspective in a note to Petty's Aunt Corinne.

> We are living happily with your Niece. She is a very good and kind lady. She makes us happy all the time and more to the sick and little babies. I am the one who pierced her ears and now she wears fine ear-rings, but one funny thing is that she nearly bit me when I wanted to beautify her the more, by piercing her ears…Although she did like this, she is the type we want in our country.[24]

Similar good-natured humor and affection prevailed among all the women. Hays and Petty teased each other over the students' elevating their historical significance. Instead of identifying Florence Nightingale as the founder of modern nursing, one student wrote on her exam that it was "Petty Matron," while another wrote that same answer, then crossed it out and substituted Hays's name.[25] Additionally, the Igbo women poked fun at their missionary friends, not only openly as in Lydia's letter, but also surreptitiously. Petty delighted in their laughter one day when they were unaware of her approach. "Eunice Ukegbu, who was a clown…was mocking Dr. Farrar walking and talking, and then me, and then Iris…It was so funny!…She said, 'And this is Sister [Petty]'s beady eye look.'" Petty made a lot of noise as she got closer, "and they just scattered."[26]

The camaraderie between the Igbo and US women flourished within a context of the nurses' limited self-consciousness. During Nigerian Republic Day, on October 1, 1965, while the missionaries listened to

---

[22]Ibid.
[23]Hays-Savio, Interview.
[24]Agbara, in Petty to Corlew, April 4, 1966.
[25]Petty to Spann, September 17, 1965.
[26]Farrar and Petty-Kraus, Interview.

speeches and celebrations as "the only white people...[in] this sea of black people," Hays recalled a moment when she moved her arm:

> It startled me because it was white! There was no distinction between being black and white. I felt as much at home and at ease being there...because I was just as happy as they were that it was their 5th anniversary of independence...I had forgotten that I was white.[27]

The nurses spoke together of how the consciousness of differing skin colors that proved inescapable in a mid-1960s US context seemed irrelevant to their relationships in Nigeria, except when the occasional Nigerian drew their attention to it. And Petty's clothing choices became an apt metaphor. "Nigerian women wear many colors together, and I am getting so I don't think a lot about it," Petty observed of herself as she returned from Aba shopping in red shoes, a brown dress, and a pink and yellow scarf.[28] Still, Petty noted, amused Nigerian strangers in the street were not hesitant to call her *onye ọcha* (white person), and missionary children bicycling through the village were often accompanied by celebratory crowds of laughing youngsters running alongside and shouting, "*Beke, beke!*" (white, white).[29]

Conclusion

Missionaries' preparation of their own nursing staff created both anticipated and unanticipated outcomes. As expected, classes drew Nigerian and US women together in nursing practice. Unexpectedly, the classes also nurtured friendships and new perspectives, as relationships transcending race, ethnicity, role, class, and culture were forged between two very different groups of women: Nigerians, who "grew up on dirt floors" with little if any education beyond eighth grade,[30] and North Americans, who were Western college-educated, licensed professionals and affluent by comparison. Affection, respect, and a willingness to laugh at themselves grew. As Igbo women evolved into nursing staff members, Petty altered communications, expectations, and dress, while Hays used comfortable secretarial skills to engage in uncomfortable teaching. The

---

27Hays-Savio, Interview.
28Petty to Spann, September 17, 1965.
29Petty to Spann, July 14, 1965; Author's recollection.
30G. Farrar, Interview.

US missionary nurses, who came intending to change Nigeria, discovered that it was changing them.

21
Revolutionaries
(1965–1966)

My angel was just workin' double overtime.
—Nancy Petty

Missionaries expected Christianity to work a religious revolution among Nigerians, but likely did not anticipate how radical their Clinic rules would be. The team's Western ideas about sliding scale billing, triaging, patient advocacy, health teaching, and law and order stood in sharp contrast to local customs. Matron Nancy Petty, however, insisted that everyone follow NCH directives, and an amused Rees Bryant assessed enforcer Petty as one "tough customer."[1]

Enforcer

Western-style patient advocacy of the missionaries quickly thrust Matron Petty into the role of cultural revolutionary. Treating the sickest first then others on a first-come-first-serve basis was utterly countercultural for locals, who expected missionaries to conform to their practice of catering to the most powerful first. Nonetheless, Petty was determined that politically important men were "not going to push these little women with babies aside."[2] The team would treat a baby dying from measles before a village chief complaining of impotence.[3]

Petty enforced that Clinic rule, and nine months later, she became the center of a story that passed into missionary lore—albeit with varying details.[4] On that day, a large, muscular soldier pushed his way to the front desk manned by "meek, little" Registrar Joseph Nwaoguegbe and menac-

---

[1] Bryant and Bryant, Interview.
[2] G. Farrar, Interview.
[3] Farrar and Petty-Kraus, Interview.
[4] G. Farrar, Interview; Kee, *African*, 45; Petty to Spann, April 4, 1966.

ingly demanded his entitlement. "I was an officer in the Nigerian army in the Congo, and I want to see the doctor," the soldier barked.[5] Quickly shifting responsibility, Nwaoguegbe explained that the soldier would have to see "Sister" and ran to get the Matron. When Petty emerged, the menacing soldier reiterated his demand. I'm "not afraid to fight," he threatened.[6] "I am so-and-so, and I came from the Congo, and I want to see the doctor."[7]

Drawing herself up to her full five feet and three-inch height, Petty countered. I'm not "afraid either," she told him.[8] "I am Nancy Petty from Bear Creek, Tennessee, and you are going to wait in line like everybody else."[9] Likely flustered by this short, resolute white woman, the soldier hastily retreated without being seen. Clinic staff were openly amused.[10] "I was not raised in a fear-based home," explained Petty later, "so I didn't operate like that there. Probably my angel was just workin' double overtime."[11]

Additionally, the team mandate for people to use the flushing latrines out of public view introduced another unfamiliar practice that required staff explanations to patients about how to use the novel equipment. Local modesty standards were not Western ones, and public urination was common practice.[12] Most used open holes in the fields behind their houses as latrines, and when they were away from home they simply availed themselves of open sewers or other convenient locations. The wraparound porch off the Clinic waiting area turned out to be convenient.

Matron Petty resolved that if the government required the missionaries to build flushing latrines before they could open, then patients and families would be required to use them. On the very first Clinic day, she took immediate action when she spied a man relieving himself off the veranda. "I grabbed me a stick, and I ran out there, and I hit him on his shoulder. I said, 'You're not supposed to do that there. These are the latrines we had to have before we could open this clinic, and you go in there.'" Having observed this incident from a distance, Dr. Farrar took the staff's

---

[5]G. Farrar, Interview.
[6]Petty to Spann, April 4, 1966.
[7]G. Farrar, Interview.
[8]Petty to Spann, April 4, 1966.
[9]G. Farrar, Interview.
[10]Petty to Spann, April 4, 1966.
[11]Farrar and Petty-Kraus, Interview.
[12]Ibid.; Petty-Kraus, Presentation to Keen-Agers.

morning tea and biscuit break as an opportunity to instruct Petty about such things.

"Now, Nancy," Farrar began, "A man can't stop like that."

"Well, he did," Petty retorted.[13]

Sheriff

The COC team's understanding of law and order also differed from Igbo ideas. Petty learned this firsthand one Tuesday in November 1966 when she faced down an angry mob intent on meting out ultimate justice. By then Dr. Farrar trusted the nurses enough to delegate Tuesday maternity and well-baby clinics to them, and Petty described her related maternal-child practice as "acting like a doctor."[14] She treated patients independently and referred to Dr. Farrar as she deemed necessary.[15] In clinic, she and Iris Hays were always surrounded by a crowd of men and their expectant wives, who arrived "sitting up regal like queens on the back of [their husband's bicycles]....straight as an arrow. Beautiful head ties on."[16]

All Nigerian bicycles looked the same to Petty, but the Nigerians knew their own, and they knew a bicycle thief when they saw one. When Petty arrived at the Clinic, a woman, about eight months pregnant, was throwing herself on the ground and crying that someone had stolen her bicycle. The US nurses proceeded to see patients, but suddenly chaos erupted: a crowd of men were stoning the suspected thief on the spot.[17] As Petty described it, the man was

> ...screaming and squirming, and I went flying out there and said, "Stop that! What are you doing? What are you doing? You can't!" They said, "He stole a bicycle." I said, "No, no. You cannot do it."... I could just see the headline: "Husband of Patient at Nigerian Christian Hospital Stoned to Death."[18]

Two staff men managed to drag the suspected thief away from the mob and into the Clinic, and Matron Petty threatened the yelling, fist-shaking mob with closing clinic for the day if they didn't stop. Still grumbling, the group backed away, and Petty sent for the police. Keeping one eye on the

---

[13]Farrar and Petty-Kraus, Interview.
[14]Petty to Spann, July 27, 1966.
[15]Ibid.; H. Farrar to Morgans, September 13, 1966.
[16]Farrar and Petty-Kraus, Interview.
[17]Petty to Spann, November 3, 1966.
[18]Farrar and Petty-Kraus, Interview.

furious crowd, she returned to patient care, but violence quickly exploded again. "The lady (whose bike was stolen)...pulled the man out the door...One minute they were talking & the next...they were beating him."[19]

A male staffer (probably Sunday Awaziama[20]) and Matron Petty "rushed out and pushed" into the crowd. Fortuitously, former native juju doctor Moses Oparah (also Opara or Oparrah), who was now a Christian and NCH chaplain, was working that day.[21] Petty and Sunday grabbed the man with help from tall, intimidating Oparah, and Petty locked the accused in the nurses' office until the police could take him away. The Nigerians, who wanted to kill him, "were really aggravated" with Petty, and they weren't the only ones. When she told cook-steward Mark Apollos about the incident after she got home, he reprimanded her: "You did a bad thing, Sister. The only good thief is a dead thief. You should never have stopped them."[22] Now realizing the danger in which she unhesitatingly put herself and anticipating her family's alarm, the twenty-six-year-old Petty boldly asserted in a letter to them that she was capable, careful, and intended to come home unharmed. "I can take care of myself," she closed. "I have *absolutely no* desire to be the first nurse martyr in Nigeria."[23] The unapologetic Matron remained a force to be reckoned with.[24]

Competitors

Although locals flocked to the COC Clinic, they probably did not fully abandon the native juju doctor, who worked in time-honored ways.[25] Most believed that the native doctor maintained constant communion with the spirit world that governed the lives of the living, and it was his "business to know what is to be done in every case." Even when people knew he was deceptive and seeking personal gain, they remained "afraid of his mysterious art."[26] When missionary medicine did not bring "magi-

[19]Petty to Span, November 3, 1966.

[20]Farrar, "Financial Report of Nigerian Christian Hospital, April 1—April 30th [1967], W-COC file.

[21]"Biographical Sketches" (Oparah), 205–06; Bryant, *Divine,* 275–76; Bryant, *Gently,* bk. 3, 137.

[22]Farrar and Petty-Kraus, Interview.

[23]Petty to Spann, November 3, 1966.

[24]P. Bryant to Mattoxes, January 17, 1967; Bryant and Bryant, Interview.

[25]Bohrer, "Narration;" Nnadi and Kabat, "Nigerians' Use."

[26]Nau, *We Move*, 181–82.

cal and instant cures," then locals assumed that "the white man's juju" was ineffective for blacks. Yet when missionary treatment brought healing, they assumed that the white man's "juju was just stronger than black man's juju."[27]

Unlike missionary health practitioners, native doctors proclaimed their omnipotence and never shared their secret knowledge. Thus while the NCH team might reasonably refer patients to experts, native doctors asserted they could treat everyone. And while missionaries sought to heal by scientific diagnosis and care, native doctors searched out who had bewitched, poisoned, or cast a spell on the patient; naming the culprit took priority over patient healing. Moreover, the cost and pain of treatments were evidence of their effectiveness, and exorbitant charges suggested that native remedies were powerful indeed.[28]

In contrast, missionaries worked to control pain,[29] and NCH billed only fourteen cents (roughly a third of a day's wages) to see the doctor, get a penicillin injection, or obtain forty aspirin.[30] Hays and Petty's personally paying those bills for the most destitute[31] must have seemed strange, and missionaries' willingness to teach all they knew about prevention and care perhaps surprised locals, who "eagerly snatched up" new learning.[32] Native doctors held on to their knowledge as power that created fear because fear created profit and job security. Better to die with knowledge than to share it, as Petty learned in encounters with an Umuahia native doctor, who was unwilling to reveal why his tetanus treatments produced better survival rates than did NCH care.[33]

Even COC preaching students were not immune to the appeal of expensive, traditional care. Although missionaries envisioned the NCH Clinic as a resource for Bible Training College (BTC) students,[34] it was not always their first choice. In one particularly tragic instance, the two-year-old daughter of a BTC student was irreversibly paralyzed from the neck down by a native doctor's injection that cost "10 times" more than missionary care. "They need so much teaching," Petty lamented.[35]

---

[27]G. Farrar to Mrs. H.C. Farrar, June 26, 1966.

[28]Bohrer, "Narration;" G. Farrar to Mrs. H.C. Farrar, June 26, 1966; Nau, *We Move*, 181–85.

[29]Farrar and Petty-Kraus, Interview; Hays-Savio, Interview.

[30]*Christian Chronicle*, "Hospital;" Farrar to Lafayette [sic] Church, September 21, 1965.

[31]Hays-Savio, Interview.

[32]G. Farrar to Johnson, June 5, 1965.

[33]Farrar and Petty-Kraus, Interview; Nau, *We Move*, 181.

[34]Lawyer, "Narrative," 37.

[35]Petty to Spann, July 13, 1966.

Conclusion

Nigerian surprise, amusement, skepticism, gratitude, anger, fatalism, and eagerness greeted the ways in which missionaries enacted their vision of a Christian clinic. As the missionaries cared for the vulnerable, faced down the powerful, and opened new doors of healing and knowledge, their mores and practices challenged traditional Nigerian ways. Meanwhile, an intrepid Matron Petty remained determined to achieve what she saw as good, right, and necessary.

22
Keeping the Mission Alive
(Fall 1965)

Dr. Farrar's health must be considered.
—Iris Hays

Dr. Henry Farrar was so impatient to open the Clinic during John Morgan's summer stay that he chalked up his own exhaustion, loss of appetite, low-grade fever, jaundice, and dark urine to stress, "tension, worry, and anxiety."[1] Nonetheless, just days before the Clinic admitted its first patients, Farrar begrudgingly admitted to "a light case" of serum hepatitis probably acquired from two infected physicians at the leprosarium in Itu.[2] Farrar convinced the Bryants that he was improving and told his wife, Grace, that he didn't have hepatitis—despite admitting symptoms to the contrary.[3]

By the time Morgan left on August 26[4] and the Clinic's first week ended, Farrar was worse. On Sunday morning, August 29, he stayed home as "the first time in 56 Lord's days for me not to preach," Farrar wrote to West End COC (W-COC), forgetting his Sunday, March 7 church absence because of malaria.[5] "I have a little infectious hepatitis," he confessed to his mother.[6] Nonetheless, he refused to rest and kept a rigorous Monday schedule; Hays's diary read simply, "We treated 133 patients in seven hours. Dr. Farrar thinks he is sick with viral hepatitis."[7] On Tues-

---

[1] Farrar, *Stand*, 88; G. Farrar to Johnson, September 13, 1965.

[2] P. Bryant to Mattoxes, August 18, 1965; Farrar to Mission Committee, August 3, 1965, W-COC file; H. Farrar to Morgans, September 5, 1965.

[3] R. Bryant to Massey and Lawyers, September 9, 1965; P. Bryant to Mattoxes, August 18, 1965; Farrar, *Stand*, 130–31; Petty-Kraus, Interview 1.

[4] G. Farrar to Johnson, September 13, 1965.

[5] Farrar to Mission Committee, September 1, 1965, *WEV*; G. Farrar to Johnson, March 7, 1965.

[6] H. Farrar to Mrs. H.C. Farrar, August 29, 1965.

[7] Hays-Savio, Interview.

day, Farrar could deny his situation no longer and sought diagnostic testing at the Port Harcourt (PH) Shell Oil Company Hospital Delta Clinic, where laboratory results were wholly conclusive: he had hepatitis. While he reported to W-COC that he would require four to six weeks of rest as the only available treatment, he told his wife and Morgans that he would need a mere two.[8]

Hays and Petty took charge. On Wednesday, before Farrar could arrive at the Clinic, the nurses closed it, telling over a hundred waiting patients[9] "to go home. The doctor is sick." The ill left, but refused referrals, preferring to wait for Farrar's return.[10] Then immediately, in a reversal of nurse-physician roles, Petty went from the Clinic to Farrar's house and forbade him to go to work. "He had bad hepatitis....yellow as a pumpkin...We didn't know if he was going to live." Without any patients to see an exhausted Farrar complied[11] and redeemed the day by writing his monthly report to the W-COC Mission Committee.[12] Grace Farrar became his private duty nurse,[13] and Dr. Farrar administered protective gamma globulin injections to her and their children.[14] He also wrote to John Morgan in the US, recommending that he be tested and receive gamma globulin as well.[15]

Meanwhile, the US nurses picked up the pace of their own work. On the same day Farrar tested positive for hepatitis,[16] Hays tested her nursing students for learning, and although Farrar failed at good health, four of Hays's six remaining students passed their first exam. Hays doubled her class time in order "to get ahead" and picked up Dr. Farrar's first-aid lectures to landowner children. "School, school, school," her diary read.[17] Petty wrote letters, lectured, and expanded her practice in the new, nurse-run, emergency-only Saturday morning clinic.[18] When one of her patients complained of swelling after her suture repair of his leg, a worried Petty consulted with Dr. Farrar. But when she removed the old bandage, she

---

[8]Farrar to Mission Committee, September 1 and October 4, 1965, *WEV*; G. Farrar to Johnson, September 13, 1965; H. Farrar to Morgans, September 5, 1965.
[9]Farrar to Mission Committee, September 1, 1965, *WEV*; Hays-Savio, Interview.
[10]Farrar, *Stand*, 88.
[11]Petty-Kraus, Interview 1.
[12]Farrar to Mission Committee, September 1, 1965, *WEV*.
[13]Farrar to Johnson, September 13, September 26, and October 18, 1965.
[14]G. Farrar to Johnson, September 13, 1965; Farrar to Mission Committee, September 1, 1965, *WEV*.
[15]H. Farrar to Morgans, September 5 and September 21, 1965.
[16]H. Farrar to Morgans, September 5, 1965.
[17]Hays-Savio, Interview.
[18]G. Farrar to Johnson, September 13, 1965; Petty to Spann, September 17, 1965.

found the man's wound healing well and thus diagnosed him as overly cautious. "That is the way it goes; they worry you too much, or they do not come soon enough," she sighed.[19]

After nineteen days of confinement, Dr. Farrar impatiently returned to Clinic practice on Monday, September 20. The missionary nurses' inability to keep him confined any longer and their own eagerness to resume work overcame any misgivings,[20] and the team treated fifty-seven patients in three hours on his first morning back—a feat that he proclaimed possible only because of Hays and Petty.[21] A still jaundiced Farrar now resumed Monday, Wednesday, Friday, and Saturday half-day clinics for about two weeks,[22] while Hays taught every afternoon. The nurses turned away waiting, "desperate" patients at noon, consoling themselves that this was necessary in order to keep Dr. Farrar, the Clinic, and their own work alive.[23] Despite his tiring quickly, Dr. Farrar reassured everyone that he was "getting stronger every day."[24] Nonetheless, he temporarily abandoned his beloved Sunday preaching in a prioritization of medical practice over sermons.[25]

Nurse Hays's concern that a recurrence of Farrar's hepatitis might force them all back to America was heightened on October 7 when the Clinic closed again because the doctor was "really sick."[26] Although his liver function tests were improved, he suffered from sinusitis, dizziness, fever, and weakness,[27] and now all Onicha Ngwa missionaries saw Dr. Farrar's refusal to rest as a danger to the entire hospital project. A frustrated Patti Bryant, whose own illness had sent the Bryants home prematurely in 1961 for three years, wrote home that Farrar "just *won't*...slow down & pace himself—thinks he's a superman or something. *Nothing* anyone says impresses him."[28] W-COC, too, recognized Farrar's hepatitis as a threat to the medical mission, and in that context gave his unique physician role ascendancy over his shared evangelistic one. Elders high-

---

[19]Petty to Spann, September 12, 1965.

[20]Hays-Savio, Interview.

[21]H. Farrar to Morgans, September 21, 1965.

[22]Ibid.; Farrar to Mission Committee, October 4, 1965, *WEV*; Hays-Savio, Interview.

[23]Hays-Savio, Interview.

[24]Farrar to Mission Committee, October 4, 1965, *WEV*.

[25]G. Farrar to Johnsons, September 26, 1965.

[26]Hays-Savio, Interview.

[27]G. Farrar to Betty and Carol Farrar, October 9, 1965.

[28]P. Bryant to Mattoxes, October 9, 1965; Bryant, *Divine*, 144–68.

lighted "the need for another doctor," and members sent numerous get-well letters.[29]

When Henry Farrar did stay home from clinic, rest was difficult. Grace Farrar and household staff constantly turned away people wanting to see him, and if any caught sight of him, they would yell into the house for his attention. Thus, Grace was delighted[30] when US relatives deposited $100 in the Farrars' discretionary account[31]—"the first time" the family received money for personal use—and she persuaded her husband to spend those funds on a family vacation. Hays "squealed with delight" as the nurses celebrated that monetary gift as God's answer to their prayers to make Dr. Farrar rest.[32]

Farrar consistently denied his need for vacations, but he could justify an Enugu trip to follow up on government review of COC hospital blueprints. Hays accompanied the Farrars to Enugu from October 12–16 so that she could share driving responsibilities with Henry.[33] In Enugu, she delighted in hot baths, "no mosquito nets," air conditioning, a trip to the zoo, and shopping at the British Kingsway department store. All enjoyed swimming, a pottery factory tour, and visits with the Keesee and Curry COC families.[34] Moreover, the working vacation paid off as Enugu's Regional Ministry of Health at last approved Nigeria's own preapproved hospital blueprints—after requiring Farrar to modify them. Farrar intended to modify them further still to his own preferences; he had thrown away his own blueprints.[35] Upon return to Onicha Ngwa, Grace Farrar recorded that her husband was "practically going full blast," and that he preached for the first Sunday in three months.[36]

By October's end Dr. Farrar had returned to his regular load "although...not *entirely* well," wrote a cautious Patti Bryant.[37] He enthused to W-COC that he preached twice in October, resulting in six baptisms and saw over one hundred patients a day during each of three Clinic days

---

[29]Elders, in Farrar to Mission Committee, October 4, 1965, *WEV*; G. Farrar to G.B. Farrars, September 26, 1965.

[30]G. Farrar to Johnson, October 18, 1965.

[31]Lauderdale to H. Farrar, September 28, 1965.

[32]G. Farrar to Johnson, October 18, 1965.

[33]Petty-Kraus, Interview 1; Farrar, "Travel Collins Diary," October 12–16, 1965.

[34]G. Farrar to Johnson, October 18, 1965; Hays-Savio, Interview.

[35]Farrar, *Stand*, 92; G. Farrar to Johnson, October 18, 1965; G. Farrar, personal communication, n.d.

[36]G. Farrar to Johnson, October 18, 1965.

[37]P. Bryant to Mattoxes, October 29, 1965.

per week. In the briefest of nods to his weariness and jaundice, he rejoiced that "the infectious hepatitis is on the way out of my own liver!"[38]

The next month, Dr. Farrar added back into his schedule both Queen Elizabeth Hospital (QEH) surgery and more distant preaching points. Petty wrote home on November 8 that NCH Clinic was back "in full swing" and their patient load was increasing; they treated 143 patients that day alone.[39] Many were critically ill, like the seizing postpartum woman brought five miles to the clinic propped up on the back of a bicycle.[40] The nurses were relieved that Dr. Farrar's strength was returning,[41] and Dr. Farrar labeled their work "marvelous." One Wednesday, he recorded that Hays administered "32 injections," including penicillin, chloroquine, diuretics, and vitamins. Moreover, under Petty and Hays's tutelage, auxiliary students were "doing excellent work."[42] Petty-apprenticed lay pharmacist Mark Peter also "exceeded…expectations."[43] Missionary nurses made the Clinic run, and its missionary physician applauded them.[44]

Conclusion

Afraid that Dr. Farrar's refusal to care for himself would undermine their own calling, Petty and Hays forced him out of his captain-of-the-ship role. Petty took the opportunity to expand her clinical practice, and Hays accelerated staff education. Soon his hepatitis led to a Farrar vacation that in turn facilitated both hospital blueprint approval and a new acknowledgement that his unique medical role was more critical to the mission than his shared evangelistic one. Farrar survived, Hays and Petty's work continued, and the missionaries' healthcare dreams moved forward.

[38]Farrar to Mission Committee, November 3, 1965, *WEV*.

[39]Petty to Spann, November 8, 1965.

[40]G. Farrar to G.B. Farrars, November 7, 1965.

[41]Hays-Savio, Interview; Petty to Spann, November 8, 1965.

[42]Farrars to Morgans, December 1965.

[43]Farrar and Petty-Kraus, Interview; H. Farrar to Morgans, October 27, 1965.

[44]H. Farrar, Interview 1; Hays-Savio and Petty-Kraus, Interview.

23

United By NCH

(October–November 1965)

It will take all of us.
—Patti Bryant

Not only did the Clinic survive Henry Farrar's 1965 health crisis, but Nigerian Christian Hospital (NCH) prospects thrived. Architectural blueprints for NCH inpatient units had been approved, landowners leased farmland to missionaries, and financial backers stepped forward. Concurrently, Onicha Ngwa preaching and teaching gained momentum with the September 22 arrival of the Underwood family: Ralph David (1928–2010) and Myra Louise Wade (1931–2019) Underwood, teenager Rebecca, preteen David, and eight-month-old Bryan.[1] Nancy Petty, who desperately missed her infant niece and preschool nephew, delighted in Bryan and joked that she should have thought to bring along a baby herself.[2]

David Underwood replaced Doug Lawyer as Bible Training College (BTC) principal, and the Underwood family moved into the Onicha Ngwa home that had been sequentially occupied by families of Nicks, Peden, Massey, Lawyer, and Morgan.[3] Grace Farrar enjoyed seeing the mission through Myra Underwood's fresh eyes,[4] and Rees Bryant happily relinquished BTC principal work to David, a handover that allowed Rees more time to help with NCH. Meanwhile, in reference to the missionaries' most-used antiseptic, Nancy Petty laughed at Bryan that a "germ-conscious…Myra was going to Dettol that baby to death."[5]

---

[1]*Huntsville*, "Ralph Underwood;" "Myra Underwood," January 1, 2018, findagrave.com no. 186285685; Farrar, *Stand*, 89.
[2]Petty to Spann, September 25, 1965.
[3]Bryant, *Divine*, 233; Farrar, *Stand*, 10.
[4]G. Farrar to G.B. Farrars, September 26, 1965.
[5]Bryant to Mattoxes, October 9, 1965; Petty, quoted in Bryant to Mattoxes, October 9, 1965.

Motives: Good and Bad

The day after the Farrars and Iris Hays returned from Enugu, bargaining over hospital land intensified.[6] Regional government approval of blue-prints was one thing, but local village politics was quite another, and ob-taining a land lease proved "a big job haunted with threats of failure right up to the very last thumbprint" on paper.[7] Doug Lawyer and Rees Bryant had already built a strong American-Igbo rapport, as illustrated in village men's teaching the royal greeting and kola nut ceremony to them—a rap-port that had resulted in a verbal agreement to lease farmland for NCH.[8] Translating that verbal assent into a legal contract, however, now required the best diplomatic skills of Bryant, BTC teacher J.O. Akandu, Dr. Farrar, and others.[9]

During earlier negotiations, Bryant had appealed to Igbos' love of drama and humor. When land-owning villages demanded a high price, Bryant "jumped up on the table and became the goose that laid the gold-en egg." Then when clan elders insisted as part of the deal that the mis-sionaries hire more of their own children regardless of examination scores, Bryant "threw himself on the floor," pretending to be sick and dying. He acted out what would happen to him under the care of "an ignorant nurse" and then under the care of "a good nurse."[10] Bringing the point home, Bryant asked if they wanted the most qualified person to care for them or "just somebody that happens to be the daughter of somebody that owns the land?...He'd have them all laughing and pretty soon they'd see the point," Patti Bryant chuckled.[11]

Now on October 17, the day before lease-signing, numerous local offi-cials visited the Farrar house throughout the day, examining every detail of the deed. Jealousy between two chiefs previously kept them from be-ing "in the same room at the same time," a necessary condition for the signing, and missionaries held their collective breath. Conversations were passionate. "Neither is a Christian," wrote Grace Farrar, "but if they

---

[6]G. Farrar to Johnson, October 18, 1965.

[7]P. Bryant to Mattoxes, October 29, 1965.

[8]Bryant and Bryant, Interview; Bryant, *Divine*, 244–45; Farrar, *Stand*, 93; Lawyer to Farrar, February 25, 1964. Lawyer letter includes his sketches of contiguous hospital land, COC compound buildings and clinic buildings.

[9]P. Bryant to Mattoxes, October 9, 1965; R. Bryant to Masseys and Lawyers, September 9, 1965; H. Farrar to Morgans, October 4, 1965.

[10]P. Bryant to Mattoxes, October 9, 1965.

[11]Bryant and Bryant, Interview.

meet…to sign over land for a Christian cause, then we can say that Christianity has brought them together in a way that nothing else could."[12]

Uncertainty prevailed late into that night. Nlagu village elders made last-minute demands for money and employment, prompting Henry Farrar and Rees Bryant to go out to them in the villages.[13] Emmanuel Onuoha, the Bryants' cook, and Effiong, the Underwoods' yardman, also trekked "all night…from house to house trying to persuade" them to agree, and Patti Bryant speculated that the chiefs and elders finally relented so they could "get some sleep."[14]

The drama continued the next day. In order to make sure that everyone arrived on time, Rees Bryant rented a bus to gather all signatories for their appointment with the lawyer and the divisional officer in Aba. One chief insisted that the bus pick him up from his doorstep and emerged only after earnest, honest persuasion that the path to his house was too narrow for the vehicle. Consequently, by the time the group arrived in Aba, the lawyer had gone home, and someone had to fetch him. Even after signing commenced, one leader became so angry at seeing the name of his brother ahead of his own on the deed that "several minutes of loud palaver" ensued before he would finally press his inked thumb to the page.[15]

And so it was that finally on October 18, 1965, a ninety-nine-year lease was signed for 119.4 acres at £24 per year[16] with a renewal option of ninety years. The deed committed missionaries to build a hospital and staff housing worth £15,000 on the land within ten years. Twenty-four village leaders confirmed their agreement with their nineteen thumbprints and five signatures representing "themselves and…the people of Nlagu, Umuwoma, and Ntigha villages of Onicha Ngwa." Dr. Farrar and the three registered trustees of the Church of Christ (Eno Otoyo,

---

[12]G. Farrar to Johnson, October 18, 1965.

[13]Bryant and Bryant, Interview.

[14]P. Bryant to Mattoxes, October 9, 1965.

[15]Bryant, *Divine*, 246.

[16]The official £24/year was higher than the original figure of £19/year cited in three sources: R. Bryant to Elders, South Park COC, August 9, 1965; Bryant, *Divine*, 246; and Bryant and Bryant Interview.

John Beckloff, and Rees Bryant) signed as witnesses.[17] Only divine intervention could explain this event, wrote Henry Farrar,[18] and Patti Bryant grew poetic: "Failure was so close…Somehow God has brought all these diverse elements together to accomplish his purposes. Chiefs that don't ordinarily speak to each other have cooperated. Competing villages have joined hands and…pagan chiefs have surrendered to an overall plan… [from] motives both good and bad."[19]

States: Texas and Tennessee

Fall 1965 brought other good news as two large COCs joined hands in financial support of NCH. The missionaries already received frequent individual[20] and group donations for NCH, but neither W-COC nor any other congregation had committed to oversight of and fundraising for NCH. Happily in September, Green Lawn COC elders, including F.W. Mattox, accepted the responsibility,[21] and on November 12, they ran a roughly half-page fundraising advertisement in the *Christian Chronicle* (Central Oklahoma Edition, 11). A black-and-white photograph of Henry Farrar with an open Bible alongside a Nigerian child painted white to ward off illness displayed a small corner caption: "Help Dr. Farrar Save Lives and Souls: Nigerians Donated Land. Building Needed," followed by an address for contributions. Almost every page of that *Chronicle* edition contained Nigeria-related articles, touting the historical success of evangelism in Nigeria and plans for the medical mission. A picture of Nancy Petty and Iris Hays in their nurses' caps and white uniforms flanking Dr. Farrar in his shirt and tie highlighted a piece on Nigeria's need for healthcare professionals (4).

---

[17]Indenture of Lease. Survey attached and signatories from top to bottom and left to right on the lease: Chief Thomas Nwaulu, Onyeike Efuribe, Daniel Nwaulu, Nwagbarar Amonye, Ota Nna, Ikonne Amata, Dickson Ikonne, Okpokoro Nwosu, Ahukanna Nwoko, Benson Nwogrugru, Awaziama Ngwogu, Nwabeke Atuegwu, Samuel Nwakpuka Dimkpa Atuegwu, Chief Thomas Ebere [signature], Dick Ebere, Paul Egege, David Ebere [signature], Samuel Inyama, Nwaonu Mgbokwo [signature], Shadrack Agbasonu [signature], Mark Nwoke, Micah Nwaonu [signature], and Rufus Nwogu. HGF (copy).

[18]H. Farrar to Morgans, October 27, 1965.

[19]P. Bryant to Mattoxes, October 9, 1965.

[20]P. Bryant to Joe Mattoxes, April 11, 1965.

[21]Farrar to Mission Committee, October 4, 1965, *WEV*; Green Lawn, *Nigerian Evangelism*. More details from W-COC file: Bergstrom to Benson, January 27, 1965; Bergstrom to Mattox, July 15 and September 24, 1965; Massey, "Green Lawn;" Mattox to Lauderdale, September 15, 1965; Minutes, Elders Meeting, May 17, 1965; Thweat to Mattox, June 11, 1965.

From Tennessee W-COC threw its fundraising support for NCH behind Green Lawn COC in Texas. Seemingly confident that member donations for the Hospital would not affect W-COC's budget, its elders more than once published a call to send hospital funds to Green Lawn.[22] The $32,000 needed for hospital construction is an "everlasting investment…saving lives, to save souls for eternity," W-COC leaders proclaimed to congregants.[23] They seemed pleased that others were building a hospital for their preaching physician.

From Nigeria Dr. Farrar delighted in this Nashville-Lubbock partnership. Having grown up in the shadow of sharp, post-Civil War, doctrinal differences between COC congregations in the two states, he found it "very encouraging…a wonderful commentary…that churches in Texas and Tennessee can work together" in renewed harmony.[24] Individual missionaries from Texas and Tennessee already did so in Onicha Ngwa.

Americans: Black and White

October 1965 also saw the first recorded financial support from a black-led US COC for the white-led medical mission. That month African American preacher Francis Frank "F.F." Carson (1909–1987) made his second evangelistic trip to Nigeria accompanied by his wife, Wilma E. Carson, and a Mrs. (possibly Faye, also Mrs. Hugh[25]) Taylor from the Carsons' Southside COC congregation in Richmond, California.[26] Accompanying them was Levi A. Kennedy Jr. (1899–1970), preacher for the "largest," black US congregation, Michigan Avenue COC in Chicago.[27] During the mid-1950s, Eno Otoyo and others had persuaded F.F. Carson to engage in Nigerian missions; Otoyo was then a student at the historically black Southwestern Christian College in Terrell, Texas.[28]

---

[22]Farrar to Mission Committee, October 4 and November 3, 1965 and June 4, 1966, *WEV*.
[23]Elders to Members, November 3, 1965, *WEV*.
[24]Farrar to Mission Committee, October 4, 1965, *WEV*. For more on Texas-Tennessee conflict, see Williams et al., *Stone-Campbell*, Chapters 5 and 8.
[25]Southside, "Financial."
[26]P. Bryant to Mattoxes, October 29, 1965; G. Farrar to Johnson, October 18, 1965; Eno Otoyo, email to author, July 1, 2017; Silvey, "Richmond's F.F. Carson."
[27]Farrar to Mission Committee, November 3, 1965, *WEV*; "Levi Kennedy, Jr.," June 28, 2011, findagrave.com no. 72180098. The discontinued webpage of Dr. David C. Penn—Robbins Church of Christ documented that Michigan Avenue COC is now Sheldon Heights COC, Google search (accessed July 1, 2018).
[28]Eno Otoyo, email to author, July 1, 2017.

Carson convinced Kennedy to travel with him to Nigeria in 1962 and now again in 1965 in the place of Richard Nathaniel "R.N." Hogan, the preacher at Figueroa COC in Los Angeles, who was reluctant to fly.[29] During their first trip, Carson and Kennedy baptized 650 Nigerians and established twenty-seven congregations,[30] and by January 1965 Carson was committed to financial support of COC medical mission facilities in Onicha Ngwa or Abak. He and Dr. Farrar corresponded,[31] and before Carson's 1965 visit Grace Farrar recorded that he had sent $675 for NCH, raised during only "1 night speaking before colored brethren in California."[32]

The Carsons, Kennedy, and Taylor spent twelve days in Ukpom and three weeks in Onicha Ngwa.[33] During that time, F.F. Carson attended the lease-signing for NCH land[34] and announced that he and the Southside COC in California would raise $40,000 for NCH.[35] Carson and Southside were already mission pioneers as "perhaps the first...predominantly black church supporting a white missionary," Tom Tune, in Hong Kong,[36] and Levi Kennedy soon pleaded for "men of my race" to go to Nigeria.[37] They stood in contrast to a sometimes otherwise limited involvement of black US COCs in foreign missions.[38]

Onicha Ngwa missionaries were delighted with Carson's decision, and he seemed pleased when told of Green Lawn COC's commitment to gather funds. Believing that "the more people working for the hospital, the better" and in "all of us working together," the missionaries encouraged Carson to meet with Green Lawn leaders after returning to the US. Perhaps momentarily forgetting John Morgan's Clinic experience, Patti Bryant wrote to her father, F.W. Mattox, suggesting that Green Lawn issue a speaking invitation to F.F. Carson, as the first US visitor to see "the clinic in operation."[39] Yet, despite these efforts, Southside and Green Lawn COCs continued contributing significantly but independently to

---

[29]"Richard Hogan," October 12, 2009, findagrave.com no. 42989652; Eno Otoyo, email to author, July 1, 2017.
[30]Kennedy, "Greetings;" Martin, "Nigeria Missionaries."
[31]Eno Otoyo, email to author, July 1, 2017.
[32]G. Farrar to Carol and Betty Farrar, October 9, 1965.
[33]G. Farrar to Johnson, October 18, 1965.
[34]Mattox, "Nigerian Hospital."
[35]P. Bryant to Keesee, September 14, 1965; P. Bryant to Mattoxes, October 29, 1965; H. Farrar to Morgans, October 27, 1965.
[36]"Biographical Information;" Silvey, "Richmond's F.F. Carson."
[37]Kennedy, "Greetings."
[38]Hooper, *Distinct*, 279.
[39]P. Bryant to Mattoxes, October 29, 1965.

the Hospital.[40] Perhaps each congregation shied away from directing their contributors elsewhere and valued controlling their own affairs, or perhaps Carson and Southside wanted to avoid the all-too-prevalent COC pattern of white paternalism.[41] Whatever the case, Southside and Green Lawn congregations each sent thousands of dollars to fund NCH.[42]

The Hospital project no doubt also benefited from US black evangelist Marshall Keeble's earlier theological support. Keeble first visited Nigeria for seventeen days in summer 1960 with Lucien Palmer, dean of Michigan Christian College and former Ukpom Bible Training College (BTC) principal. During that visit, Keeble preached, met with village leaders, and taught in BTC classes, open-air markets, and village schools.[43] Despite some white COC missionaries' self-confessed and later-repented concerns about how Nigerians might receive an African-American preacher, Keeble drew scores of Nigerians who came to hear the missionary that "looks like us,"[44]—a phenomenon that Carson and Kennedy also experienced.[45] "Some of his illustrations were not understood," Patti Bryant wrote, "but Bro. Keeble, the man, the spirit, the message, crashed right through the wall of differences…They loved him."[46]

In 1962 Keeble made his second visit to Nigeria, accompanied by Palmer and Houston Ezell, a contractor and Vultee COC elder in Nashville.[47] Many Nigerians wept because they were so moved that Keeble as a black American of advanced age would "care enough about them to" return. They begged him to bring a hospital to them, and Keeble responded that "he would see about it." Although Ezell told Keeble this meant he would "build them one," and "Palmer and Ezell tried to get Keeble to go easy on that point…it didn't do much good," and soon Keeble was promoting the hospital idea among US COCs.[48] He was now convinced that healthcare delivery was necessary to fulfill the commands

[40]P. Bryant, email to author, May 23, 2017; *Christian Chronicle,* "Three Facets;" Mattox, Nigerian Hospital.

[41]Robinson, "Conversation with."

[42]Farrar to Mission Committee, September 1 and October 4, 1965, December 27, 1966, January 20 and June 8, 1967, *WEV.*

[43]Choate, *Roll,* 128–34; Goff, *Great,* 45.

[44]P. Bryant to Mattoxes, July 16, 1960.

[45]Martin, "Nigeria Missionaries."

[46]P. Bryant to Mattoxes, July 16, 1960.

[47]Goff, *Great,* 51–52.

[48]Choate, *Roll,* 136, 138.

of Jesus. "The first parts of our commission," Keeble observed, are to preach and teach, but the church is also responsible "to heal."[49]

Conclusion

Progress toward NCH united many. The coming together of Petty and Hays as "the nurses" and their subsequent relationships with Nigerian women represented important alliances. Now chiefs and landowners, animists and Christians, Texas and Tennessee congregations, Nigerians and Americans, black and white joined hands to provide financial, material, and theological support for the Hospital. Onicha Ngwa missionaries rejoiced.

---

[49]Keeble, quoted in Robinson, *Godsend*, 100.

24

Out with the Old; In with the New

(December 1965–January 1966)

"Here We Are But Straying Pilgrims"
—Nancy Petty

The turn of the year was a time of change. Empty Nigerian Christian Hospital (NCH) construction coffers filled, emptied, and refilled. Buildings rose from farmland, and a military coup d'état rattled the country. As these events swirled around them, Iris Hays found a home in Nigeria, and Nancy Petty longed more than ever for her US one.

Manna

Nigerians hand-cleared Hospital land with hoes and machetes, and missionaries anticipated gratis construction help from contractors Houston Ezell and John Dedman. Beginning in November, the two supervised construction at the Nigerian Christian Secondary School (NCSS) in Ukpom and stood ready to assist with building the Hospital if Onicha Ngwa missionaries could pay for materials.[1] Unfortunately, NCH cash on hand totaled $2.75.[2] Rees Bryant penned an urgent plea for funds on the morning of December 10 to F.W. Mattox: Please borrow $5,000—to be paid back from Green Lawn COC's NCH fundraising—and please ask West End (W-COC) to solicit funds. "The land is ours. The need is here. Doctors and nurses have come. Now we need MONEY for buildings." Onicha Ngwa missionaries themselves, he wrote, had "advanced NCH £300 ($1,000.00)" from their campus congregation. Pledges were appreciated, but cash was essential.[3]

---

[1] R. Bryant to Mattoxes, December 10, 1965(A); G. Farrar to Johnson, October 18, 1965; H. Farrar to Morgans, December 9, 1965.
[2] H. Farrar to Morgans, December 9, 1965.
[3] R. Bryant to Mattoxes, December 10, 1965(A).

Mattox's response was quicker than anyone expected. When David Underwood returned from mailing Bryant's request in the Aba Post Office, he brought back with him a just-arrived letter from Mattox containing a $2,500 check for NCH. Bryant celebrated in his second letter to Mattox that day: "I wish you could see the rejoicing on this compound!!" "Like *manna*," Patti Bryant biblically described this infusion of just-in-time dollars,[4] and a delighted Henry Farrar immediately drove to Ukpom to recruit Ezell.[5] He found Ezell and Dedman still occupied with NCSS work, and so Onicha Ngwa missionaries decided to proceed with their previous plans for Rees Bryant to serve as contractor for the maternity and kitchen-laundry structures.[6] Bryant possessed Nigerian construction experience, including the Lawyer/Farrar house.

Immediately, however, a zealous, take-charge Dr. Farrar began countermanding Bryant by directing workers himself, and the dismayed Bryants decided privately that soft-spoken Rees must talk "faster...louder and longer than Henry." This Rees Bryant did, although it was "quite outside his comfort zone," insisting that either he would do the job without Dr. Farrar or Farrar could do it without him. The strategy worked, and trust was restored, leading to Patti Bryant's conclusion that Farrar's combined strong will and humility were "perfect...for building a hospital from nothing."[7] Goodwill returned.

December's construction began,[8] and buildings grew "slowly but surely,"[9] block by block under Rees Bryant's direction alongside foreman Anthony Agali. Missionaries hoped to finish external walls of all seven Hospital buildings before the spring rainy season began,[10] and Dr. Farrar appealed to W-COC for additional funds, declaring that everything could "easily be finished by the end of 1966 as the Lord provides the money."[11]

---

[4]Bryant, *Divine*, 247.
[5]R. Bryant to Mattoxes, December 10, 1965(B).
[6]Bryant, *Divine*, 247–49; P. Bryant to Joe Mattoxes, May 24, 1965.
[7]Bryant, *Divine*, 248.
[8]Farrar to Mission Committee, January 1, 1965 [sic], *WEV*. Correct citation year is 1966.
[9]H. Farrar to G.B Farrars, January 31, 1966.
[10]Bryant, *Divine*, 248–49; Farrar to Mission Committee, March 16, 1966, *WEV*.
[11]Farrar to Mission Committee, January 1, 1965 [sic], *WEV*.

Missionary Identity

During this time, Iris Hays consolidated her identity as a missionary in her own and others' eyes. Colleague Rees Bryant lauded Hays to her supporters without mentioning nursing.

> Dear Brethren, I am writing you to commend you for sending Sister Iris Hays to Nigeria and for supporting the outstanding work she is doing here. I think Iris is one of the finest missionaries we have ever had on this field. She is a hard worker. She is dedicated and capable. She is unselfish and generous to those who are in need. Her sweet personality and unselfish service make it a real joy to serve with her on the same compound…You can take justifiable pride in the way that she is representing you and Christ in this place.[12]

Hays, too, conscious of her transformation to missionary, remembered one African evening "sitting on the front porch…[with] such a feeling of contentment, satisfaction, joy, happiness. 'Well, Iris, after all those years

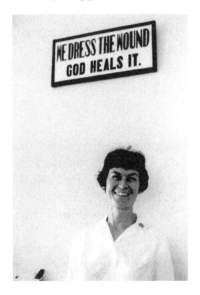

Photograph 24. Iris Hays, RN,
under posted motto at NCH. ca.
1966. (Author collection).

---

[12]R. Bryant to College Avenue Church of Christ, December 15, 1965.

of work…you are here. You finally made it!"' Her African dreams, family background, and the team's warm welcome made Nigeria the place she most wanted to be.[13]

In contrast, Nancy Petty's missionary identity remained more tentative, and the Christian hymn "Here We Are But Straying Pilgrims" expressed her lingering sense of being a stranger in a strange land. During the nurses' first Nigerian Christmas (1965), an ambivalent Petty, who was recovering from malaria,[14] especially missed her "wonderful home" and close-knit family. She remembered Christmas as "a big deal at home"[15] and reassured her family that her Christmas was good, too,[16] by filling an aerogram letter with cheery holiday details, denials of homesickness, and declarations of love for them. The nurses on Christmas eve were "just as excited as the smallest child" as Onicha Ngwa missionaries "sang every Christmas song they knew"[17] and watched the missionary children's self-produced, nativity play.[18] On Christmas morning, cook-steward Mark Apollos and the nurses exchanged gifts, and the Onicha Ngwa missionaries visited each other's houses, which "looked just like America" with wrapping paper from opened gifts strewn everywhere. Then all except the Farrars traveled to visit the isolated John and Dottie Beckloff family in Ikot Usen for more gift-giving and a potluck dinner with US families from all three southeastern Nigeria COC compounds.[19] "One of my best Christmasses," Petty wrote home of that rare day without work. Yet she wept over time missed with preschool nephew John.[20]

New Year

January 1966 marked a transition to the nurses' only twelve-month calendar year in Nigeria. Hays, Petty, and the Bryants greeted the new year with an Enugu vacation, while the Farrars and Underwoods celebrated with a Port Harcourt (PH) trip and firecrackers. Grace Farrar covered one day of clinic work for the nurses during their Enugu trip—her first

---

[13]Hays-Savio and Petty-Kraus, Interview.

[14]Ibid.; Petty to Spann, December 8, 1965.

[15]Hays-Savio and Petty-Kraus, Interview.

[16]Petty-Kraus, phone call to author, July 6, 2015.

[17]Petty to Spann, December 29, 1965.

[18]Ibid.; Author's recollection; Untitled photographs of nativity play, Bryant house, December 24, 1965, AUTH.

[19]R. Bryant to Mattoxes, December 10, 1965(A); G. Farrar to Folks, January 1, 1966; Petty to Spann, December 29, 1965.

[20]Petty to Spann, December 29, 1965.

time to give direct care beyond her backdoor in twelve years—and the experience reminded her how much more she enjoyed home and home-schooling.[21] Annual, dry Harmattan winds distributed fine Sahara sand across West Africa, and Grace Farrar reveled in the change to cooler air. For many others, however, the dust triggered miserable asthma and upper respiratory infections.[22]

A change in the compound staff also came with the new year. The Far-rars' steward, Monday John Akpakpan, whom Grace Farrar called "the sweetest, most dedicated Christian I ever met and…a symbol of all we have accomplished here,"[23] graduated as valedictorian from the Onicha Ngwa Bible Training College (BTC) and began secondary school at Ukpom's NCSS.[24] Americans of all ages loved energetic, cheerful Mon-day,[25] and as Petty observed, "a lot of sunshine" left the compound with his departure.[26] She and her US family sent him £2/month for food after she learned that Monday John was going hungry in order to pay his younger siblings' school fees; the Farrars and their relatives helped with his tuition.[27] Meanwhile, Grace Farrar's workload rose as she oriented Monday's replacement, steward Clement Ahiakwo—a BTC student rec-ommended by Monday for the job.[28]

Political change came, too, in a violent military coup d'état. A combina-tion of twentieth-century British land amalgamation in 1914 and gover-nance that favored some religio-ethnic groups over others ensured Nige-ria's foundation was built on historically divided tribal loyalties, not na-tional identity.[29] Thus, post-independence conflicts grew between people in Nigeria's four regions: East (majority Igbo), West (majority Yoruba), North (majority Hausa-Fulani), and the smallest Mid-West (majority mi-nority). The outcome was a January 15, 1966, coup that began what Igbo intellectual Chinua Achebe called "The Dark Days,"[30] and triggered a

---

[21]G. Farrar to Morgans, January 16, 1966.

[22]G. Farrar to Folks, January 1, 1966.

[23]G. Farrar to G.B. Farrars, January 24, 1965.

[24]G. Farrar to G.B. Farrars, January 5, 1966; G. Farrar to Johnsons, August 23, 1966.

[25]Author's recollection; Farrar, *Stand*, 100; Joyce Massey, email to author, March 11, 2018.

[26]G. Farrar to Folks, January 3, in January 1, 1966.

[27]Farrar, *Stand*, 95; G. Farrar to G.B. Farrars, January 5, 1966; G. Farrar to Wiemhoffs, January 22, 1967; Petty to Spann, February 15 and March 8, 1966.

[28]Farrar, *Stand*, 95.

[29]Madiebo, *Nigerian Revolution*, 3–5.

[30]Achebe, *There Was*, 65.

shift in Henry Farrar's prayers for peace in Vietnam to gratitude for US prayers for peace in Nigeria.[31]

The coup began when a group of mostly Igbo, junior army officers, who represented the unhappiness of many with government corruption, vote rigging, and Northern dominance, overthrew Nigeria's citizen government. Rebels murdered perhaps fifty prominent officials, whose bodies were found in shallow graves and beside the roads, and Major Chukwuma Nzeogwu took power in the northern city of Kaduna. Quickly, however, in a relatively smooth transition of power from Nzeogwu, military command unified in Lagos under Igbo-born, Northern-raised Army Commander Maj. Gen. Johnson T.U. Aguiyi-Ironsi,[32] who gained swift backing from conspirators, army units, political groups, students, youth groups, labor unions, and self-preserving politicians. Concurrently, Northerners seethed at the rise of this Southerner whom they saw as a threat to their own dominance. Nonetheless, his ascendency ushered in calls for an end to months of ongoing riots in the West, and the *West African Pilot* newspaper articulated widespread public optimism: "This great country has every reason to be proud of the military which has taken over the fumbling feudal and neo-colonialist regime. Today independence, which is said to have been granted by the British five years ago, is really won."[33]

The "emergence of a new Nigeria free from corruption, tribalism and nepotism" was widely and prematurely celebrated throughout Nigeria.[34] In an effort to maintain Nigeria's unity, Aguiyi-Ironsi centralized power "to restore law and order,"[35] revoked the constitution, and eliminated civilian offices. Additionally, he appointed dynamic young military leaders in each region, including the assignment of thirty-three-year-old Igbo Lt. Col. Chukwuemeka Odumegwu Ojukwu to the East.[36]

Igbo and missionary hopes soared that Ojukwu would put all things right, despite Ojukwu's labeling expectations of "miracles overnight [… as] our greatest enemy."[37] Missionaries saw gasoline prices drop, inordinate postal customs recede, and NCH government hospital approval gain

---

[31]Farrar to Mission Committee, January 1, 1965 [sic], *WEV*; Farrar to Mission Committee, February 7, 1966, *WEV*.

[32]Garrison, "Power;" Madiebo, *Nigerian Revolution*, 18–28; *Time*, "The World."

[33]Garrison, "Army;" Garrison, "Power;" Ojukwu, *Biafra*, 1–3; *West African Pilot*, quoted in Garrison, "Power."

[34]Madiebo, Nigerian Revolution, 27.

[35]Garrison, "Army."

[36]Garrison, "Army;" Reuters, "Nigeria Army Chief;" Garrison, "New Dynamism;" Madiebo, *Nigerian Revolution*, 26.

[37]Garrison, "New Dynamism."

speed.[38] Yet they were unable to recruit Ojukwu's help in connecting NCH to existing power lines. In a brief encounter at Nwaigwe Police Station near NCH, Ojukwu told Rees Bryant that prayers were Nigeria's greatest need, shook the missionary children's hands, and ran his fingers through five-year-old Lee Farrar's shock of white hair.[39] Subsequently, Lee began all his prayers with what he thought most important: petitions for God to help the family's pet genet and "the new military governor."[40] (The genet was a small, ring-tailed, nocturnal, cat-like mammal sold to them by locals.)

International optimism rose. US newspapers reported that the military government ran smoothly[41] and highlighted Aguiyi-Ironsi's three goals: "to stamp out corruption, to expose those who indulged in it, and to re-chart Nigeria's economic planning."[42] Spring 1966 saw many former officials tried, convicted, and stripped of property that was liquidated "for the good of the people."[43] COC missionaries worked unhindered within the new government context as they had within the old.[44]

Missionaries at Onicha Ngwa received most of their news from *Voice of America* radio and universally wrote home reassuring families that negative fallout from the coup d'état seemed confined to Nigeria's West and North.[45] Using the post-independence Congo uprising as a benchmark for anti-white sentiment and the Peace Corps as their barometer of safety, Dr. Farrar wrote to his brother and W-COC elder, George Farrar, that their prayers were keeping the East calm, the Peace Corps planned to stay, a central Nigerian government was in control, and local law and order were unchanged.[46] A concurring Grace Farrar penned that missionaries lived in the most politically stable of Nigeria's seemingly "three separate countries" of North, West, and East,[47] and former missionary Jim Massey in the US downplayed the coup as national "growing pains," free from animosity to whites, and with a Lagos epicenter hundreds of miles

[38]G. Farrar to Johnson, May 17, 1966; Shannon, "Indefinite."

[39]Bryant, *Divine*, 261–62; G. Farrar to Johnson, April 10, 1966.

[40]G. Farrar to Johnson, April 10, 1966.

[41]Garrison, "Idealistic;" Shannon, "Indefinite."

[42]*Chicago Defender*, "Nigeria."

[43]G. Farrar to G.B. Farrars, March 27, 1966.

[44]Bryant, *Divine*; Farrar, *Stand*.

[45]Bryant to Mattoxes, January 17, 1966; G. Farrar to G.B. Farrars, January 16, 1966; G. Farrar to Johnson, February 13, 1966; H. Farrar to G.B. Farrars, January 31, 1966; Petty to Spann, January 21, 1966.

[46]H. Farrar to G.B. Farrars, January 1, 1966; Farrar to Mission Committee, February 7, 1966, *WEV*.

[47]G. Farrar to G.B. Farrars, January 16, 1966.

from Onicha Ngwa.[48] Concurrently, Petty reassured concerned Igbo neighbors that Nigerians were not angry with whites, and to family she declared the overthrown as interested in "lining their own pockets" and the coup "for the best."[49]

A hopeful Henry Farrar speculated that firm military rule might even be good for Christian evangelism by creating national stability with more opportunities to spread the faith in the mainly Muslim North.[50] And he wondered in surprisingly nondemocratic terms whether Nigerians might not be better off under a benevolent authoritarian regime than under "self-rule." The new leaders, Farrar opined in Cold War era terms, were patriotic, "not Castro-like…[and they wanted to save] their country from dishonest politicians." Still, he noted, "the turn of events cannot always be predicted."[51]

Conclusion

The new year brought change within change. In Onicha Ngwa, Hays's missionary identity, team relationships, funding, and Hospital buildings advanced. National upheaval seemed far away and, despite some uncertainty, missionaries anticipated that the new government might be better for Christian evangelism, for their Hospital, and for Nigeria itself.

---

[48]Massey, "Nigerian Disturbance."
[49]Petty to Spann, January 21, 1966.
[50]Farrar to Mission Committee, February 7, 1966, *WEV*.
[51]H. Farrar to G.B. Farrars, February 7, 1966.

25

Walls Up; Missionaries Down; Nigeria Uncertain

(February–June 1966)

> The Lord used a lot of our mistakes.
> —Rees Bryant

Missionaries moved forward with their plans for NCH as a scaled-down version of Queen Elizabeth Hospital (QEH) in Umuahia. QEH was a low-cost, British-originated hospital,[1] and Henry Farrar was initially impressed by its collaborative funding from the local government, regional government, Church of England, Scottish Presbyterian Church, and Methodist Church. QEH, too, benefited from expatriate volunteers like US Peace Corpsman Irwin Cohen, who established a blood bank, and John Garland, a Scottish senior medical student, who set up a bacteriology lab.[2]

"Hospitals here go out, not up," observed Grace Farrar,[3] and such were plans for NCH. Land was more plentiful than money, and the single-story QEH consumed expansive acreage in order "to offer the most care to the most people at the smallest expense." The campus was a sprawling maze of concrete block buildings with abundant geckos, cement floors, and corrugated metal roofing all connected by paved, covered walkways. Inpatient areas included several multi-bed open wards alongside ancillary buildings for laboratory, pharmacy, X-ray, kitchen, and clinic. The operating room held two tables employed simultaneously by physicians using "general anesthesia...where necessary; spinal anesthesia...when possible." QEH buildings also included student and staff housing with unscreened windows "in the English tradition."[4]

---

[1]H. Farrar, Interview 1; Farrar, "Heroes" Interview.
[2]Morgan, "Report," 14–15.
[3]G. Farrar to Wiemhoffs, January 22, 1967.
[4]Morgan, "Report," 15, 17.

Visiting COC medical student John Morgan wrote of QEH as "modern by Nigerian standards" with a nursing school and an annual workload of "about 7,000 inpatients, 150,000 outpatients, 6,000 operations, and 2,000 deliveries" handled by six physicians alongside numerous nursing students and staff. Morgan classified outpatients into two groups, similar to those he would see at NCH before his departure: those with less threatening headaches, fever, and malaria and the seriously ill who should have received care "months or years earlier."[5]

Morgan also contrasted QEH with two other hospitals. The first, "the most modern hospital facility in the Eastern Region," was "the orthopedic unit at the government hospital in Enugu....built by [expatriate organization] Medico, and...staffed by [volunteer] American and Canadian orthopedic surgeons on a rotational basis."[6] The second in Aba was a private, physician-owned, two-story, concrete structure surrounding a muddy courtyard where families cooked over an open fire. The narrow stairs, bed coverings, shared hospital room, and the one nurse's uniform were "dirty." Beds were "split bamboo without any sort of mattress or padding," and the three unscreened windows in a room with five postoperative women were not enough to rid the space of its "foul, musty odor."[7]

The COC team had no funds for a Medico-like hospital and no stomach for the Aba-like one. QEH best matched COC resources and ideals. Unlike QEH, however, NCH would be self-supporting, begin with fewer beds, and have neither nursing school nor collaborative funding. Staffing would start with one physician, two expatriate RNs, a few Nigerian Registered Nurses (NRNs), and a small cadre of ancillary staff who had been educated in-house. NCH buildings, connected by covered walkways, would be similar.[8]

Walls Up

In February 1966 contractors Houston Ezell and John Dedman finally arrived to supervise significant NCH construction over three days, while

---

[5]Ibid, 14–15.

[6]Ibid, 13. According to Spray's *Nigeria Orthopedic Project*, expatriates established Medico in 1962, it became affiliated with Cooperative for American Relief Everywhere (CARE), and its last expatriate to Nigeria before the Nigeria-Biafra conflict was Dr. Douglas MacInnis of Encino, California, in February 1967.

[7]Ibid, 13–14; Morgan, "John's Journal," June 11, 1965.

[8]G. Farrar to G.B. Farrars, March 27, 1966.

their wives sewed clothing for each Onicha Ngwa missionary.[9] Thirty construction workers almost completed the maternity ward and started the men's ward and laundry-kitchen buildings before Ezell and Dedman left for the US with plans to return in October.[10] Unfortunately, in his haste, Ezell laid the men's ward foundation as slightly trapezoid not square, a problem that Rees Bryant discovered later during ceiling tile installation. Remediation was impossible, and an amused Bryant reflected on God and missionaries that "the Lord used a lot of our mistakes and corrected them and went on; and let us go on."[11]

Missionaries hoped to open at least one inpatient unit within months, and US construction funds arrived erratically. In February, the team received $7,000 from an estate bequest[12] that was almost exhausted by April 4; six days later, another $1,000 arrived to missionary rejoicing and more construction.[13] Inflation increasingly devoured funds, but every time money ran low, more funds always seemed to be waiting in the Aba post office.[14] Construction was mostly paid for as it was completed.

The first building finished on hospital land was a staff house that was promptly occupied on May 2 by novice missionaries and young, new college graduates, Raymond "Ray" Leonard and Charlotte Ann Green Lanham, friends of missionary Mike King in Ukpom.[15] Prior to the Lanhams' arrival, COC missionaries had not known what the self-recruited Lanhams would do or where they would live, but Ray soon engaged with NCH construction and Charlotte provided secretarial support and children's Bible classes.[16] Their move into the new house, a home perhaps ultimately intended for a missionary physician,[17] reduced their miles-long, daily commute from other COC compounds to a short walk, and Rees Bryant and Ray Lanham divided construction oversight. Lanham took on the more nearly completed maternity and kitchen-laundry structures,

---

[9]G. Farrar to Johnson, February 13, 1966.

[10]G. Farrar to G.B. Farrars, January 16, 1966; Farrar to Mission Committee, January 1, 1965 [sic], *WEV*.

[11]Bryant and Bryant, Interview.

[12]H. Farrar to Mrs. H.C. Farrar, February 19, 1966.

[13]R. Bryant to Mattoxes, April 13, 1966.

[14]Bryant, *Divine*, 247, 259; P. Bryant to Mattoxes, July 26, 1966; G. Farrar to G.B. Farrars, March 27, 1966.

[15]P. Bryant to Mattoxes, April 4, 1966; G. Farrar to Johnsons, April 10 and May 4, 1966; *Tennessean*, "Don't Quote."

[16]P. Bryant to Mattoxes, August 18, 1965; Hillsboro, "Report."

[17]R. Bryant to Mattoxes, December 13, 1966; Farrar to Lafayette [sic] Church, September 21, 1965.

while Bryant focused on the operating room and one large ward. Bryant also maintained his full-time preaching and BTC teaching.[18]

On June 11, construction funds ran out again, "the work stopped dead," and missionaries sent laborers home. Then, same-day mail brought $5,000 in two separate checks: $2,000 from F.F. Carson and $3,000 from W-COC. Missionaries enthusiastically summoned workers back.[19]

Sickness

As NCH buildings rose, Grace Farrar fell prey to homesickness triggered by family accounts of Tennessee winter snow. The dry season was upon them in Nigeria, and while two and a half months without rain facilitated construction, it exacerbated the wistful longings of Grace Farrar and Nancy Petty for home. "Send us a snowball," Grace closed a February letter.[20]

Meanwhile, Petty, who was tired of taking baths in "3 cups of water," planned her future US remedy: drink all the cold water that she could hold and then soak for hours in a full bathtub. Nonetheless, her Onicha Ngwa time passed quickly, and only the team's accomplishments convinced her that she had lived there almost a year.[21] Moreover, despite her longing for American conveniences, she was ambivalent about furlough, and after one particularly long clinic day, she reflected on her passion for Nigeria. "I really do love these people," she wrote. "There are times I think if I ever get home, I'll never stir out again but most of the time I feel like I cannot stand to leave & never see them again."[22]

Beyond the challenge of homesickness, a "raging measles epidemic" in February plagued both missionaries and locals.[23] Vaccines were limited, and the deaths of many Nigerian children from this "white man's disease"[24] grieved the team. Iris Hays and Petty rescued measles-infected cook-steward Mark from native doctor treatments in the village and brought him to the mission compound, where they nursed him through dehydration, skin loss, and near death.[25] Missionary children did not es-

---

[18]G. Farrar to Johnsons, May 4, 1966.

[19]G. Farrar to Mrs. H.C. Farrar, June 11, 1966; H. Farrar to Morgans, July 11, 1966.

[20]G. Farrar to G.B. Farrars, February 13, 1966; Petty to Spann, January 10, 1966.

[21]Petty to Spann, March 8, 1966.

[22]Petty to Spann, May 19, 1966.

[23]Farrar to Mission Committee, February 7, 1966, *WEV*.

[24]G. Farrar to Johnson, February 13, 1966.

[25]Hays-Savio and Petty-Kraus, Interview.

cape the epidemic's misery, with David Farrar and Becky Underwood developing telltale symptoms, and Tonya Keesee, daughter of Dayton and Ruth in Enugu, surviving a serious case. The Farrars speculated that a particularly dangerous strain coupled with poor population health worsened the outbreak.[26]

Vacation Thwarted

With no regular days off, Hays and Petty eagerly anticipated a two-week February vacation. During the first week, they relaxed in Owerri, possibly with nurse friend Rosemary Sweetham from QEH.[27] During the second, they joined the Farrars at the Obudu Cattle Ranch on Nigeria's northeastern cool plateau. While Dr. Farrar presumably worked solo during the first week of the nurses' absence, he closed the Clinic for the Obudu week.[28]

Unhappily, the overdue vacation disappointed. In Obudu everyone except Grace Farrar developed typhoid-like symptoms, probably related to unsanitary food preparation at the British rest house where they stayed. Farrars speculated that Grace escaped the illness because of a childhood bout with typhoid,[29] but, as she put it, "Another 'vacation' like [that]… might send us home" to America.[30] Mercifully they had come prepared with medicine to which all but the nurses responded, with Petty's symptoms dragging on into late March.[31] Petty, however, did not tell her family about being ill, but instead laughingly observed of Obudu that the British were "just plain odd," an impression fueled in part by the nurses' struggles with unfamiliar-to-them breakfast egg cups. Nonetheless, before getting sick, Petty had enjoyed the ranch's morning tea in bed, tasty meals, afternoon tea, outdoor sports, and evenings cool enough to sit by a fire.[32]

The still-recovering team returned March 6 to their rigorous schedule and Onicha Ngwa's high heat and humidity.[33] The miserable weather was

---

[26]G. Farrar to Johnson, February 13 and May 4, 1966; Farrar to Mission Committee, February 7, 1966, *WEV*.

[27]Petty to Spann, January 10, February 15, February 25, and April 19, 1966; Hays-Savio and Petty-Kraus, Interview.

[28]G. Farrar to Johnson, February 13 and March 15, 1966; H. Farrar to Mrs. H.C. Farrar, February 19, 1966; Petty to Spann, February 25, 1966.

[29]Farrar, *Stand*, 104; G. Farrar to G.B. Farrar, April 9, 1967.

[30]G. Farrar to G.B. Farrars, March 27, 1966.

[31]G. Farrar to Johnson, March 15, 1966.

[32]Petty to Spann, March 8, 1966.

[33]G. Farrar to Mrs. H.C. Farrar, March 15, 1966; Hays-Savio, Interview.

accentuated by the loss of evening fans and lights, caused by a lightning strike on the compound generator, and while missionary children enjoyed lamplight as an adventure, Grace Farrar and Myra Underwood compensated by retiring early and sleeping directly on their cool, Colorcrete floors. "Now I know why civilization made so much progress after electricity," Grace Farrar wrote after a US friend from PH loaned them a generator. Still, they found cause to rejoice that Dr. Farrar's liver function tests finally returned to normal. The family was happy, Dr. Farrar wrote to W-COC, and they looked "forward to the next 1 ½ years for the Lord in Nigeria."[34]

No National Peace

Displays of the country's widespread optimism after the January 15 coup proved only a calm before the storm. Despite many Nigerians' initial welcome of Aguiyi-Ironsi's military government, his shared Igbo heritage with coup perpetrators generated abundant rumors that the coup was an Igbo ploy to dominate Nigeria. Northern Hausa-Fulanis wanted Aguiyi-Ironsi to execute the young Igbo officers who assassinated Northern leaders, while Eastern Igbos considered the same men heroes and thought Aguiyi-Ironsi too friendly to the North.[35]

Caught in the middle, Aguiyi-Ironsi hesitated, and his selective inattention to ethnic tensions escalated them. His perhaps well-intended but unpopular attempts to strengthen Nigeria's central government, reduce regions to provinces, unify civil service, and ban political parties likely accelerated his failure,[36] and Northern demonstrations on Sunday, May 29, quickly devolved into violent, well-organized, Islamic Hausa mobs, who hunted "the roughly one million 'strangers' of the Ibo tribe"[37] living in their midst. Thousands of Igbo men, women, and children were slaughtered in Northern cities of Kano, Kaduna, Sokoto, and Gusau;[38] the beginning of waves of 1966 pogroms in which "hundreds of thousands" would be "wounded, maimed and violated."[39] Unrestrained rioters de-

---

[34]G. Farrar to Johnson, March 15, 1966; Farrar to Mission Committee, March 16, 1966, *WEV.*

[35]Achebe, *There Was,* 79–80; Garrison, "Army;" Garrison, "New Cry;" Garrison, "Rioting."

[36]Achebe, *There Was,* 80; Baxter, *Biafra,* 12–13; Garrison, "New Cry;" Madiebo, *Nigerian Revolution,* 47–62.

[37]Garrison, "New Cry."

[38]Ibid.; Baxter, *Biafra,* 13–14; Garrison, "Crisis;" Special, "Weekend Rioting."

[39]Achebe, *There Was,* 82.

stroyed Igbo property and burned alive people taking refuge in their homes and Christians praying for peace in their churches. Narratives that calm was returning on May 31 were belied by foreign allegations of the ongoing torching of Igbo-owned businesses and roaming gangs. Some police joined rioters, and military response was tepid. Survivors fled for their lives to tribal homelands in the East,[40] and scholar Achebe gave voice to many: Only premeditation and "careful coordination" could have generated anti-Igbo riots on the same day in cities over a hundred miles apart.[41]

Reasons given for the attacks were overlapping and varied. Some said they were revenge for January's coup, others described them as a call for Northern secession, and still others thought they were a way for the North to maintain economic and political power. Islamic Hausa-Fulanis resented their economically disadvantaged position created by their rejection and Igbos' concurrent embrace of missionary-delivered Western education. In a modernizing Nigeria, better-educated Igbos held over half of the jobs in the national Nigerian Railway Corporation, Foreign Service, and Port Authority, but meritocratic arguments were unpersuasive to Northerners in a context of persistent political, tribal, and religious divisions.[42]

On the Doorstep

Fallout from the massacre landed on the Farrars' doorstep on June 11, when Igbo refugee and BTC graduate Moses Oparah and family arrived "bruised, exhausted, and hungry" from the Northern Muslim-majority city of Gusau. Hausa-fluent Moses served as a Christian missionary in Gusau, and on May 29 a Muslim mob had burst into COC Sunday services where he was preaching and demanded, "Is the name of Allah known here?" When he replied, "The name of Jesus Christ is known here," the crowd attacked. Church members ran for their lives, and the Oparahs' youngest child was killed. The mob ripped the family's clothing from their backs and looted and burned their property.[43] A Hausa woman pulled their fleeing children off the streets into her home until she could return them to their parents by night, and Comfort Oparah hid

---

[40]Ibid.; Garrison, "Crisis;" Special, "Weekend Rioting;" Madiebo, *Nigerian Revolution*, 35–45.

[41]Achebe, *There Was*, 83.

[42]Achebe, *There Was*, 74–80; *Daily Defender*, "Nigeria's School Problem."

[43]Farrar, *Stand*, 117–18; G. Farrar to Mrs. H.C. Farrar, June 11, 1966.

under a neighbor's bed praying "while Muslims entered and demanded to know where the 'Igbo Infidel' was." The neighbor told them Comfort had left, and the mob moved on.[44]

The police protected the Oparahs long enough for them to flee East on a train, and when they arrived at Onicha Ngwa, Grace Farrar offered them boiled eggs, peanut butter, and whatever she "thought might taste good to a Nigerian. As he sat there…[Moses] kept repeating, 'I must go back. You cannot change a nation until you change its spirit. They must be taught.'"[45] US COC missionaries already admired Moses for his several conversions from feared juju doctor to Christian after hearing Jim Massey preach in the marketplace, to BTC student after hearing 82-year-old Marshall Keeble preach, to domestic missionary, and they now received his family as Christian heroes. For them, the Oparahs' partial martyrdom in Gusau was not merely a story of ethnic hatred, but one of genuine faith, and in Moses they saw a brother in Christ and symbol of evangelistic success. "A giant among men," Patti Bryant called him,[46] and missionaries subsequently hired Moses to teach Bible classes to NCH construction workers, making him arguably the Hospital's first chaplain.[47] A few months later, it was this same Moses Oparah who waded into an angry NCH Clinic mob with Matron Petty to save a bicycle thief from stoning.[48]

Grace Farrar and Nancy Petty, who had been quick to reassure US families of their own safety, did not hesitate to share the Oparahs' story of persecution.[49] Petty's sister was touched by the murder of the family's daughter—the same age as her own—and penned a letter directly to Comfort Oparah. Petty relayed home how much that letter meant: "Some people have the idea that these people don't love their children as much as we love ours but it isn't true."[50]

Yet even in the face of Northern brutality, many Nigerians and Americans remained confident in the stories they told themselves about Nigeria's stability. Patti Bryant reassured her family that the country's unrest would "soon be completely under control," the violence seemed far away,

---

[44]Bryant, *Divine*, 275. A captioned picture of Comfort Oparah and 7 "surviving children" is in HGF clippings, and the clipping's picture of an anonymous Ekpo dancer is inaccurately labeled, "Moses as a witchdoctor."

[45]Farrar, *Stand*, 118; G. Farrar to Mrs. H.C. Farrar, June 11, 1966.

[46]Bryant, *Divine*, 276; R. Bryant to Friends, August 1, 1965; G. Farrar to Mrs. H.C. Farrar, June 11, 1966.

[47]Bryant, *Gently*, bk. 3, 137.

[48]Farrar and Petty-Kraus, Interview.

[49]G. Farrar to Mrs. H.C. Farrar, June 11, 1966; Petty to Spann, June 20, 1966.

[50]Petty to Spann, June 5, 1966 [sic] (probably July).

and day-to-day work went on as usual. By Chinua Achebe's own account, he was one of the last to leave his Lagos home for safety in the East, even after helping his wife and children flee and witnessing state acquiescence to the systematic and random murder of Igbos. Achebe himself fled only after a group of drunken soldiers unsuccessfully searched for him in order to test whether his pen really was mightier than their guns. At that point, he could no longer deny the anti-Igbo pogrom taking place around him.[51]

Conclusion

NCH buildings went up as unpredictable funding allowed, but homesickness, physical illness, and oppressive weather lowered missionary spirits. Yet, while violence escalated in Nigeria, the relative calm in the missionaries' immediate area bolstered their optimism that national peace would return. If peace survived, so could their dreams. None were ready to consider the alternative that would soon be upon them.

---

[51]Bryant, *Divine*, 276; Achebe, *There Was*, 64-72.

26
The Wider Workforce
(Spring–Summer 1966)

Could American women equal that?
—Grace Farrar

The lives of Iris Hays and Nancy Petty were dominated by patient care, NCH operations, and hiring or educating nursing staff. The nurses left to the missionary men all fundraising, NCH construction, and recruiting of US nurse and physician replacements. Meanwhile, many paid and unpaid, Nigerians and Americans, adults and children worked alongside the COC healthcare team to complete NCH stage two: an inpatient facility.

Nursing Expansion

Clinic staff-in-training continued to gain independence, but more personnel were needed for the soon-to-open NCH maternity and surgical services.[1] Because Matron Petty was immersed in Hospital logistics, Hays selected a second nursing auxiliary cohort on her own—a task so stressful that she developed painful neck and back tension.[2] Years later, she remembered little of the process other than giving more examinations.[3] Each of the newly selected seven women came from a different village,[4] and those villages studiously maintained their representation. When the village of Abala couldn't contact Hays-selected Gloria Ekwenye, they sent Abala daughter Hellen Enyinna.[5] Such local participation may be

---

[1]G. Farrar to Johnson, April 1, 1966; Hays-Savio, Interview.
[2]G. Farrar to Morgan, March 27, 1966; Petty-Kraus, Interview 1.
[3]Hays-Savio, Interview.
[4]Chi Ekwenye-Hendricks, personal communication in June 2011.
[5]Chi Ekwenye-Hendricks, personal communication, May 5, 2012; Ekwenye-Hendricks, Interview 1.

why there is no record of grievances like those generated by the first cohort's selection.

Hays began classes on March 28 for this second, newest cohort of Rachel Akwarandu (or Anyano), Mercy (or Mary) Ekanem, Hellen Nna Enyinna, Clara Maduike, Rose Ngwakwe, Zilpa (or Oti) Onwuchekwa Nwadibia, and Eunice Uzuegbu Uche.[6] Running simultaneous cohorts meant that Hays prepared two sets of weekly lessons and accommodated twelve students at twelve dissimilar skill levels during her clinical teaching. Torrents of rain on the classroom roof still intermittently drowned out her lectures, and high daytime humidity between rains prevented cooling evaporation of the sweat that drenched her body and hair.[7]

Meanwhile, Matron Petty engaged staff and auxiliary students in triaging 180 to 250 patients each Clinic day. They identified the 100 to 150 most ill for Dr. Farrar to examine at roughly three minutes per patient. Team lunch breaks diminished from two hours to one, and their quitting time of 4:00 p.m. sometimes stretched to 6:30 p.m.[8] Petty grieved when seriously ill patients were seen at day's end and then forced to walk or cycle ten to fifteen miles home.[9] The Clinic ran five days a week[10] with Tuesdays and Thursdays likely limited to emergencies, those requiring daily treatments, and the maternal-child clinic. The team treated 2,143 individuals in June alone.[11]

On May 10, 1966, the visiting regional Minister of Health granted on-the-spot permission to open the Hospital at Dr. Farrar's discretion, assuring them that he would personally attend its grand opening. Missionaries marveled at the speed of this military government approval in contrast to the earlier, months-long civilian government authorization of their clinic, and they hoped to open the six-bed maternity unit in June.[12] "Strike while the iron is hot," declared Dr. Farrar, and construction moved as fast as

---

[6]Ngwakwe and Ukegbu, quoted by Chi Ekwenye in email to author on December 3, 2012, listed names and their memory of the cohort of each. Corrected using "Capping Ceremony," February 1967; alternate names from Farrar "Financial Report...April 1—April 30th [1967]."

[7]G. Farrar to Johnson, April 1, 1966; Hays-Savio, Interview.

[8]P. Bryant to Mattoxes, March 18, 1966; G. Farrar to Johnson, February 13, 1966; H. Farrar to Mrs. H.C. Farrar, May 22, 1966; G. Farrar to G.B. Farrars, May 17, 1966; H. Farrar to G.B. Farrars, January 31, 1966; Hays-Savio and Petty-Kraus, Interview; Petty to Spann, May 19, 1966.

[9]Petty to Spann, May 19, 1966.

[10]H. Farrar, Interview 1.

[11]Petty to Spann, July 1, 1966.

[12]G. Farrar to Johnsons, May 17, 1966; H. Farrar to Mrs. H.C. Farrar, May 22, 1966.

money allowed.[13] They also hired their first four NRNs,[14] and by November 1966, six NRNs were on staff, including some or all of these Grade one and Grade two midwives: Miss Bibina (or Bibena) John, Mrs. Pauline Eduok, Miss Ima (Usua) Ebong, Mrs. Jemimah Nwakanma (or Wakanma), and Miss Mabel Solomon.[15] Petty mentioned especially NRNs Eduok and Ebong for their "great sense of humor," indispensable help, and willingness to speak up as needed.[16] She already appreciated the first two qualities in the auxiliaries and may have found the last a refreshing contrast.

Roller Coaster

In the US, West End COC (W-COC) unsuccessfully pursued recruitment of additional missionary health professionals beginning as early as 1964.[17] One nurse from Long Island, New York, envisioned coming in 1966 but did not,[18] while two others made plans. Nurse Elizabeth Burton, the widowed daughter-in-law of wealthy Nashville COC member A.M. Burton, planned to come with the Ezells in October,[19] and student nurse Becky Nicks, the daughter of Bill and Gerry Nicks and fiancé of missionary Mike King, prepared to arrive in 1969 after her graduation and marriage. In the end, neither came. Becky neither completed nursing school nor married King,[20] and the outcome of Burton's plans were unrecorded.

Concurrent physician recruitment also yielded mixed outcomes. W-COC appealed for a physician replacement for Farrar, pointing to him as a model in foregoing a lucrative US salary for a place in heaven,[21] and whether from those or other efforts, three physicians expressed interest: Ken Yearwood, MD, from Nashville;[22] Damon Martin, MD, from Ola,

---

[13]G. Farrar to Johnson, May 17, 1966.
[14]Petty to Spann, July 1, 1966.
[15]Farrar, "Financial Report, Nov. 13–Dec. 15, 1966," W-COC file.
[16]Petty to Spann, September 9, 1966.
[17]Elders to members, October 5, 1964, *WEV*.
[18]G. Farrar to Mrs. H.C. Farrar, September 25, 1966; Farrar to Mission Committee, October 4, 1965, *WEV*; P. Bryant to Mattoxes, September 28, 1966.
[19]G. Farrar to Mrs. H. C. Farrar, February 13, 1966; G. Farrar to Morgans, November 5, 1966.
[20]G. Farrar to G.B. Farrars, January 5, 1966; G. Farrar to Johnson, April 10, 1966; Jeanie Nicks Crocker, Facebook Messenger to author, October 17 and October 23, 2019; Petty to Spann, April 19, 1966.
[21]Farrar to Mission Committee, October 4, 1965, *WEV*.
[22]G. Farrar to G.B. Farrars, January 5, 1966.

Arkansas;[23] and Don Thomas, MD, from Houston, Texas.[24] Green Lawn COC began raising funds for Martin, who intended to move to NCH in March 1967,[25] while Dr. Yearwood planned to arrive after completing his internship at Nashville's Baptist Hospital in December 1967.[26]

At the same time, however, three previously interested physicians withdrew: F.B. Coleman, MD, from Indiana, John Morgan, MD, from Tennessee, and intern Robert E. White, MD, in Galveston, Texas. Dr. Coleman abandoned his plans to spend two years in Nigeria because of the expense of moving his large family, opting instead to use his skills in short medical mission trips to Mexico.[27] In a further disappointment to the Farrars, Drs. Morgan and White canceled Nigeria plans in order to avoid the Vietnam draft. Morgan accepted a pediatric residency,[28] and White joined the National Guard.[29] Dr. Farrar suggested to Morgan that he recruit Nashville pediatrician Dr. Dorothy Turner for NCH,[30] but her name did not reappear in preserved correspondence.

Women and Children

In Nigeria women and children—some of whose names are no longer remembered—volunteered time and energy to NCH. One group of 150 to 200 women from nearby COCs labored for days clearing more Hospital land with hoes and machetes. They removed weeds, dug up stumps, and leveled the ground. Many came on foot or bicycle from ten or more miles away, and Dr. Farrar drove one exhausted older woman thirteen miles home after she toiled all day. "Could American women equal that for a desire to have a hospital?" marveled Grace Farrar.[31]

Missionary children also raised funds and supplied extra hands in their own ways. They ran a lemonade stand to gather coins (probably from their parents as customers) for purchase of a Hospital bed.[32] Additional-

---

[23]H. Farrar to G.B. Farrars, February 7 and November 13, 1966.

[24]Bergstrom to Fromberg, April 18, 1966, W-COC file; G. Farrar to Johnson, May 17, 1966; Fromberg to Elders April 9, 1966, W-COC file.

[25]Farrar to Mission Committee, December 27, 1966, *WEV*.

[26]G. Farrar to G.B. Farrars, January 5, 1966; H. Farrar to McInteer, February 19, 1967.

[27]Coleman, "Challenge;" Lawyer, Untitled.

[28]H. Farrar, July 11, 1966; Morgan, Morgan, and Farrar, Interview.

[29]G. Farrar to Morgans, October 3, 1965; H. Farrar, September 21, 1965.

[30]H. Farrar to Morgans, September 13, 1966.

[31]Farrar to Mission Committee, June 4, 1966, *WEV*; G. Farrar to Mrs. H.C. Farrar, June 11, 1966.

[32]Bryant, *Gently*, bk. 3, 117.

ly, Sara Bryant and Marty Farrar initiated a fundraising set of fishing and guessing games for a penny each from US children, in an effort that garnered several shillings. Elementary-age Hank and Lee Farrar raised three shillings and nine pence (~forty-eight cents) by picking, packaging, and selling seeds—an effort that Grace Farrar called "the children's 'mite.'"[33]

Moreover, when the US Agency for International Development (US-AID) sent several 100-pound bags of wheat and powdered milk for free distribution to NCH Clinic patients, Grace Farrar promptly engaged all missionary children, except infant Bryan Underwood, in that effort. She "set up an assembly line" of delighted youngsters who divided the food into accompanying, smaller bags premarked "Donated by the people of the United States of America. Not for Sale or Exchange." Nurse Farrar wondered how many recipient parents sold those filled bags in order to purchase *gari*, their nutrient-poor, cassava staple.[34]

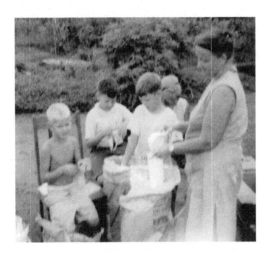

Photograph 26. Grace Farrar, RN, with (left to right) Lee, David, Hank and Marty Farrar packaging USAID wheat and powdered milk nutritional supplements for NCH distribution. June 1966. (Author collection)

[33]Farrar, *Stand*, 105, 144–45. Grace reference to Mark 12:41–44.
[34]Ibid., 110; G. Farrar to Emery Johnsons, June 11, 1966.

27
Saving Evangelism
(May–July 1966)

Each person I baptize will be indebted to Henry Farrar, Miss Iris Hays, and Miss Nancy Petty.
—David Underwood

In Onicha Ngwa, COC team members traveled freely, vacationed, socialized, and celebrated holidays. Nigerian and expatriate friendships flourished, mail delivery continued, and healthcare missionaries treated both Nigerians and American colleagues. A hard-working Dr. Farrar described his Nigerian clinic practice as like "trying to dip the ocean dry with a teaspoon."[1]

Native doctor treatments, neglect, and lack of follow-through on NCH-prescribed care made some patients worse. Words like "pathetic," "worst I have ever seen," "terrible," "poison," and "horrible" peppered missionary case descriptions.[2] "Doctors especially will understand my frustration," Henry Farrar wrote about a woman in premature labor who cycled ten miles to clinic, was seen near day's end, and then cycled home with instructions to rest. A bulging necrotic tumor replaced one six-year-old's eye,[3] and other parents brought their three-year-old daughter eight miles by bicycle and waited six hours only to be told that she would be permanently blind from lime juice put in her eyes by a native doctor. Juju doctor slashes in another child's foot created infected skin sloughing,[4] and native doctor injections destroyed the foot of a young man who had wanted simply to experience a shot.[5] "So go...our efforts," sighed Grace

---

[1]Farrar, *Stand*, 180.
[2]Ibid., 120; Farrar to Mission Committee, April 12, 1966, *WEV*; Petty to Spann, July 13, 1966.
[3]Farrar to Mission Committee, April 12, 1966, *WEV*.
[4]G. Farrar to Johnson, June 26, 1966.
[5]Petty to Spann, July 13, 1966.

Farrar.[6] Additionally, Nancy Petty estimated that each maternity patient with four to five living children had lost two to three more before they were a year old.[7] Reflecting on such cases, Petty observed wryly that July's "Friday the 13th comes on Wed this month, [and] that must be a good sign of some kind."[8]

The COC team encountered those with mental health issues, too, but provided no related care. One woman wandered naked, dusty, shouting, and talking to herself outside a church building where Dr. Farrar preached,[9] and a mentally ill man living near NCH looked well-fed, reportedly from stolen chickens. He often waved and smiled at missionaries and gathered NCH empty pill bottles to sell.[10] The paucity of mental health care, Dr. Farrar wrote to W-COC, reminds "us of how much we need to do."[11]

Self-Care

Missionaries took holidays away from the compound, supported each other, and were encouraged by guests in their homes. Sometimes the nurses spent an afternoon in the Port Harcourt (PH) Shell Oil Company compound pool with missionary girls or their friend Dianne North from QEH.[12] Additionally, the Bryants and the two nurses regularly vacationed,[13] and Grace Farrar enforced her family's vacations when a relief physician was available, recognizing that otherwise her husband would labor nonstop.[14] Younger team members, including Petty, Iris Hays, Mike King, Don and Joyce Harrison, and Ray and Charlotte Lanham enjoyed a spring group retreat in Owerri,[15] and missionaries from the three compounds and Enugu gathered for occasional spiritual retreats of worship and Bible study.[16]

Outside visitors also renewed missionary spirits. Hays and Petty enjoyed hosting and being hosted, and Grace Farrar welcomed dinner

---

[6]G. Farrar to Johnson, June 26, 1966.

[7]Petty to Spann, June [sic] 5, 1966. (Correct likely July)

[8]Petty to Spann, July 13, 1966.

[9]Farrar to Mission Committee, March 16, 1966, *WEV*.

[10]Petty to Spann, May 31, 1966. Live chickens left as sacrifices belonged to no one and perhaps provided his meals.

[11]Farrar to Mission Committee, March 16, 1966, *WEV*.

[12]Petty to Spann, June 9 and June 20, 1966.

[13]Bryant, *Divine*; Hays-Savio, Interview.

[14]Petty-Kraus, Interview 1.

[15]Petty to Spann, February 25, April 28, and May 19, 1966.

[16]G. Farrar to Johnson, October 18, 1964 and June 16, 1965.

guests from many denominations,[17] as well as a surprising number of COC visitors from the US who "boost...our own zeal."[18] Among those were Eugene Peden in January, and Patti Bryant's brother, Joe Mattox, MD, and her teenage cousin, Matt Young, during summer 1966. Dr. Mattox ran the Clinic for a week under Matron Petty's tutelage so that the Farrars could vacation in cooler Jos on Nigeria's western plateau,[19] and Petty taught Matt Young how to administer injections, draw blood, and explain prescriptions to patients; Matt's Clinic assistance proved invaluable to her and Dr. Farrar.[20]

During one Clinic day in July 1966, Petty saw fifty-two pregnant women and thirty-four mostly ill babies. "It is called a maternity & *well* baby clinic," Petty asserted, but all the babies were either too ill for vaccinations or mothers refused injections for their healthy children.[21] Dr. Mattox saw no babies healthy enough for immunization during his time in the Clinic, but he was so impressed with Petty's work that he invited her to join him in his Arkansas practice. Given Petty's make-do and expanded Clinic practice, she jokingly responded that when she finished two years in Nigeria, she "would not be fit for a US hospital."[22]

During summer 1966, the nurses also enjoyed tennis, movies, and interactions with thirty to thirty-four US short-term evangelists and other visitors led by three former COC evangelists to Nigeria under the auspices of Green Lawn COC: Jim Massey, Jimmy Johnson, and Leonard Johnson. Hays and Petty especially relished time with group member Bonnie Beaver, a home economics teacher from Freed Hardeman College in Henderson, Tennessee.[23] Beaver's daily "health, nutrition, sewing, and Bible" classes for Nigerian women showcased COC missionary women's evangelistic work, and so pleased the local chief that he personally visited the compound to ask—in vain—if someone could continue classes after her departure. Even Beaver's male colleagues recognized that preaching might be more about practice than audience gender, as revealed in their good-natured jabs about "women evangelists" among

---

[17]Petty to Spann, April 28 and August 8, 1966; Farrar, *Stand*, 108-09.
[18]G. Farrar to Johnson, May 17, 1966.
[19]G. Farrar to Folks, July 22, 1966; Farrar to Mission Committee, *WEV* ; Petty to Spann, July 1 and August 8, 1966.
[20]Bryant, *Divine*, 278-79; R. Bryant to Mattoxes, August 4, 1966; G. Farrar to Folks, July 22, 1966.
[21]Petty to Spann, July 27, 1966.
[22]Bryant, *Divine*, 278-79; Ibid.
[23]Chronicle News, "Months-long;" Petty to Spann, August 8, 1966.

them.[24] Nonplussed Patti Bryant and Grace Farrar already long described their own women's classes as "preaching appointments."[25]

During the Farrars' vacation in Jos, courtesy of relief physician Joe Mattox, an always busy Dr. Farrar kept working. He established a new COC congregation at Bukoru near Jos, but the ten-day change in venue so refreshed him that he compared it favorably to a US furlough.[26] The Sudan Interior Mission (SIM) rest house, where the family stayed served American (not British) food that cost less per day than their Onicha Ngwa meals, and most other guests were US missionaries from various denominations. Cooler weather, hiking, the zoo, an art museum, cave paintings in Bauchi, a tin smelting plant, and a cobra charmer contributed to the family's sense of getting away. As Boyd Reese and Eldred Echols had observed in 1950, white expatriates found it "healthful and invigorating" to spend a few weeks relaxing in cooler locations. The fourteen-hour drive home, which included an unexpected 600-mile detour, however, nearly undid the Farrars' rest.[27]

Colleague Care

The missionaries' health care for Nigerians took center stage in the US COC public eye, but the mission team insistently drew supporters' attention to the equally important task of keeping evangelists healthy and working.[28] The spring and summer of 1966 unfortunately provided ample such opportunities. Patti Bryant returned from an Obudu Ranch vacation with serious amoebiasis, the same disease that had forced her family back to the US in 1961. This time, however, on-site physician Farrar confined her to bed for thirteen days with daily emetine injections from Petty and Hays. Additionally, future RNs Marty Farrar and Sara Bryant wished her a thousand prayers by folding the same number of tiny origami storks that Patti Bryant said "rivaled…the emetine."[29] She recovered, and the Bryants' work continued uninterrupted.[30] The US healthcare team treated others, too: four Bryants for malaria, a visiting US

---

[24]G. Farrar to Folks, July 22 and August 7, 1966; Farrar, *Stand*, 135.

[25]P. Bryant to Family, September 28, 1958; Farrar, *Stand*, 139; G. Farrar to Johnsons, August 23, 1966.

[26]Farrar to Mission Committee, July 22, 1966, *WEV*.

[27]G. Farrar to Folks, July 22, 1966; Reese and Echols, *Report*, 5.

[28]Ray Lanham, quoted in Hillsboro, "Report."

[29]Bryant, *Divine*, 262.

[30]G. Farrar to Johnsons, May 17, 1966; Underwood to McInteer, June 13, 1966, *WEV*.

preacher for a recurring leg wound that required packing and penicillin, Patti Bryant for gas gangrene, and Sara, David, and Rees Bryant for amoebiasis. Drs. Mattox and Farrar collaborated with Hays, Petty, and Patti Bryant to treat all successfully at home in Onicha Ngwa.[31]

David Underwood's health crisis, however, threatened life, health, and the mission more than any other. In May 1966 Underwood drove himself to NCH Clinic with chest pain,[32] and Dr. Farrar immediately sent Underwood to Queen Elizabeth Hospital (QEH), where they admitted him for a "small" heart attack.[33] Adding to Underwood's trepidation was a person with rabies in the bed on one side of him and another with active tuberculosis on the other. Matron Petty or Dr. Farrar checked on him daily, Myra Underwood stayed at times, and three weeks later an improved Underwood returned to Onicha Ngwa with stronger body, but lower spirits—his long-term dream of mission work in doubt.[34] Marty and Sara delivered another set of origami prayers.[35]

In June, David Underwood asserted in a very personal way the value of COC medical missions to missionaries themselves. Using physician Farrar as both person and a proxy for the healthcare team, he wrote to W-COC:

> If Henry Farrar never: (1) edified a single congregation on Sunday, (2) handed out a single gospel tract, (3) preached, debated, or answered one question in the crowded marketplaces, (4) treated any Nigerian medically in Christian compassion, (5) raised a lone dollar for mission work and oversaw a building program to bless generations to come, (6) trained one nurse, (7) taught health classes, (8) or taught in the Bible training college—he does all of this, however—all of your interest and support would be more than justified purely in terms of evangelistic investments.
>
> How? Simply because of the time, money, energy, travel, and even lives he saves for all the missionary families here. Formerly, even a simple headache among missionaries...meant a

---

[31]Bryant, *Divine*, 299; P. Bryant to Mattoxes, July 21 and September 28, 1966; R. Bryant to Mattoxes, December 13, 1966; G. Farrar to Folks, July 22, 1966.

[32]Bryant, *Divine*, 264.

[33]Farrar to Mission Committee, June 4, 1966, *WEV*.

[34]Farrar, *Stand*, 113; G. Farrar to E. Johnsons, May 17, 1966; Petty to Spann, May 31, 1966.

[35]G. Farrar to E. Johnsons, May 17, 1966.

day lost to the work in order to take a long, hot, dangerous, and rough trip for a single malaria blood test. It takes ten minutes now! Think what the new hospital will do! ...

Recently, I suffered severe chest pains and had Henry not been here would have probably dismissed it as acute indigestion...Without his advice I might have died. If I recover fully, every congregation God establishes through me, every church I edify, and each person I baptize will be indebted to Henry Farrar, [and to] our nurses Miss Iris Hays, and Miss Nancy Petty.[36]

Dr. Farrar remained optimistic about Underwood's recovery,[37] but unfortunately, the chest pain returned, Hays initiated care, and David was readmitted to QEH. Drs. Mattox and Farrar now recommended that Underwood return to the States for best care, and this "cast a gloom" over the mission compound.[38] Grace Farrar grieved the family's impending departure as a "loss for the mission and missionaries." Not only would David Underwood's leaving vacate the BTC principal position, but she would miss his unique ability to get her husband to take regular evening breaks with David's cries of "Emergency!"—his coded summons for a Farrar versus Underwood chess match.[39]

Conclusion

The relationship between evangelism and healthcare had shifted. In 1953 evangelism brought incidental healthcare to Nigeria. A decade later, intentional health care saved evangelism.

---

[36]Underwood to McInteer, June 13, 1966, *WEV*.
[37]Farrar to Mission Committee, June 4, 1966, *WEV*.
[38]G. Farrar to Folks, July 22, 1966.
[39]Author's recollection; Farrar, *Stand*, 121.

28
Joining Forces and Families
(Summer–Fall 1966)

"Our" baby is just beautiful.
—Nancy Petty

Calls to equip the Hospital and drill its water well were answered by Christians on both sides of the Atlantic. Prices for medical equipment in Nigeria were "outrageous,"[1] and Dr. Farrar appealed to US supporters for used devices.[2] Grace Farrar invited her family to ask their personal physicians to donate old technology when they upgraded to new, and Patti Bryant's mother, Mildred Formby Mattox, recruited twenty individuals each willing to buy a $35 NCH bed.[3] A COC teen group in Florida sent $14 for bed money, and Proctor Street COC was inspired to purchase the remaining beds ($900).[4] Dr. Joe Mattox brought and shipped materials to NCH,[5] and more money and pledges came in the bags of the short-term evangelists led by Jim Massey.[6] One W-COC member sent funds for a Hospital stove, another contributed the cost of its washing machine, and two more pledged bed money;[7] earlier Farrar's mentor, Dr. John S. Cayce, had donated an X-ray machine.[8]

Donations bolstered missionary hopes of opening a few NCH beds soon, and they spent excess bed money on other Hospital needs.[9] We plan "to open THE hospital August 1," Nancy Petty enthused. "It gets

---

[1]G. Farrar to Johnson, May 17, 1966.
[2]Farrar to Brethren, October 5, 1964, *WEV*.
[3]G. Farrar to Johnson, May 17 and June 26, 1966.
[4]Brown to McInteer, September 13, 1966, W-COC file; Qualls to Farrars, June 27, 1966.
[5]G. Farrar to Mrs. H.C. Farrar, June 26, 1966; G. Farrar to Johnson, August 7, 1966.
[6]Bryant, *Divine*, 278.
[7]G. Farrar to Folks, July 22, 1966; Johnson to H. Farrar, June 27, 1966, W-COC files.
[8]Farrar to Brethren, October 5, 1964, *WEV*.
[9]G. Farrar to Folks, July 22, 1966; G. Farrar, personal communication, n.d.

more exciting all the time and more rushed and more…to be done."[10] Although that date proved unrealistic, Joe Mattox's hand-delivered cash infusion of $1,500 took missionaries from "flat broke" to finishing most of the six-bed maternity unit, a delivery suite, another ward, and the kitchen-laundry building.[11] Other donations flowed in, too. Physician F.B. Coleman sent a check for equipment, and US women shipped hand-sewn hospital gowns, including "some…very cleverly made from discarded shirts," along with rolled bandages from sheets torn in strips.[12] Moreover, the congregation in Una, Tennessee, in collaboration with COC-affiliated *Action* newspaper raised $2,000 from their special, June 1966 Nigeria-focused edition and nationwide call for individual COC members to contribute $1 each for NCH.[13]

Mildred Mattox and other Lubbock women gathered and packed 275 flat sheets and 140 pillowcases—based on Iris Hays and Patti Bryant estimated NCH needs—and Jim Massey arranged their shipping in three barrels. Unexpectedly, Nigerian officials demanded $180 in customs for these linen donations labeled "hospital use only," and a frustrated Grace Farrar took some consolation only in knowing that NCH wasn't singled out for such unwarranted charges. Customs officials also levied high customs on USAID free shipments of nutritional supplements, prompting USAID to halt donations. Yet when missionaries finally opened their linen barrels at NCH "their fragrance must have reached to Heaven—a sweet aroma to God," wrote Patti Bryant.[14] Every missionary recognized the smell of America.[15]

Drilling

New NCH water access came when J.R. Lewis, a US manager with the International Drilling Company in Port Harcourt (PH), fulfilled his promise to drill a Hospital water well. Although he had previously voiced his intention to do so, "I never really believed it," confessed Grace Farrar.[16] Now COC-member Lewis delivered.

This was no small contribution. Private companies estimated drilling costs at $3,000, yet "just out of love and a desire to help" Lewis and oth-

---

[10]Petty to Spann, July 1, 1966.
[11]G. Farrar to Mrs. H. C. Farrar, June 26, 1966.
[12]G. Farrar to Johnson, August 7, 1966.
[13]G. Farrar to Johnson, August 23, 1966; Lovell, "Editorial."
[14]Bryant, *Divine*, 260; G. Farrar to Folks, July 22, 1966.
[15]Farrar, *Stand*, 27.
[16]G. Farrar to Folks, July 22, 1966.

er expatriates covered full expenses. They hauled rig equipment fifty miles inland over less than ideal roads, paid overtime wages to a Nigerian crew, donated their own labor,[17] and presumably gained necessary company approvals or pardons. On Saturday, July 16, Lewis and US colleague John Freeman arrived on NCH land with crew and rig. By 4:00 p.m. they were set up, by midnight they struck water at 107 feet, and by 12:30 a.m. they placed a pipe. Missionaries supplied meals and coffee on site, and Dr. Farrar stayed throughout to watch. After 3:00 a.m., Lewis and workers grabbed two hours sleep in their PH beds, and then returned at 7:00 a.m. Sunday to drill a second borehole. To their dismay, however, they were forced to work unsuccessfully all day to unclog the first. Then in an astonishing display of commitment over many weekends, a determined Lewis and coworkers returned repeatedly to drill over almost a year until they finished a functioning NCH water well in May 1967.[18]

Gaining Ground

Bible teaching and preaching remained an NCH priority with morning devotionals and distribution of tracts to all patients, staff, and construction workers. Some baptized patients reported that NCH "kindness and teaching" led them to conversion,[19] thus bolstering missionary claims of preaching in word and deed. Clara Maduike and Zilpa Nwadibia from Iris Hays's second nursing auxiliary cohort were baptized, and Dr. Farrar delighted in what he saw as fulfillment of missionary responsibilities toward these women leaders. Thirty-six of fifty-six NCH staff were now COC members,[20] although one auxiliary converted from the COC to Seventh Day Adventist after her marriage.[21]

Missionaries also expected NCH to empower the COC to prevail against religious rivals. The Roman Catholics possessed what Grace Farrar saw as an "unlimited quota, [...] the best schools, the finest hospitals...the largest churches," and the most influence. She looked forward to a day when both locals and missionaries could receive COC-delivered

---

[17]Ibid.

[18]Ibid.; P. Bryant to Mattoxes, July 23 and August 21, 1966; G. Farrar to Johnsons, September 6, 1966; G. Farrar to G.B. Farrar, May 25, 1967. Author's recollection of Farrar conversations: Freeman was raised Seventh Day Adventist (SDA); he tithed significant amounts to NCH and was generous to missionaries in time and resources.

[19]G. Farrar to Johnson, August 7, 1966.

[20]Farrar to Mission Committee, February 7 and November 13, 1966, *WEV*.

[21]Ekwenye-Hendricks, Interview 1.

healthcare, rather than continuing their dependence on Medical Missionaries of Mary (MMM) hospitals and the Protestant QEH. A COC hospital, she penned, might also counter both the religious threat of a growing ethnocentric African National Church, as well as the political threat of Nigeria's increasing immigration preference for healthcare professionals and educators. NCH could attract expatriate COC physicians, nurses, and teachers, who could freely evangelize once in the field.[22]

Interwoven Families

As with other missionaries, US nurses Hays and Petty were integrated into a "huge extended family" of Nigerians, who shared their most private concerns related to work, family, domestic abuse, religious, and reproductive issues. Petty was reluctant to be so involved,[23] but nonetheless found herself dealing with issues such as reassuring the Clinic janitor that his wife, who had already delivered five living children, would not be sinning by taking birth control pills.[24] At the same time, missionaries faced contention over whom to hire into the NCH staff family. The US team considered the best qualified to be those with either healthcare knowledge or an aptitude to learn; but locals disagreed with missionaries and each other. Landowners argued that NCH positions should go to their village sons and daughters,[25] while COC leaders maintained that jobs should go to COC members. The latter group angrily asserted that if missionaries persisted in hiring non-members, the Nigerian Christian Hospital would become the "Nigerian Heathen Hospital."[26] Rees Bryant's diplomacy prevailed, however, and the missionaries continued hiring as before. Thus, when political violence drove Eastern Nigerians home, NCH hired a number of well-educated, Seventh Day Adventist nurses and midwives and an anesthetist. Missionaries welcomed these opportunities both to fill Hospital positions despite low NCH salaries and potentially to convert Nigerian professionals to the COC.[27]

---

[22]G. Farrar to Mrs. H.C. Farrar, June 26, 1966. A transcribed news clipping of an October 18, 1958 debate between COC missionaries and a National Church priest is with R. Bryant to Mattoxes, October 23, 1958.
[23]Farrar and Petty-Kraus, Interview.
[24]Petty to Spann, January 21, 1966.
[25]Bryant and Bryant, Interview.
[26]Bryant, *Divine*, 280.
[27]G. Farrar to Johnson, March 5, 1967; Petty report, Minutes, Mission Committee, May 28, 1967, W-COC file; Petty-Kraus, personal communication, November 15, 2018.

Petty also created new family relationships by mothering the motherless. When local women died in childbirth, their dependent newborns usually died shortly thereafter because baby formula, refrigeration, supplies, and related knowledge were not readily available. When one local preacher sought help for his newborn after his wife's death, Patti Bryant and Nancy Petty learned too late that their good intentions could be dangerous. They supplied the father with a bottle, powdered milk, and instructions, but he returned days later with an unwashed, sour-milk-encrusted, moldy bottle and a three-week old baby dying from diarrhea. Bryant and Petty's intense rehydration efforts proved too late, and the infant died in Nancy's arms. She wrapped the baby in a blanket and, along with Charlotte Lanham and an interpreter, returned the infant to a grieving father.[28]

Patti Bryant and Matron Petty determined not to repeat this mistake, and their opportunity to save a different child soon came. In early fall, the wife of a Nigerian COC preacher died,[29] and as was customary, the family buried the mother but left the grave partly open to bury the baby with her when she also perished. Instead, three days later, the family brought the "very dehydrated but very spunky...[and] cute," tiny girl to the missionaries.[30] Bryant and Petty took the baby, named her Virginia, hired a daytime nanny, and rotated nighttime care until NCH opened and a twenty-four-hour nursing staff could help. A thriving Virginia thus became the Hospital's first inpatient, often staying in the nursery for premature and sick infants. There, Petty would dutifully place Virginia on her tummy to prevent SIDS, and Nigerian nurses would determinedly flip her onto her back to protect her from murderous spirits.[31]

Petty's fostering of Baby Virginia changed both their identities and revealed Igbo ones. Virginia's association trumped her biology and set her apart from local staff. They affectionately nicknamed her Ginny[32] and delightedly told Ginny that she would be "an American Negro," while insisting to a mystified Petty that they were not "Negros at all," but Nigerians.[33] Meanwhile, Petty enjoyed her new maternal role, including elaborate, middle-of-the-night routines of going in and out from under mos-

---

[28]Bryant and Bryant, Interview; G. Farrar to Folks, August 7, 1966; C. Lanham to [missing], n.d., RPB.

[29]Bryant and Bryant, Interview; G. Farrar to Johnson, August 7, 1966.

[30]Petty-Kraus, Interview 1.

[31]Ibid.; P. Bryant to Mattoxes, September 2, 1966; Bryant and Bryant, Interview; Petty to Spann, October 24, 1966.

[32]Petty to Spann, October 4 and 24, 1966.

[33]Petty to Spann, September 13, 1966.

quito net and lighting lamps, candles, and stove to feed and change Virginia.[34] Before long, Ginny turned her head to the nurses' voices, and Petty thought her beautiful. "All mothers [must] feel this way," she mused. Petty started Virginia's routine vaccinations, and Ginny spent her days in the village with nurse-maid Victoria, the wife of a BTC student.[35]

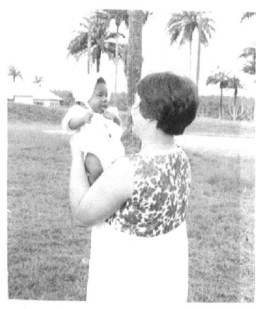

Photograph 28. Nancy Petty with Igbo foster daughter, Virginia. Onicha Ngwa mission compound. ca. 1966. (NPK collection with permission).

Petty's love for Virginia also presented a dilemma. She struggled with whether she as a white, single woman should bring black, Igbo infant Virginia home to Tennessee during furlough. Despite her deep love for Virginia and confidence that the Petty family would wholeheartedly welcome Virginia,[36] as had the missionaries,[37] she worried that Ginny might become "a misfit," who identified as neither American nor Igbo. Virginia's emigration would place her at risk for becoming what has since become known as a third culture kid: a child from everywhere but

---

[34]Petty to Spann, August 17 and 28, 1966.
[35]Petty to Spann, October 24, 1966.
[36]Petty to Spann, September 9, 1966.
[37]Farrar, *Stand*, 81.

nowhere; one with a sense of belonging neither to the culture of birth nor the culture of residence.[38]

Second Coup d'État

Sadly as these missionaries and local Nigerians grew closer, the country's regions moved further apart. Suspicious Northerners began to move against Aguiyi-Ironsi,[39] ultimately leading to a July 29 military counter-coup, in which he and scores of Eastern soldiers stationed in the North were murdered. This brought Northerners back to power under thirty-two-year-old, minority tribesman Col. Yakubu "Jack" Gowon, who in response to British urging reversed his calls for Northern secession, tried to appease the Western region with a prisoner release (already planned by Aguiyi-Ironsi), and pledged to keep the country together.[40] Meanwhile, both Eastern and Western regions considered declaring their own independence, and in Enugu, leader Lt. Col. Ojukwu surrounded himself with heavily armed Igbo policemen.[41]

The earlier massive repatriation of Igbo refugees to the East in summer 1966 already represented one step toward secession, as Eastern residents saw the federal government as unwilling or unable to protect them.[42] Still, Gowon and Ojukwu maintained communications, engendering feeble hopes of unity in the face of intertribal slaughter. The federal government hesitated to jettison the "prosperous," oil rich East,[43] and Gowon's announcements that he feared Eastern secession while concurrently taking actions that distanced and alienated the East were counterbalanced by Ojukwu's assertions and actions directed toward a unified Nigeria. Ojukwu hoped that unity might be possible under a loosely constructed confederacy of its very different constituencies.[44]

Missionaries hoped in Gowon's promises of safety for foreigners and civilian rule,[45] but the immediate effects of the counter-coup were fur-

---

[38]Pollock and Van Reken, *Third Culture*.

[39]Baxter, *Biafra*, 13; Garrison, "Crisis;" Garrison, "Nigeria Peaceful;" Madiebo, *Nigerian Revolution*, 29–35.

[40]Garrison, "Nigeria: Wounds;" Garrison, "Political;" Garrison, "Nigeria Outwardly;" Madiebo, *Nigerian Revolution*, Chapter 3.

[41]Garrison, "Head;" Garrison, "Political;" Garrison, "Nigeria: Wounds;" Ojukwu, *Biafra*, 1–5, 30–34.

[42]Achebe, *There Was*, 82–83; Madiebo, *Nigerian Revolution*, 81–91; Ojukwu, *Biafra*, 41.

[43]Garrison, "Nigeria: Wounds."

[44]Achebe, *There Was*, 86–87; Ojukwu, *Biafra*, ix–xiii, 101–13.

[45]G. Farrar to Johnson, August 4, 1966; Garrison, "Nigeria to Name;" Special, "Army Aid."

ther violence, closure of domestic airports, and cessation of mail. On August 5, the departing Jim Massey group, was unable to fly out of PH and so found it necessary to charter taxis to the Lagos airport 600 miles away, carrying with them hurriedly penned reassurances from resident missionaries to their US families.[46] Becky Underwood went with them in order to begin fall school in the US.[47] "I am sure that newspapers will make it sound as sensational as possible...All is calm where we are," Grace Farrar wrote, and her husband agreed. "We do not expect any trouble in this part of the country...We are all well and the work continues," he reassured family.[48]

Not all, however, were so optimistic. Although the country's troubles had previously escaped comparisons to violence elsewhere in Africa, an August 3, 1966, *Los Angeles Times* editorial author ominously observed of Nigeria, "We have seen this sort of thing before..., notably in the Congo" (A4).

---

[46]R. Bryant to Mattoxes, August 5, 1966; G. Farrar to Johnson, August 4, 1966.
[47]G. Farrar to Johnsons, August 7, 1966; Becky Underwood, personal communication, n.d.
[48]G. Farrar to Johnson, August 4, 1966; H. Farrar to Mrs. H.C. Farrar, August 5, 1966.

29

Launching the Hospital

(August–October 1966)

A lot of "firsts" are happening to us.
—Nancy Petty

Missionaries chose Tuesday, August 23, 1966, as the date for their grand opening celebration of NCH's first inpatient unit: a six-bed, maternity ward. The unit wouldn't be ready to admit patients until a few days later, but that date accommodated the schedule of Dr. M.T.D. Braide, the regional senior medical officer.[1] Braide's insistence on an official ceremony overcame Dr. Henry Farrar's desire not to bother,[2] but Braide also advised against newspaper publicity. Although he had approved NCH's opening, the Eastern military governor had "not yet signed the necessary papers"[3]—papers that didn't arrive until November.[4] Accordingly, the US team "widely distributed" printed invitations to the ribbon-cutting ceremony "on land donated and freely given by the villages of Ntigha Onicha Ngwa, Nlagu, and Umuwoma. 'The churches of Christ salute you.' Romans 16:16," closed the invitation.[5]

NCH staff were in varying stages of readiness. Iris Hays's first auxiliary cohort would soon graduate, and her second was almost halfway through their program. NRN midwives were hired,[6] and lay laboratory and pharmacy staff possessed a year of experience. Matron Nancy Petty was still completing "about 2 million things," on her own because Hays was sick.[7] She was receiving pharmaceutical representatives, hiring staff, procuring

[1]Farrar to Mission Committee, September 8, 1966, *WEV*; R. Bryant to Mattox, August 27, 1966.
[2]P. Bryant to Mattoxes, August 21, 1966.
[3]P. Bryant to Mattoxes, September 12, 1966.
[4]G. Farrar to Morgans, November 5, 1966.
[5]Bryant, "Reflections," 25.
[6]G. Farrar to Johnson, May 17, 1966.
[7]Petty to Spann, August 17, 1966.

supplies, and purchasing sixty yards of material for (probably surgical drapes and) towels. Bed frames arrived at the last minute, and missionary families set up the unit.[8] In PH, Petty splurged on her first fifty-five-minute, £1:2:0 ($3.08) hairstylist appointment since arrival and bought "plastic pants with ruffles" for Virginia; she was thankful that Virginia slept longer at night.[9]

Finally, on the one-year anniversary date of opening the "Cracker-box" Clinic, the Onicha Ngwa missionaries formally celebrated "the great day" for which Petty, Hays, and the Farrars had come to Nigeria.[10] Held on an NCH covered walkway to shield dignitaries from a rainy season down-pour, the ceremony was steeped in Christian proclamation, political posturing, and cataloguing of contributions. It seems unlikely that proceedings adhered to the published 10:30–11:15 a.m. timeframe. Rees Bryant, David Underwood, and Eno Otoyo led a short worship service followed by J.O. Akandu's introduction of speakers—Chiefs F.O. Ahukanna, Thomas Ebere, Awazieama Nwaogu, and Nwosu Ukpom, followed by Dr. Farrar, who each addressed the audience in turn. Dr. M.T.D. Braide (introduced by Farrar) then spoke and cut the ribbon, Bryant led a hymn, and COC missionary, John Beckloff, closed the event with a prayer.[11]

Missionaries welcomed the coming together of chiefs, supporters, and government officials, but were dismayed that each local chief in turn proclaimed himself the central actor in establishing NCH. When Dr. Braide spoke last, however, he declared it his personal privilege to work alongside Dr. Farrar and expressed both his admiration for Farrar's compassionate medical expertise and his own disappointment that none of the dignitaries had thanked Farrar. Braide's recognition of her husband's work pleased a grateful Grace Farrar.[12]

After the ceremony local people sought NCH admission immediately, but the team referred them elsewhere. Petty was still sterilizing instruments and wrapping up innumerable details. Monday, August 29, remained the target date for admissions. "It won't be long now," wrote Grace Farrar, as missionaries rejoiced in all that August 23 represented.[13]

---

[8]Ibid.; P. Bryant to Mattoxes, August 21, 1966; Hays-Savio, Interview.

[9]Petty to Spann, August 17, 1966.

[10]Petty to Spann, May 16, 1965; G. Farrar to Folks, August 23, 1966.

[11]Photograph of missionaries watching Dr. Braide cut ribbon, HGF; "Programme," August 23, 1966.

[12]G. Farrar to Folks, August 23, 1966.

[13]Ibid.

Firsts

Uncharacteristically, plans did go according to schedule, and the night before the maternity ward was to open, a self-described "thrilled, tired, apprehensive, scared, nervous and happy" Petty wrote home to her sister: "The Hospital will open TOMORROW!...I think most of the important things are ready...You wondered what I would find to do at home after this, well, I believe I will seek the dullest job with the least responsibility that I can find."[14]

Thus, six days after the grand opening, the team began admitting uncomplicated deliveries to the maternity unit. Dr. Farrar rose at 5:00 a.m. to attend the first NCH birth, welcoming the infant whose father was the Hospital laundryman. Missionaries celebrated, taking pictures and show-

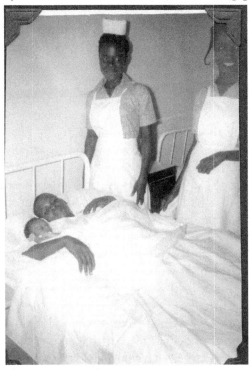

Photograph 29.1. First NCH couplet with graduated auxiliaries Lydia Agbara and Elizabeth Egbu. August 29, 1966. (Author collection)

---

[14]Petty to Spann, August 28, 1966.

ering the family with gifts. Within the week NRNs assumed management of uncomplicated deliveries with the first midwife-attended birth probably on Sunday, September 4, while Farrar was away preaching. Thereafter, Farrar limited his care to complicated cases, and NCH maternity beds remained full even with patient-preferred, next-day discharge.[15]

The unit provided opportunities for Dr. Farrar to use new obstetrical skills, gained under tutelage of Irish nuns at Medical Missionaries of Mary (MMM), including teaching from Farrar-admired "Dr. Sweeney" (probably Leonie McSweeney). He delighted in using British vacuum extraction of infants during prolonged labor—a safety improvement over American forceps.[16] In one case of difficult labor, Farrar applied vacuum extraction successfully during care of a woman with no living children, a much older husband, multiple miscarriages, and faithful attendance at NCH antenatal clinic. The newborn, however, needed immediate oxygen, and NRNs had left the delivery room tank empty. Circulating nurse Hays "flew" to and from the laundry room to retrieve a full tank, the baby was saved, and the grateful couple later invited Hays to their home for warm orange soda. "Compatible" coworkers and seeing the difference that she brought to such patients' lives generated in Hays a sense of deep satisfaction and made the work seem "easy…I knew what I was there for. I didn't have to wonder about what I am doing here."[17]

Only days later the first surgical case came unexpectedly on September 9, 1966. Petty assisted Farrar with the emergency Cesarean section (C-section) performed with "a little sedation" and local anesthesia in the delivery room.[18] The baby had died in utero, and the mother's life was in danger from the resulting severe infection. NCH had no blood bank or transfusion equipment,[19] and post-operatively the mother's blood pressure dropped to "*nothing* for 2 hours." Matron Petty spent most of the day with that "very tiny little woman" and was moved by her resilience, courage, and survival in a land where a woman's value was proportional to the number of her progeny. Of her six children, none lived.[20]

Unlike that tragic case, their probable second, also unplanned surgical case, another C-section, ended in joy. In that undated, nighttime emergency, the baby was too large for vaginal delivery, and Dr. Farrar's symphysiotomy performed to enlarge the birth canal failed to help. Having

[15]H. Farrar, Interview 1.

[16]G. Farrar to Johnsons, September 6, 1966; Wall, "Changes in Nursing."

[17]Hays-Savio, Interview.

[18]H. Farrar, Interview 1; Petty to Spann, September 9, 1966.

[19]H. Farrar to Morgans, September 13, 1966.

[20]Petty to Spann, September 9 and 13, 1966.

begun surgical intervention with perhaps his first symphysiotomy (also learned at MMM), Farrar realized that he must choose between either performing a C-section himself or transporting the woman over miles of rough roads either to MMM or to Aba General Hospital with its limited resources; the family wanted to stay at NCH. Petty, Farrar, and Hays had no electricity, no surgical packs, and no surgical drapes; they did have sterile towels, sterile instruments, flashlights, and a delivery room table.[21] The nurses "put five or six towels around" the surgical site[22] and set up kerosene lamps. An assisting Petty thought a tense "Dr. Farrar was going to eat me alive" during the case, while NCH's own "lady with the lamp" Iris Hays held their torch (flashlight). The infection-free mother and newborn did well, and Farrar was "so grateful" to Hays and Petty.[23] COC team cohesion grew.

Blood and Treasure

During this time, missionary children and women continued supporting NCH in sacrificial or fun ways. Probably at Grace Farrar's urging, daughter Marty sewed two to three hospital sheets per day on her mother's treadle machine. When US-donated gowns arrived, missionary girls joined Petty in stamping them with the NCH logo, and Sara Bryant's father trusted her to make at least one auspicious hand delivery to Dr. Farrar of an unexpected $1,000 mailed donation.[24]

Additionally, Grace Farrar gave uniquely of her own blood and treasure. Having recently sent valued steward Monday John Akpakpan off to secondary school, she now relinquished her cook, Tom Ibe, to the Hospital kitchen. Dr. Farrar wanted to hire Ibe because he was honest, knew safe food preparation, and was "the best and most experienced cook around,"[25] but this left Grace Farrar teaching both new steward Clement Ahiakwo and her older children to cook in her Nigerian kitchen, and she longed for "the electric servants and processed food of America."[26] She was grateful for Monday John's help during his school breaks, and she sped up her children's homeschool lessons in case the nation's political

---

[21]H. Farrar, Interview 1; Petty-Kraus, Presentation to Keen-Agers; Petty-Kraus, Interview 1.

[22]H. Farrar, Interview 1.

[23]Petty-Kraus, Interview 1.

[24]S.J. Bryant, "Diary," January 21, 1967; Sara Bryant, personal communication, n.d.; G. Farrar to Mrs. H.C. Farrar, September 25, 1966.

[25]G. Farrar to Mrs. H.C. Farrar, September 25, 1966.

[26]G. Farrar to Folks, August 23, 1966; Ibid.

turmoil compelled an abrupt departure.[27] She also faced papers to grade, lesson plans to prepare, and classes to teach, and because everything in her unmanageable workload seemed essential, Grace decided that anything she achieved was worthwhile.[28] She reminded herself that she could do only what time and energy allowed and took comfort in reciting to herself the kind and common Nigerian reassurance: "You have tried, Madam."[29]

Not only did she relinquish treasured staff, but Grace Farrar also gave of her universal donor, type O negative blood. Dr. Farrar had obtained transfusion equipment, but NCH, like most hospitals in the area, was without a blood bank.[30] Many Nigerians thought of blood donations as impotence-inducing or life-threatening in depleting their body's finite blood supply and potentially subjecting them to witchcraft.[31] Thus, most were understandably reluctant to give, a situation that became too much for Dr. Farrar in his first loss of a maternity patient to post-partum hemorrhage on September 17. The woman had accessed no antenatal care and was already severely anemic before delivery, and she died while her husband and Dr. Farrar desperately searched for a willing, matching donor.[32]

Dr. Farrar, who already identified the healthy Bible Training College (BTC) students as a "walking blood bank,"[33] now called on his wife for help. The next week during BTC chapel, Dr. Farrar talked about "the significance of blood in the Bible and the Hospital's need," and then Grace Farrar stretched out on a table in front of the audience of forty, mostly young men.[34] Dr. Farrar spoke:

"All of you know this is my wife."

"Yes," came the answer in unison.

"My only wife."

"Yes."

"Do you think I would do anything to hurt her?"

"No."

---

[27]G. Farrar to Folks, August 23, 1966; G. Farrar to Johnson, October 9, 1966.

[28]G. Farrar to Folks, August 23, 1966.

[29]Farrar, *Stand*, 136; Author's recollection.

[30]G. Farrar to Mrs. H.C. Farrar, September 25, 1966.

[31]Farrar and Petty-Kraus, Interview; Savio, "Nigerian Christian Hospital;" Umeora, Onuh, and Umeora, "Socio-Cultural."

[32]G. Farrar to Mrs. H.C. Farrar, September 25, 1966.

[33]Farrar, *Stand*, 140.

[34]Ibid.; G. Farrar to Mrs. H.C. Farrar, September 25, 1966.

Total silence gripped the transfixed students as Dr. Farrar withdrew a pint of Grace's blood[35] and then "held up the blood for all…to see."[36] He noted his wife's health as she stood and walked around and then offered each student an orange drink and a can of meat in exchange for a pint of blood. Fearing that his sales pitch might be ruined if she demonstrated anything less than perfect fitness, Dr. Farrar insisted on driving a stable Grace the short, uphill walk home. That afternoon nine students added their pints to hers for the first ten units of an NCH blood bank.[37] Farrar waited to take Petty's type O negative blood in case it was needed for a future emergency.[38] Having a little and doing what they could was the best there was.

Marking the Transformation

On the same humid Monday that the first NCH newborn entered the world, the first NCH auxiliary students graduated. An August 29, US-style capping ceremony with candles, speeches, prayers, and certificates marked the transformation of five Igbo women from students to qualified nurse auxiliaries. The capping served as a poignant marker, not only for the students, but also for Hays and as meaningful to her as her own graduation. Americans and Nigerians jointly planned the ceremony, invited anyone interested, and held the celebration in the BTC as the only place with enough seating. Hays and Petty enjoyed watching students dress up for the ceremony in the nurses' home, but the two were less happy with their own appearances. Hays had no clean uniform because an all-day rain prevented washing and line drying, and Petty was soaked by the same rain when she ran outside to see a full, double rainbow[39]—a sight perhaps reminding her of biblical promises (Genesis 9:16).

"Impressive," Grace Farrar called the ceremony that began as tropical darkness descended. Wearing white bib aprons over their student uniforms, the women entered carrying lighted candles and walking in step with their "softly"[40] chanted Igbo hymn. Rees Bryant offered an invoca-

---

[35]Farrar, *Stand*, 140.

[36]Bryant "Reflections," 27.

[37]Ibid.; Farrar, *Stand*, 139-40; G. Farrar to Mrs. H.C. Farrar, September 25, 1966.

[38]Farrar and Petty-Kraus, Interview.

[39]Hays-Savio, Interview; Petty notes on back of photograph of the five auxiliary graduates in BTC building with Petty, August 29, 1966, NPK; Petty-Kraus, Farrar, and Farrar, Interview; Savio, "Nigerian Christian Hospital."

[40]G. Farrar to Johnsons, September 6, 1966.

tion, and Henry Farrar then spoke "on the quality of mercy,"[41] Patti Bryant presented each graduate with a Bible, and Rees Bryant or Farrar probably reminded graduates of their persistent theme: the most important person in the hospital is the patient. Friday Onukafor translated proceedings from English to Igbo, an honor likely assigned because of his cheerful encouragement, shopping, chauffeuring, and service as a go-between with chiefs that helped to make NCH possible.[42]

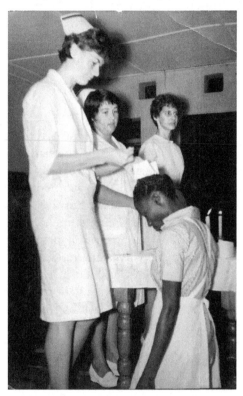

Photograph 29.2: Iris Hays, RN, capping graduate auxiliary Eunice Ukegbu with Nancy Petty, RN, and Patti Bryant in BTC Chapel, Onicha Ngwa. August 29, 1966. (Author collection.)

---

[41]Ibid.

[42]P. Bryant to Mattoxes, September 2, 1966; Bryant and Bryant, Interview; Farrar, *Stand*, 137; Hays-Savio, Interview; Hays-Savio and Petty-Kraus, Interview; Petty notes on back of black and white photograph of Iris presenting award to Lydia Agbara, August 29, 1966, NPK. Unremembered is whether R. Bryant spoke at both capping ceremonies or only the second.

Awards and capping followed. Lydia Agbara received a book and money for highest grades, and then each student knelt as Hays crowned her with a nursing cap similar to her own and Petty's.[43] Each also received a completion certificate "rolled up with a little ribbon" and signed by Farrar as Chief Medical Officer, Petty as Matron, and Hays as Sister Tutor.[44] Petty relit their candles, and the five graduates recited the Nightingale pledge in unison.[45] After a benediction and recessional, the graduates, their families, and the missionaries celebrated together with local favorites: kola nuts, oranges, peanuts, and Pepsi-Colas.[46]

Missionaries rejoiced. The capping represented one more step toward their medical mission dreams,[47] and Grace Farrar lauded "our" nursing students. She praised Hays and the auxiliaries in achieving this milestone toward an NCH future that would "of course" be Nigerian, with locals prepared to "carry on without us someday." The five, bright graduates, Grace Farrar intimated, might be called nurses if only NCH possessed the right training facilities. Hays had "taught them as earnestly as if they were registered nurses," she observed, and without them, the missionaries "could not operate the clinic or the hospital."[48] Matron Petty, to whom they were now accountable, viewed the five as functioning "on a high level of the best LPN you ever saw,"[49] and Dr. Farrar remained "pleasantly surprised" by their skills and efficiency.[50] Hays was disappointed only that she found no time to continue any structured education with them.[51]

Conclusion

Within eighteen months of the two missionary nurses' spring 1965 arrival, the COC team completed, equipped, staffed, and opened a clinic, hospital, blood bank, laboratory, and pharmacy. Personnel included both

---

[43]Bryant and Bryant, Interview; Hays-Savio, Interview; Petty (footnote 42); Untitled black and white photograph of Iris Hays capping Eunice Ukegbu in BTC building, August 29, 1966, HGF.

[44]Hays-Savio, Interview. Petty, Hays and Farrar's titles are recorded in 1967 "Capping Ceremony."

[45]Petty notes (footnote 42).

[46]G. Farrar to Johnsons, September 6, 1966; Hays-Savio, Interview.

[47]Bryant and Bryant, Interview.

[48]G. Farrar to Johnsons, September 6, 1966.

[49]Petty-Kraus, Interview 1.

[50]H. Farrar to Morgans, September 13, 1966.

[51]Hays-Savio, Interview.

professionally educated NRN midwives and missionary-educated auxiliary nurses. Hays had turned the NCH team's weakness into strength when an inability to afford NRNs sparked her preparing a cost-effective, LVN-equivalent staff, whose practice matched US expectations. A capping ceremony brought the five Igbo women into nursing sisterhood with the Americans.

And while an always-unassuming Hays never thought her classes flawless, their outcomes "amazed" her. NCH auxiliary graduates had grown up in "mud houses without knowing a lot of sanitation," and—like Hays in her younger years—probably never imagined they would become nurses. Yet, within twelve months, not only did Hays trust these auxiliaries to care for her if need be, but her work and theirs would soon go on to withstand tests of time and war into the twenty-first century. "So," Hays modestly supposed decades later, "That does make you feel like maybe the work wasn't all in vain."[52]

---

[52]Ibid.

30

Growing Pains

(September–December 1966)

It's good.

—Iris Hays

It's horrible.

—Nancy Petty

"I've been sewing while Nigeria fell apart," Patti Bryant observed of her furlough preparations.[1] The May 29 massacre of Igbos in the North was followed by another on July 29 and a third on September 29, and the ethnic brutality provoked October retaliatory genocide in the East. In September, when wounded and bleeding Easterners returned by "air, land, and sea"[2] through Enugu and Port Harcourt (PH), enraged residents killed innocent Northern beggars, traders, and others in their midst.[3] Police reportedly tried to protect non-Easterners, but headless bodies on PH streets mirrored the Igbo headless body returned to Enugu that spawned like images on gruesome propaganda posters.[4]

Even in the face of this violence, however, new COC workers continued to arrive in southeastern Nigeria, and the Bryants speculated that the only danger to white missionaries might be an anti-Christian, Islamic invasion of the East[5] or their getting "caught in the cross-fire."[6] A temporary PH airport closure stranded US first-time missionaries, teacher Lorraine Cussick and secretary Mary Cathy Newberry, in Lagos, but the two

---

[1]P. Bryant to Mattoxes, October 14, 1966.
[2]Madiebo, *Nigerian Revolution*, 84–85.
[3]Ibid.; Bryant, *Divine*, 295; P. Bryant to Mattoxes, October 14, 1966; G. Farrar to Johnson, October 9, 1966.
[4]Author's recollections; G. Farrar to G.B. Farrars, October 9, 1966; Farrar and Petty-Kraus, Interview; Madiebo, *Nigerian Revolution*, 84.
[5]P. Bryant to Mattoxes, October 14, 1966.
[6]R. Bryant to Kees, October 7, 1966.

taxied safely from there to their Ukpom COC compound destination,[7] and on October 1, Gid and Ruth Walters with preschooler son Alan entered through the reopened PH airport to work with the COC Bible Correspondence School in Aba.[8] Additionally, Rees Bryant's letters to the soon-to-arrive Kee family also focused on ordinary work and life,[9] and COC evangelists still traveled to distant preaching appointments on Sundays without fear. Henry Farrar spoke in nearby COCs in case of NCH emergencies,[10] and business-as-usual Nancy Petty took a six-day, October holiday in Enugu.[11]

Underwoods Depart

When David Underwood was well enough to travel, the Underwood family left Nigeria on October 27 through the reopened PH airport. Albeit only thirteen months at Onicha Ngwa.[12] David Underwood transformed into an outspoken advocate for healthcare missions, as his health crisis brought new attention to the contributions of COC physicians and nurses to evangelism.[13] Too, his cries of "Emergency!" were permanently etched into 1960s missionary laughter, lore, and language. The potential "catastrophe" of the Underwood family exodus was averted only by arrival of replacements, novices Gaston Dwayne and Jan Tarbet with baby Debbie, who arrived five days before the Underwoods' departure.[14] In a final act of caring, Rees Bryant surprised the Underwoods by accompanying them on the plane to the edge of the country in Lagos, where he then successfully followed up on visas for contractor Houston Ezell, Ezell's electrician son-in-law Doug Sanders, and the Kee family, who would replace the Bryants. For the first time, missionaries now filled the COC immigration quota of twenty-two, inspiring optimism about the future[15]—if only missionaries could ignore concurrent "reports of ethnic killings and rumors of war."[16]

---

[7]P. Bryant to Mattoxes, September 12 and October 14, 1966; G. Farrar to Mrs. H.C. Farrar, September 25, 1966.

[8]Bryant, *Divine*, 291.

[9]R. Bryant to Kees, October 7, 1966.

[10]G. Farrar to Mrs. H.C. Farrar, November 19, 1966; H. Farrar to G.B. Farrars, November 13, 1966.

[11]Petty to Spann, October 24, 1966.

[12]Bryant, *Divine*, 292.

[13]Underwood to McInteer, June 13, 1966, *WEV*.

[14]Bryant to Mattoxes, October 28, 1966.

[15]Bryant, *Divine*, 291–92; R. Bryant to Kees, November 2, 1966.

[16]Bryant, *Divine*, 291.

After returning to the US, David Underwood fully recovered, and the family entered fulltime mission work in Liberia and the Caribbean. They eventually returned to Florence, Alabama, where he served as both an elder at the Chisolm Hills COC for twenty-five years and a professor of Bible at Heritage Christian College for thirty-five years until his death at the age of eighty-two. Myra Underwood wrote and taught COC Bible curricula for women and children, retiring a few years before her death at eighty-eight years of age.[17]

NCH Nursing Image

Meanwhile, at NCH, Matron Petty designed new nursing uniforms after learning that NRNs customarily wore colored dresses, white aprons, and a hospital-specific cap. In September 1966 Petty wrote proudly of her handiwork that defined an NCH image for the all-women nursing work-force. Grade-one NRN midwives' uniforms were navy dresses with white collars, cuffs, aprons like Petty's student ones, and caps that were "smaller versions" of Petty's with a blue band on the corner. Grade-two NRN dresses were light blue with white aprons and the same style caps with light blue band. "Ward maids" (nursing auxiliaries) would wear new aqua head ties (scarves) and new aqua dresses with a white collar and half-apron that tied in back.[18]

No one recorded details of the transition to the new, NCH-provided attire, and a photograph of nursing auxiliaries in their previous style caps and uniforms suggests the change-over occurred during the US nurses' final weeks in the field. (See Photograph 31). Moreover, although the new uniforms may have pleased NRNs, NCH-educated auxiliaries objected to exchanging their awarded caps for scarves. After Matron Petty furloughed in March 1967, they secretly convinced tailor Irondi to make green nursing caps for them, but their plan failed when Windle Kee, the new US NCH administrator, discovered and forbade it.[19]

Months later after Hays and Petty left Nigeria, the titles of nursing staff seemed also in flux. Perhaps in-house NCH titles reflected staff functions rather than credentials, or perhaps Dr. Farrar wrote in his own professional shorthand. In his April 1967 payroll report, Dr. Farrar listed names of six NRNs, now including Miss Rose Ikonna, fourteen Assistant

---

[17]"Ralph David Underwood," findagrave.com no. 48041968; *Commercial Appeal,* "Myra Underwood."
[18]Petty to Spann, July 1 and September 13, 1966.
[19]G. Farrar to Petty and Hays, May 1, 1967.

Nurses, four Ward Maids, and five "Clinic" positions. Among the Assistant Nurses were Hays's eight graduates, three auxiliary students still in training when Hays furloughed, and three other names. One auxiliary student (Miss Helen) was listed among Ward Maids alongside three new Ward Maid names. Farrar did not record qualifications and titles of the five women holding "Clinic" positions.[20]

Infrastructure Grows

From September through December 1966, NCH added beds, welcomed new mission staff, benefited from professional builders, and saw progress toward a US fundraising board. The maternity unit quickly became self-supporting, at the same time that several other buildings neared opening: a thirty-bed women and children's ward, a surgical suite, and a laboratory and X-ray structure.[21] Just-in-time construction funds trickled in, and missionaries reallocated funds or sent workers home to control debt.[22] On Thanksgiving Day, Onicha Ngwa missionaries welcomed Hazel Buice, a US Registered Medical Technologist (RMT) at the reopened PH airport.[23] Faith Corps volunteer Buice arrived a day later than expected, but Hays was there to greet her[24] in keeping with her promise to meet every missionary.[25] Supported by the West Islip COC in New York,[26] Buice improved NCH's laboratory, provided skilled care, taught NCH's lay lab technicians, expedited nighttime emergency transfusions,[27] and possessed a "sunny disposition."[28]

---

[20]Farrar, "Financial Report…April 1—April 30th [1967]," W-COC file; Farrar, "Nigerian Christian Hospital, Payroll," April 1967, W-COC file.

[21]G. Farrar to Mrs. H.C. Farrar, November 19, 1966.

[22]P. Bryant to Mattoxes, September 28, 1966; Bryant, "Reflections, 27–28."

[23]Farrar to Mission Committee, December 27, 1966, *WEV*. According to Hazel Buice's daughter, Dorothy Buice, in email to author, August 21, 2017, Hazel Bickle (1912–1983) married Hugh Buice in 1940, and they divorced in 1949. In 1963 she moved from Texas to New York to become a member of Long Island's Exodus Bay Shore urban COC mission movement, and from there she moved to Nigeria as part of the Faith Corps in West Islip, NY. When evacuated from Nigeria, she began work with other evacuated COC missionaries in Republic of Cameroon, returned to Texas in 1976, and remarried Hugh Buice in 1979. Hazel was born and died on US Thanksgiving Days.

[24]P. Bryant to Mattoxes, November 25 [sic], 1966 (likely November 27); G. Farrar to Mrs. H.C. Farrar, November 19, 1966.

[25]Hays-Savio, Interview.

[26]Farrar to Mission Committee, December 27, 1966, *WEV*.

[27]G. Farrar to Mrs. H.C. Farrar, November 19, 1966.

[28]P. Bryant to Mattoxes, November 25 [sic], 1966.

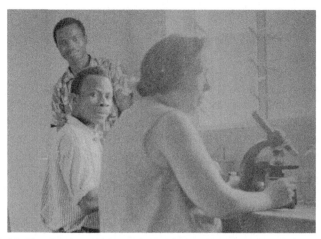

Photograph 30. Hazel Buice, RMT, with lay laboratory technicians, Sylvanus Nwagbara and Peter Uhiara in NCH laboratory. ca. 1966. (Bryant collection with permission).

Other US workers came, too, and more prepared to come. The day after Buice arrived, contractor Houston Ezell and electrician Doug Sanders arrived for three months of construction work at Ukpom's Christian Secondary School (NCSS) and at NCH.[29] Robert Windle (1930–) and spouse Barbara Oteka McFarland Kee (1930–), with preteens Paul and Alicejoy, were still scheduled to arrive in January 1967,[30] bringing with them four barrels of hospital supplies,[31] as well as funds to connect NCH and missionary houses with a nearby power line. Grace Farrar imagined "it would be like a dream" to have twenty-four-hour fans, as well as ice-making and daytime laundry capabilities. "We can understand how the people felt at the advent of the Industrial Revolution,"[32] she wrote, and with the heat of dry season upon them, she vowed not to return from US furlough until air conditioning cooled at least one room in her Nigerian house.[33]

Meanwhile, in the US, Green Lawn COC elders selected two of their own, Dr. F.W. Mattox and anesthesiologist Dr. Jesse Paul, "to take the lead" in identifying members of a proposed NCH board modeled after the Nigerian Christian Schools Foundation (NCSF).[34] Prompted partly by

---

[29]Farrar, *Stand*, 143; G. Farrar to Mrs. H.C. Farrar, November 19, 1966.

[30]Bryant, *Divine*, 263; R. Bryant to Mattoxes, December 26, 1966; Barbara Kee, Facebook Messenger to author, August 25, 2017.

[31]Bryant, *Divine*, 298.

[32]G. Farrar to Mrs. H.C. Farrar, November 19, 1966.

[33]G. Farrar to G.B. Farrars, November 5, 1966.

[34]R. Bryant to McInteers, October 19, 1966.

Rees Bryant's August 1966 proposal to F.W. Mattox, involved parties likely expected the board to be more efficient than a single congregation in raising money, expanding a COC fundraising base, providing "continuity" of NCH oversight, and managing recruitment and administrative issues, all while preventing direct financial entanglement of congregations in a hospital.[35] Mattox drafted a board charter, and a few months later in January 1967 held an organizing meeting in his home with Jim Massey, Hugh Rhodes, Jesse Paul, and Ray Wilson. During that meeting Wilson suggested that the board solicit funds only from individuals rather than congregations, possibly in order to avoid any appearance of being a mission society. Their efforts began what is today the nonprofit International Health Care Foundation/African Christian Hospitals.[36]

Concurrently in the field, care for missionaries and Nigerians continued. On Thanksgiving weekend, Dr. Farrar was called into service for an acutely ill Bill Curry, a COC evangelist living 150 miles away in Enugu. Within hours of learning that Curry had been hospitalized for a ruptured appendix complicated by dehydration and the often-fatal malarial black water fever, Henry Farrar and Rees Bryant made an emergency trip to check on him. Farrar determined that Bill Curry probably did not have black water fever, reassured his family about medical care and his likely recovery, and then returned to Onicha Ngwa the next day.[37] Doubtless Farrar ran a full NCH Clinic schedule the day after his return that helped to bring the total number of NCH patients treated in November to an estimated 2,735.[38]

Always eager to illustrate how the healthcare team's work facilitated evangelism, Farrar framed that number as the equivalent of a "campaign

---

[35]Bryant, *Divine*, 281, 325–26; R. Bryant to Mattoxes, August 4, 1966; G. Farrar to Mrs. H.C. Farrar, November 19, 1966; Mitchell, "Position Paper," January 3, 1984. Per Bryant in *Divine*, R. Bryant's proposed Board structure would include wealthy Christian donors with a nimbler small administrative group (281). Years earlier, in R. Bryant to Lawyers and Masseys on August 2, 1961, Rees stated that non-institutional Sewell Hall, would accept a Board as a scriptural way to fund a physician; and Mitchell in 1984 Position Paper, defends medical benevolence as an extension of the work of the Christian home. Mitchell also cites ACHF identification of its original functions as described in 1972 minutes of ACHF's first post-incorporation meeting: (1) appoint an "executive secretary" to carry out will of the Board, "(2) provide medical benevolence to Christian families in Nigeria, 3) assume oversight of the Nigerian Christian Hospital at Onicha Ngwa, (4) screen, recruit, and seek support for expatriate medical personnel for the hospital, (5) furnish medicine and other needed support, (6) originate appropriate written materials which would serve to promote the work of the Board."

[36]Bryant, *Divine*, 325–26.

[37]Bryant, *Divine*, 298–99; P. Bryant to Mattoxes, November 25 [sic], 1966.

[38]Farrar to Mission Committee, December 27, 1966, *WEV*.

for Christ" that reached 2,735 Nigerians at a total cost of $4,598.40, a figure that included costs for fifty-eight staff, medications, printed religious tracts, and building maintenance and construction. He reassured supporters that Nigerians themselves covered an estimated forty-four percent of those expenses, and his reporting of the Hospital's current debt as $5,500 perhaps was an implicit appeal for funds.[39]

Team Challenges

During Fall 1966, Petty complained that her Matron operational responsibilities forced her into becoming an administrator and no longer a nurse.[40] Meanwhile, she was happy to find NRNs willing to work for low NCH salaries and likely invested time in their orientation, while Hays continued educating the second auxiliary cohort.[41] Yet despite her complaints about paperwork, Petty alongside Hays and the NRNs treated a significant number of patients. Petty might see over one hundred patients weekly in maternal-child clinic, as well as take care of high-risk individuals, such as the three-pound, hospitalized newborn whose mother had infectious hepatitis.[42] Farrar-written protocols guided Nigerian nurses in assessing, treating, and admitting Clinic patients to the Hospital and in referring more difficult cases to Hays and Petty. By now NRNs and US RNs daily treated all but about ten of the most complex cases, whom Dr. Farrar would see.[43] Thus, in fall 1966 when Rees Bryant wrote to W-COC that Dr. Farrar was seeing 500–600 patients per week,[44] his use of "Dr. Farrar" is best understood as a proxy for the full team. Farrar had transitioned from his initial mistrust of others' seeing patients[45] to reliance on a diverse team.

Nonetheless, delegating remained difficult for Dr. Farrar, and at some point, Matron Petty reached her breaking point. Just as Farrar earlier usurped contractor authority delegated to Bryant,[46] he also usurped re-

---

[39]Ibid.

[40]Petty to Spann, December 1 and 29, 1966.

[41]Petty-Kraus, personal communication, November 15, 2018; Hays-Savio, Interview.

[42]Petty to Spann, October 24, November 3, and December 1, 1966.

[43]Hays-Savio and Petty-Kraus, Interview; Petty to Spann, July 27, 1966; Petty-Kraus, personal communication, April 10, 2017. After Hays and Petty's departure, H. Farrar to G. Farrar, June 15, 1967, documented midwives seeing 75 of 103 maternity clinic patients, assisting in 5 surgical cases, and delivering 3 babies of primiparas.

[44]R. Bryant to McInteer, October 19, 1966.

[45]Farrar and Petty-Kraus, Interview.

[46]Bryant, *Divine*, 248.

sponsibilities delegated to Petty. Repeatedly, Farrar would ask her to do a necessary task, and she would pray, plan, and present her ideas to him, only to have Farrar respond, "Don't worry about it; I've already done it."[47] These intrusions into her professional space finally became too much when he assigned Hays and Petty the work of designing and pricing inpatient furniture. Ten days later, the nurses brought their well-researched plans to Farrar, only to learn that he "had already done it!" A furious Petty rejected Farrar's proposal that the nurses could work on other furniture, suggesting that he do so himself.[48]

Before long, Rees Bryant gently confronted Petty. Dr. Farrar won't come to apologize to you, he counseled; she would have to take the initiative. The Matron accepted Bryant's advice, and as an exasperated, younger, and less powerful team member, she called a meeting to confront in-charge Farrar.[49] "Dr. Farrar," she asserted bluntly during the meeting, "I'm going home." You are doing everything yourself, and you don't need me.[50] Farrar was stunned; and he tearfully repented, begging Petty not to leave and promising never to interfere again. He kept his word, the Matron stayed, and the two reconciled. Nonetheless, from then on Petty took minutes at every meeting and, despite Farrar's protestations, required him to sign them, later coming to see these events as a therapeutic intervention. The two regained their strong, truth-telling friendship that lasted a lifetime.[51]

While Petty unswervingly appreciated Farrar's energy, creativity, skills, and heavy workload in preaching, teaching, seeing patients, and organizing NCH, she felt disrespected when he took over tasks delegated to her. The missionary nurses loved and admired Farrar, mused Petty years later, but he didn't always understand either what things meant to them or the work they did; but he knew "that it was more than he could do."[52] Onicha Ngwa men and women missionaries, she observed, were strong-willed "with a common goal and common vision" to spread the Christian faith and to alleviate physical suffering. Their different ideas about how to achieve those goals resulted in many "big...loud" arguments, yet the team concluded every meeting by praying for each other on their knees.

---

[47]Petty-Kraus, phone conversation, July 7, 2009.
[48]Hays-Savio and Petty-Kraus, Interview.
[49]Ibid.
[50]Petty-Kraus, phone conversation, July 7, 2009.
[51]Ibid.; Hays-Savio and Petty-Kraus, Interview; Petty-Kraus, personal communication, February 21, 2010.
[52]Hays-Savio and Petty-Kraus, Interview.

"You can't be angry with somebody that's praying for you very long," she conceded.[53]

"Good" and "Awful"

The thirty-bed women and children's ward opened on December 5, 1966, but it was too late to save its first patient, a protein-deficient little boy who died within hours of admission. Grace Farrar lamented that his perhaps fatalistic family did not seek care sooner. Conscious of the need to document NCH work, she regretted that no one took the boy's photograph.[54]

Yet other very ill children survived, sometimes unexpectedly, creating joy for parents and missionaries alike. In one case, the nurses administered intravenous (IV) medications to a preschool, comatose child with cerebral malaria. They anticipated his likely death, but "all of a sudden this child sits up in bed and tells his mom, 'I'm hungry,'" Hays laughed. "Just like that! It was wonderful!"[55]

Hays also expressed deep satisfaction in engaging nursing staff beyond the work of saving lives and later remembered a quieter morning when she modeled "care for the whole patient." The result was a woman, "happy as a lark," after Hays and Nigerian staff soaked and trimmed the patient's quarter inch thick, nails that extended beyond her toes. "It was one of those little things that you can...do...that makes somebody happy," Hays reflected. "It's good. It's good."[56]

The two US nurses covered shifts, supervised staff, and monitored women in labor. A nursing auxiliary might pass medications, but Hays or Petty started IVs and did anything needed. One night Hays attended a woman in labor—something she had never done before. Dr. Farrar had prepared her to manage an uncomplicated delivery, but she discovered that the infant was a breech or shoulder presentation and sent the night watchman to summon Farrar. Hays said that she "could've hugged Farrar's neck" when he arrived to relieve her and was thankful when NCH finally hired enough Nigerian midwives to deliver all babies.[57]

---

[53]Petty-Kraus, Presentation to Keen-Agers.

[54]G. Farrar to Mrs. H.C. Farrar, December 10, 1966; Petty to Spann, December 1, 1966.

[55]Hays-Savio, Interview.

[56]Ibid.

[57]Ibid.

In other care instances, sometimes a patient died and the family was not present. This meant that the Matron was responsible for transporting the body to NCH's unelectrified, hence unrefrigerated morgue in the field some distance from the wards, and the first time this happened was in the wee hours of the morning. The stretcher and body were too heavy for Hays and Petty and too long for their tiny car, so they borrowed the Farrars' Peugeot. Hays drove slowly while Petty walked behind in flip-flops holding onto gurney poles protruding from the car. "No snakes! No snakes! No snakes!" was all Petty could think until the trip was safely over.[58]

Matron Petty also made sure that deaths did not threaten NCH linen count. Once when a young woman and an old matriarch died on the same day, neither the families nor the hospital staff removed the sheets to check patient identity. The family of the young, childless woman buried her with little fanfare, but when the matriarch's relatives began preparing for her auspicious funeral, they discovered they had the wrong body. The family was understandably upset, and Petty was "furious." "It's your own fault," the Matron scolded the family and likely staff as well. "You knew you weren't supposed to take my sheets." The young woman's family dug up the matriarch's body, and driver Onukafor spent the day making sure that each set of relatives received their own family member. For Petty "it was horrible...It was awful." But she did get her sheets back.[59]

Homesick Holidays

The missionaries celebrated not only US holidays, but British Guy Fawkes Day and Dutch Queen Juliana's birthday, and Grace Farrar reveled in them all.[60] The Americans took care to explain to staff the details behind their Halloween décor, including Petty's carved "paw-paw" (papaya), which made each home "look like a 'juju' house," and Grace Farrar swiftly removed decorations before Halloween-naïve Nigerians visited.[61] The Farrars' third Thanksgiving in Nigeria was enhanced by her discov-

---

[58]Farrar and Petty-Kraus, Interview.

[59]Ibid. Petty-Kraus did not remember whether the sheet incident occurred pre-war or post-war.

[60]Farrar, *Stand*, 93, 99, 144, 163; Hays-Savio, Interview.

[61]G. Farrar to Johnson, October 18, 1964; G. Farrar to G.B. Farrars, November 5, 1966; G. Farrar to Morgans, November 5, 1966.

ery of a cranberry-like native fruit,[62] and she enjoyed leisure time for family and letters in December, instead of being "plagued by Christmas parties" as in America.[63] An especially high point was her husband's Christmas gift: a phone call to her parents in celebration of their fiftieth wedding anniversary. The Farrars' prearranged telephone-radio communications from the US Peace Corps Office in Aba went through London to a ship and then on through New York to Indiana, 9,000 miles away. The significant space dedicated to that happy call in Grace's letters suggests that she felt equally what she hoped for her parents: "Africa will not seem so far away now."[64]

Petty's preparations for her second African Christmas heightened her longings for home, and she experienced US holiday cards and letters as powerful reminders of beloved friends.[65] At the same time, she expected her remaining fourteen weeks in Nigeria to "fly by," and she nurtured a Christmas spirit, sitting barefoot in the oppressive heat and humidity beside her artificial tree, listening to American carols on the record player.[66] Later, Hays and Petty probably gathered with other missionaries for a December 23 holiday meal in the Ukpom Secondary School Dining Hall; there were too many missionaries now to fit in anyone's home. Then they may have spent a quieter Christmas Eve and Day relaxing in Onicha Ngwa.[67] Cool Harmattan winds brought in "perfect" December 25 weather, and Petty delighted in watching "bouncing happy" Virginia[68] chew open gifts during their only Christmas together.

Vocational Call Continued

BTC teacher J.O. Akandu closed out 1966 with a petitionary letter colored by his Christian faith. Echoing C.A.O. Essien years before,[69] his letter reflected a dream come true: the long expected Hospital had arrived. Akandu greeted, congratulated, and thanked missionaries by name. Then, instead of calling them to action based on a reciprocal Igbo-American

---

[62]P. Bryant to Mattoxes, November 25 [sic], 1966; G. Farrar to Mrs. H.C. Farrar, November 19, 1966.

[63]G. Farrar to Mrs. H.C. Farrar, December 10, 1966.

[64]G. Farrar to Johnsons, December 26, 1966.

[65]Petty to Spann, December 16 and 29, 1966.

[66]Petty to Spann(s), October 24 and December 16, 1966; Petty to John Spann, [1967]; Nancy Petty to Nancy Beth Spann, December 16, 1966.

[67]R. Bryant to Mattoxes, December 13, 1966.

[68]Petty to Spann, December 1, 1966.

[69]Goff, *Great*, 18.

relationship,[70] he petitioned all NCH staff to honor their shared religious obligation to God. Addressed to Rees Bryant, as secretary of the COC trustees, and closed with a signed blessing, the transcribed letter read in full:

> Much Congratulation to Dr. Henry Farrar, the Medical Superintendent of the Nigerian Christian Hospital, Box 823, Aba, To Miss Nancy Petty, Miss Iris Hays and the entire Hospital Workers, both white and black, for their good works in the Hospital throughout this year, 1966.
>
> Thank you for your sacrifices and successes. Many thanks to both Americans and Nigerians, who contributed towards the establishment of this Hospital. May Glory be to God.
>
> I hope you will be encouraged to continue taking part in Christian conduct according to the highest standards of conduct. Remembering the words of our Lord Jesus, "I was sick, and you visited me," (Matt. 25:36) And also the [Apostle] Paul's instruction, "So then every one of us shall give account of himself to God." (Rom. 14:12)
>
> May God grant all of you His richest blessings, throughout the New Year.
>
> Yours in His Service, J.O. Akandu[71]

---

[70]Korieh, "May it please."
[71]Akandu to Bryant, December 27, 1966.

31
Replacement-less
(December 1966–March 1967)

We are replacement-less.
—Henry Farrar

Nancy Petty enjoyed NCH patient care, citing a smooth-running C-section that added an infant son to one woman's six daughters. "I do enjoy scrubbing with Dr. Farrar," she penned a few days after Christmas.[1] Then, Petty's letter-writing pen fell almost silent under her heavy workload, furlough preparations, and accompanying exhaustion.

Missionaries Petty, Iris Hays, and Mike King planned to leave March 29, sightsee in Europe, and arrive in the US in April.[2] During 1966 the nurses had helped to care for 25,601 outpatients and to hire and prepare about sixty Nigerian staff. After inpatient beds opened in August, the team presided over ninety-five deliveries, five C-sections, and care for 233 inpatients, with an average six-day stay that yielded 1,396 patient days from September through December 1966.[3] By January 1967 the NCH team managed thirty-six beds[4] that kept Dr. Henry Farrar fully occupied and "his spirits…soaring." No longer did he send critically ill women and children home from the Clinic with stop-gap interventions; he admitted and treated them.[5]

[1]Petty to Spann, December 29, 1966.
[2]Farrar, *Stand*, 154–55; G. Farrar to Mrs. H.C. Farrar, March 14, 1967; Petty-Kraus, Interview 2.
[3]Bryant, *Gently*, bk. 3, 159; Farrar to Mission Committee, January 20, 1967, *WEV*.
[4]G. Farrar to Wiemhoffs, January 22, 1967.
[5]G. Farrar to G.B. Farrars, February 26, 1967.

Glass Half Empty

Hays and Petty intended to furlough as planned after two years even if US replacements didn't come. Hays, whom Rees Bryant called "a real jewel," intended to return to Nigeria after six months of rest; a burned-out Petty envisioned never coming back,[6] although she later agreed to relieve Hays during furloughs.[7] Meanwhile, US missionary Charley Bridges, RN, expected to arrive in Nigeria during April 1967 with financial support from the COC in Meadow, Texas, where Jim Massey preached.[8] Onicha Ngwa missionaries hoped that Bridges would arrive before Hays and Petty departed, but Matron Petty now prepared for Bridges to begin without them.[9] Additionally, Bryant asked F.W. Mattox to advertise for another nurse.[10]

How the absence of Hays and Petty would affect NCH work was unknown and received little attention in preserved correspondence. Many Nigerian staff were not COC members[11] and so did not share the US nurses' evangelistic aims. Moreover, none projected how novice Bridges might fill a space vacated by two now experienced missionary nurses. Petty and Hays had been pioneers, tackling their work with a faith commitment to do what they could. They built complementary work roles that fit their talents and energy, just as Nurse Glenna Peden had created a 1950s work that fit hers. Petty, Hays, and Farrar functioned as a team, and the nurses' departure would shrink the team by two-thirds. Perhaps missionaries hoped that just-in-time expatriate nurses would arrive in the same way that construction money came. But this was not to be. Bridges's arrival date became a matter of mere conjecture when the missionaries learned that her visa application was not submitted until March 31—days after Hays and Petty departed. Expected visa approval time was at least two months.[12]

Unlike Hays and Petty, by the end of 1966 the Farrars decided to wait on their replacement. They originally intended to serve three years

---

[6]R. Bryant to Mattoxes, December 26, 1966; Hays-Savio, Interview; Hays-Savio and Petty-Kraus, Interview; Petty to Spann, December 1, 1966.

[7]Petty, quoted in Minutes, Mission Committee, May 21,1967, W-COC file.

[8]G. Farrar to Mrs. H.C. Farrar, March 14, 1967; Hays-Savio, Interview; Minutes, Mission Committee, March 8, 1967, W-COC file. Per cited minutes, Meadow (misspelled Meador) COC requested West End COC help with costs of nurse Bridges.

[9]Petty to Spann, March 20, 1967.

[10]R. Bryant to Mattoxes, December 26, 1966.

[11]Bryant, Divine, 280; G. Farrar to Johnson, March 5, 1967.

[12]G. Farrar to Petty and Hays, May 1, 1967.

(1964–1967), furlough for one to two years,[13] and then return to Nigeria for a second tour. Dr. Farrar, however, was unwilling to leave without stewarding his much-loved NCH to a new physician, and when Dr. Damon Martin committed to come to NCH in spring 1967 and Dr. Ken Yearwood made plans to arrive in early 1968, Dr. Farrar decided to stay until both were in the field. By 1968, Farrar thought that NCH might require two physicians.[14] Rees Bryant urged F.W. Mattox to use the fledgling, still unincorporated NCH Board to help finance Martin's coming, and Nashville's Hillsboro COC joined W-COC in calling for a relief physician.[15]

Despite these efforts, the physician replacement situation worsened, when in January 1967, Martin declined to come for three reasons: fear of impending war in Nigeria, personal health, and potential church conflict because he was not a preacher.[16] The West End congregation (W-COC)[17] and Farrar did their best to persuade Martin that medical care itself was preaching through actions, with Farrar using "I Peter 3:1–2 to show that people may be won to Christ without saying a word,"[18] but Martin remained unmoved.

Moreover, the US government conscripted into military service "every young doctor" planning to serve in Nigeria as soon as each finished medical school, and now in support of the Vietnam War the draft board called up intern Yearwood for a physical. At Yearwood's request, Dr. Farrar petitioned the board to grant him a two-year deferral. Yearwood remained missionaries' "best prospect,"[19] and as Farrar's exhaustion grew, the Onicha Ngwa team prayed for Yearwood's coming.[20] In NCH, "Henry had a 'tiger by the tail,'" and could not or would not let go, observed Patti Bryant.[21]

---

[13]G. Farrar to Betty Johnson, in G. Farrar to Johnson, December 26, 1966.

[14]R. Bryant to McInteer, October 19, 1966; G. Farrar to Lashley, January 3, 1967; H. Farrar to G.B. Farrars, November 13, 1966; H. Farrar to McInteer, February 19, 1967.

[15]R. Bryant to Mattoxes, December 13, 1966; Hillsboro, "Dr. Henry Farrar;" Hillsboro, "Dr. Farrar."

[16]Bryant, *Divine*, 309; G. Farrar to Wiemhoffs, January 22, 1967; H. Farrar to McInteer, February 19, 1967.

[17]Minutes, Mission Study Committee, February 19, 1967, W-COC file.

[18]H. Farrar to McInteer, February 19, 1967.

[19]G. Farrar to Mrs. H.C. Farrar, March 14, 1967.

[20]R. Bryant to Mattox, February 14, 1967; H. Farrar to McInteer, February 19, 1967.

[21]Bryant, *Divine*, 309.

Glass Half Full

Grace Farrar adopted a positive spin on plans for the family's extended stay. First, Rees Bryant would soon be in the US raising NCH funds that an on-site Dr. Farrar could use to build NCH according to his specifications.[22] Second, an increased COC immigration quota created a need for more missionary housing, and that enabled her dream of building a home according to *her* specifications. Nevertheless, she announced unequivocally that the Farrars would leave "as soon as another doctor" arrived.[23] She loved Nigerians but missed US family and climate.[24]

She also felt the pinch of family finances. The Farrars deeply appreciated W-COC's ongoing, enthusiastic generosity in supporting them, and they considered themselves fortunate that a single congregation was willing and able to meet their financial needs.[25] After two and a half years in the field, however, Grace Farrar struggled to feed and clothe a family of seven on Dr. Farrar's unchanged salary. Their wages began low, did not keep up with inflation, and covered everything from voluntary church tithes to US insurance, household expenses, clothing, and a doubling of both teenage appetites and food prices. Before coming to Nigeria, Dr. Farrar had insisted that his income should match those of evangelists, so W-COC paid him exactly what Rees Bryant earned. While this strengthened Henry's status as a preacher and facilitated peace among missionaries, home budget manager Grace faced a different inequity: the Farrars, who had more and older children made less per family member than anyone else.[26]

Consequently, when Grace Farrar heard that W-COC had learned from Douglas Lawyer of their strained budget, she took family finances into her own hands. While not asking for a raise, she documented the rationale for it in a letter to her Nashville sister-in-law, Evelyn Farrar, whose husband George Farrar was a W-COC elder. Writing out "a little more exact information" to pass on to W-COC, Grace insisted that the family was not destitute, detailed their line-item budget, supplied a food price list, and noted that clothes were wearing thin. To make ends meet, Grace continued, she fixed local food in new ways, accepted second-hand

---

[22]G. Farrar to Lashley, January 3, 1967.

[23]G. Farrar to Johnson, March 5, 1967.

[24]G. Farrar to E. Farrar, February 26, 1967.

[25]Farrar to [missing], May 16, 1967.

[26]Bryant and Bryant, Interview; G. Farrar, personal communication, August 1, 2011; G. Farrar to E. Farrar, February 26, 1967; H. Farrar, personal communication, n.d.; Lawyer to W-COC, July 4, 1964.

clothes from departing missionaries, sewed for herself, bought used US children's clothing in Aba's market, and hired a tailor for Henry's wardrobe. She thanked Evelyn for gifting a shirt to each Farrar boy and reported that each owned "nice" church clothes and their clothes were no more patched than in the US. An always thrifty Grace Farrar proudly explained that she spent less money on groceries for her five children than did some other missionary families with two, adding that while she did not want the family's situation "exaggerated," they did "need more money."[27] Concurrently, a sympathetic Rees Bryant assumed that Dr. Farrar feared appearing ungrateful, and so privately wrote a direct request to W-COC asking them to increase Farrar's income.[28]

Their letters, however, proved more confirmatory than necessary. Before Farrar and Bryant had even penned them, W-COC, in a demonstration of their commitment, raised Dr. Farrar's salary by twenty percent and his working fund by thirty percent.[29]

Meanwhile, newly arrived fulltime evangelist Windle Kee and wife Barbara Kee arrived in January and applied their considerable business skills to NCH administrative work.[30] Farrar was thrilled and consequently increased his patient load, often going to the Hospital "several times a night." His health was at its best since his hepatitis,[31] although he relied on daily asthma medication to counteract Harmattan dust.[32]

Nigerian nursing personnel also increased after the February 15 graduation of more nursing auxiliaries.[33] Hays evaluated three of the seven students in the second cohort as fully prepared after eleven months of instruction, and the graduation of Clara Maduike, Rose Ngwakwe, and Zilpa Onwuchekwa Nwadibia[34] brought the total of fully qualified nurs-

---

[27]G. Farrar to E. Farrar, February 26, 1967.

[28]R. Bryant to McInteer, February 20, 1967; Bryant and Bryant, Interview.

[29]Minutes, Mission Committee, February 1, 1967, W-COC file.

[30]G. Farrar to Johnson, March 5, 1967; G. Farrar to Johnsons, April 16, 1967; H. Farrar to Mrs. H.C. Farrar, May 20, 1967; Minutes, Mission Committee, March 26, 1967, W-COC file.

[31]G. Farrar to E. Farrar, February 26, 1967.

[32]G. Farrar to G.B. Farrars, February 2, 1967.

[33]A surviving document ("Onicha Ngwa Bible Training College, Health Class Examination -1st Quarter," taken by Bernice Ugboyo, April 11, 1967, HGF) raises questions. Test items are complex (e.g., "b.i.d," and "pterygium"), but Hays-Savio and Petty-Kraus on May 16, 2012, denied knowing either Ugboyo or anything about the exam or any 3rd auxiliary cohort. Scores on the back of exam are in H. Farrar's handwriting, and calculations of average scores in the author's childhood handwriting; this suggests that the back of an old exam may have been used as scrap paper to record unrelated scores.

[34]"Capping Ceremony."

ing auxiliaries to eight. Their capping was like the first: a student processional, Gaston Tarbet's invocation, program introduction by Henry Farrar, "honor students" recognized by Iris Hays as "Sister Tutor," a capping address by Rees Bryant, "presentation of caps," students' recitation of the Nightingale pledge, a benediction by their "Bible Tutor" Gid Walters, and recessional. Again, Friday Onukafor interpreted, and refreshments followed.[35] Earning top grades was thirty-year-old Ngwakwe.[36] No one mentioned scarves versus caps.

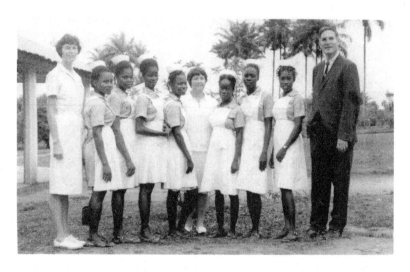

Photograph 31. NCH nursing auxiliary graduates from 1965 and 1966 cohorts, taken after the second NCH auxiliary class capping at the Bible Training College chapel, Onicha Ngwa, February 15, 1967. (left to right) Iris Hays, Comfort Amuta Nwosu, Lydia Agbara, Elizabeth Egbu, Esther Nwaghaghi Uzuogu, Nancy Petty, Zilpa Onwuchekwa Nwadibia, Rose Ngwakwe, Clara Maduike, and Henry Farrar. Graduated auxiliaries not pictured: Rachel Akwarandu, Mercy Ekanem, Hellen Nna Enyinna, Eunice Uzuegbu Uche, Nnebuihe Ugorji, and Eunice Ukegbu. Photograph by Rees Bryant or Grace Farrar. (Bryant collection with permission).

Knowing that he would soon leave Nigeria for many years, Rees Bryant used the capping address to articulate his convictions about COC healthcare. The auxiliaries' work, he proclaimed was

---

[35]Ibid.

[36]Chi Ekwenye-Hendricks, personal communication, April 30, 2014; Rose Ngwakwe, personal communication, March 3, 2018.

...a service in which the strong help the weak, a service of gratitude, a service of cooperation, and a service of love... Every patient at NCH is a soul of infinite value. No matter how poor, dirty, illiterate, old or weak, every patient is worth serving. You are not there to serve yourself. The patients are the most important people in the hospital.[37]

The missionaries celebrated, and the Bryants saw their medical mission dreams flower. Newly-arrived Barbara Kee was moved to tears,[38] while preteen Sara Bryant wrote matter-of-factly that "the capping ceremony was very good, except hardly anyone came. Also, Rose's candle went out during the benediction" (February 15, 1967). Hays regretted that her and Petty's increasingly busy schedules kept them from spending the same time in building friendships with the second cohort as they had with the first.[39] How education continued for the remaining four auxiliary students after her departure is undocumented, but Dr. Farrar's April 1967 NCH financial report showed all four still employed: three as Assistant Nurses and one as Ward Maid.[40]

Conclusion

In spring 1967, Rees Bryant asserted what all thought: NCH needed another missionary doctor and more nurses.[41] Arrival of new personnel, however, was at best uncertain, and Hays, Petty, and the Farrars responded differently. The US nurses would leave, and the Farrars would stay. Important to Petty was going home; important to Hays was returning to Africa; important to Grace Farrar was practical family support; important to Henry Farrar was living his medical mission dreams.

---

[37]Bryant, *Divine*, 314.
[38]Bryant and Brant, Interview; Kee, *African*, 65.
[39]Hays-Savio, Interview.
[40]Farrar "Financial Report...April 1—April 30th [1967]," W-COC file.
[41]R. Bryant to Mattox, February 14, 1967.

32
Fully Engaged: "Boots Feel Better Than Shoes"
(January–April 1967)

> If Nancy Petty would go with them…they felt safe.
> —Rees Bryant

"Boots feel better than shoes." So learned Nancy Petty from her dad, Albert;[1] and she wasn't the only one who valued hard work. All missionaries engaged fully in the mission until they boarded their flights to US homes. Even then, they took with them a commitment to keep the mission going.

Oil Palms & *Ọmu*

During Petty, Hays, and Bryants' remaining spring 1967 days in the field, an explosion of local animosity eclipsed missionary concerns about national conflict. The little stream where NCH, missionaries, and locals got their water also served as a tribal border between Igbos on the NCH side and Annangs (Ibibios and Efik-speakers) on the other, but a recent change in its course took both land and the land's oil palms from Igbos and delivered them to enemy Annangs.[2] The resulting ownership dispute was no small matter given the commercial significance of oil palms, and the quarrel quickly devolved into violence.[3] Perhaps worsening the situation was a historical pattern of bored young men sometimes initiating

---

[1]Nancy Petty Kraus, "Things I Learned From My Daddy," December 30, 1989, NPK.

[2]Bryant, *Divine*, 304. In letters COC missionaries often referred to Annangs as Ibibios or Efiks— the larger group of which Annangs were members.

[3]Basden, *Among*, Chapter 31; Basden, *Niger Ibos,* Chapters 14 and 29; Korieh, *The Land.*

inter-tribal conflicts "as almost a pastime" during dry season while farm-ing paused.[4]

Skirmishes between villages of Ikot Ineme on the Annang/Ibibio side and Onicha Ngwa on the Igbo side intensified in early January 1967 after Ibibio men stole water pots from Igbo women at the stream. Machete-armed Igbos, including some of the missionaries' household staff, lined up against armed Annangs on the opposite bank. Afraid of all-out con-flict at the compound's edge, outsiders Rees Bryant, Gaston Tarbet, and Henry Farrar with insider "Nigerian brethren"[5] physically stepped be-tween parties. Their pleas for peace provided a face-saving opportunity for both sides, generating the men's assertion that Bryant wouldn't let them fight. Igbos and Annangs put down their weapons and returned home.[6]

Sadly, within days the fragile peace erupted in murder. A young Igbo boy was killed, and only his head was left behind as an Annang threat or insult. Adding to the tension, two Igbo men bicycling to NCH for care were slaughtered where the Onicha Ngwa dirt road met the Aba-Ikot Ekpene highway, but they were not dragged across the border only be-cause Igbo women reportedly rushed out and threw themselves on the bodies. Local police refused to intervene in the conflict.[7]

The three murders added intratribal to intertribal fury, and as soon as the slain Igbos were buried, their villages of origin prepared to attack Onicha Ngwa Igbos because they had not protected their fellow Igbos.[8] Moreover, warring Annangs and Igbos again gathered on opposing sides of the stream "with slings, clubs, machetes, bows and arrows, home-made muzzle loaders, and every conceivable home-made weapon."[9] Again Rees Bryant and Henry Farrar, with interpreter Moses Oparah, sought peace. For three days they traveled among Igbo and Annang vil-

---

[4]Basden, *Niger Ibos*, 195, 377.

[5]Farrar to Mission Committee, January 20, 1967, *WEV*.

[6]Ibid.; Bryant, *Divine*, 304; P. Bryant to Mattoxes, January 17, 1967; Bryant and Bryant, Interview; Farrar to Mission Committee, January 20, 1967, *WEV*.

[7]P. Bryant to Mattoxes, January 17, 1967; Bryant, "Bloody;" Bryant and Bryant, Interview; Farrar to Mission Committee, January 20, 1967, *WEV*. Basden in *Niger Ibos* describes early 20th century possibilities that finding only the head suggested cannibalism (126–27) or threat of "eternal enmity" (260). Also in his 1940s *We Move*, Nau described Annangs' cannibalism as an outgrowth of animistic "belief that in eating a man's flesh the eater appropriates to himself the other man's soul and his vital power" (174); the Annang clan was feared even by other Ibibios (84–85, 174).

[8]Bryant and Bryant, Interview.

[9]G. Farrar to G.B. Farrars, February 2, 1967.

lages,[10] "preaching, praying, and persuading" everyone to disarm and call in the police for negotiations.[11] One angry man demanded to know what Bryant would do if an enemy murdered his child, and when Bryant hesitated, Oparah answered: The people of Gusau killed my daughter; "I want to...teach them the gospel."[12] Taking his cue from Oparah, Bryant recounted the Christian story of God's forgiving those who crucified his son, Jesus, and as he concluded, a lorry full of Aba riot policemen summoned by BTC teacher J.O. Akandu arrived. Conflict halted, evangelists' shuttle diplomacy ended, and a relieved Patti Bryant recorded a return to normalcy: "Missionaries could now go home and eat their supper."[13]

The dispute subsided, most likely through the combined effect of unarmed missionaries, armed policemen, and the imminent start of farming season. This allowed neutral parties Bryant and Tarbet to serve as emissaries for the quarreling groups by taking young palm fronds (*omu*) between villages as traditional Igbo "expressions of peace" and of a "desire to settle differences" between villages.[14] Grateful village elders presented an honorary machete to Bryant and assigned a corollary duty: If future trouble arose, he was to show the machete and "that will settle it."[15] Moreover, local chiefs came to the Hospital to thank missionaries for their part in restoring peace and saving lives. Dr. Farrar remembered it as the first time they had thanked him for anything.[16]

Bodyguard

The conflict also affected the missionary nurses. The three murders scared patients away from NCH in part because of false rumors that the two murdered men were pulled from the Hospital before their deaths. NCH daily census dropped from roughly two hundred outpatients to seventy or less for weeks.[17] Local Igbos, including NCH staff, were also afraid to go to the stream and instead filled their water pots at the mission. Moreover, on only one condition would frightened Hospital staff go to the stream to turn the NCH water pump on in the morning and

---

[10]Bryant, *Divine*, 305; Bryant and Bryant, Interview.
[11]G. Farrar to G.B. Farrars, February 2, 1967.
[12]Bryant and Bryant, Interview.
[13]Bryant, *Divine*, 305.
[14]Ibid.; Basden, *Niger Ibos*, 408-09.
[15]Bryant and Bryant, Interview.
[16]G. Farrar to G.B. Farrars, February 2, 1967.
[17]P. Bryant to Mattoxes, January 17, 1967; G. Farrar to G.B. Farrars, February 2, 1967; Farrar to Mission Committee, January 20, 1967, *WEV*.

off in the evening—Matron Petty must come with them. When she did, "they felt safe."[18] Petty thus became a Nigerian-recruited protector, unlike missionary men, who volunteered as peacemakers, and twice daily she walked with staff to the stream past where men were murdered to where water pots were stolen and tribes readied to kill each other. Locals on either side likely watched unarmed Petty and entourage to see what would happen on their trek to and from the contested border, and Petty joked to US colleagues that she would likely faint in the face of violence.[19] Fortunately, no one raised a hand against them, and the Matron's reputation as a determined white woman—one with a "beady-eye" glare who could snatch a thief from the hands of a murderous mob[20]—kept both peace and NCH water flowing.

Engaged

Rees Bryant worked hard until his departure. In February, he made a final trip to Lagos with the aim of increasing the COC immigration quota, and on his last Sunday, he preached with Messrs. Kee and Tarbet in distant Mballa to a crowd of four hundred, resulting in twenty-seven baptisms.[21] Then three days later, on February 22, 1967, after happy yet emotional farewell celebrations, the Bryants departed PH airport for a night in Lagos at the home of US COC members J.D. and Icy Thomas, to be followed by a trip through the Holy Land and Europe; planned US arrival was in early April.[22] Seeing the Bryants off were numerous Nigerians and Americans from Ikot Usen, Onicha Ngwa, and Ukpom compounds and COC women from PH.[23]

The Bryants 1958–1967 legacy of servant leadership included helping to replace fragmented COC first aid with a hospital—a change that brought education, employment, and Western healthcare to a corner of underserved Nigeria. There would have been no NCH without Rees Bryant, Dr. Farrar often declared.[24] After arriving in the US, Rees Bryant

---

[18]Bryant and Bryant, Interview.

[19]Ibid.; P. Bryant to Mattoxes, January 17, 1967.

[20]Farrar and Petty-Kraus, Interview.

[21]Bryant, *Divine*, 313–15.

[22]Ibid., 319–20, 292; P. Bryant to Mattoxes, February 8, 1967; Featherstone speech, February 17, 1967, RPB. The Thomases came with Nigerian Gulf Oil Company to serve as vocational missionaries in Lagos. He previously was an elder in Garden Oaks COC in Houston (R. Bryant to Mattox, February 14, 1967)

[23]P. Bryant to Mattoxes, February 22, 1967.

[24]Author's recollection.

taught at Lubbock Christian College, raised thousands of dollars in NCH funds, recruited healthcare professionals for NCH,[25] and preached part-time. The Bryants did not plan to return to Nigeria until all four children entered college, and their youngest had yet to begin elementary school.

In Nigeria, as Matron Petty counted down her own days to furlough, neither she nor NCH colleagues slowed their paces. Dr. Farrar performed his first surgery, a tumor resection, in the new Hospital operating room (OR) on February 5, 1967,[26] and he eagerly anticipated a Peace Corps regional blood bank nearby.[27] Staff moved their one large light back and forth between delivery room and OR as needed, and fascinated missionaries watched Farrar at work in the OR.[28] Matron Petty provided surgical support: running logistics of sterilization and instrument pack assembly while teaching Nigerians to do the same.[29] Although during nursing school, Petty thought it "a foolish waste of time" to spend a week "assembling packs for all kinds of surgeries," she now found that experience invaluable.[30]

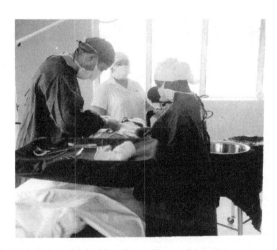

Photograph 32.1 Original label by Grace Farrar RN: "Henry operating in our new surgery. Nancy Petty is circulating nurse and Gertrude Mbong is the Nigerian nurse— She is a Christian and her father is one of our best preachers." (Author collection).

[25]R. Bryant to McInteer, February 20, 1967; Farrar to Mission Committee, May 16, 1967, *WEV*; McDaniel, "Nigeria;" Minutes of Mission Committee, March 8, 1967, W-COC file.

[26]Bryant, *Divine*, 310; R. Bryant to Mattox, February 14, 1967.

[27]G. Farrar to Mrs. H.C. Farrar, March 14, 1967.

[28]R. Bryant to Mission Committee, April 14, 1967, W-COC file; M. Farrar to B. Farrar, March 30, 1967.

[29]Farrar and Petty-Kraus, Interview.

[30]Petty-Kraus, Interview 1.

Petty also purchased family gifts[31] to carry home and delighted in serving NCH patients. Just a month before furlough she thrilled at two sets of twins delivered via C-sections and attributed one mother's lack of enthusiasm to her already having nine children.[32] In reality, the mother may have been more concerned about her own and her twins' well-being.[33] Mothers of multiples still sometimes died "mysteriously in hospitals," and in other cases husbands would no longer maintain marital relationships with them because they were "spoiled" (tainted).[34] Like Efiks in Ikot Usen, Igbos held twin taboos and might leave the infants in leaf-plugged water pots in the "bad bush" (evil forest) in order to avoid bringing supernatural wrath on the community. Some believed that normal human births occurred singly and that mothers of multiples demonstrated degradation to animal status.[35] Missionaries hoped that the Christian message would eventually undermine these beliefs[36]—a hope still not fully realized decades later as manifested in twin neglect.[37]

Meanwhile, Grace Farrar, who never intended to fill the nursing gap created by the departure of Hays and Petty, nonetheless enjoyed patient rounds with her husband and relished acting as Bible teacher for the youngest NCH patients. One Sunday she distributed "Bible pictures" and played Igbo-language "Bible stories and songs" for them, describing her audience thus:

> The first patient I came to is a tiny, emaciated little fellow who has neither mother nor father and is being cared for by his brother about 11 years old. He is in for malnutrition and bloody dysentery, making slow but steady progress. The next was another tiny fellow who had severe anemia and convulsions from malaria. After hovering between life and death for days he is making a gradual come back. The next is a darling little girl about 9 named Patience, and rightly so. She has been there for weeks in a plaster cast around her neck and spine for T.B. of the spine. It pushes her chin up high, and she cannot move so you think she would be very hot and unhappy and miserable, but she is so happy because her neck

---

[31] Petty to Spann, February 19, February 22, and March 20, 1967.
[32] Petty to Spann, February 19, 1967.
[33] Asindi et al., "Brutality."
[34] G. Farrar to Folks, August 11, 1965.
[35] Achebe, *Things*, locations 748, 1507, 1590, 1774, 2010; Basden, *Niger Ibos,* 180–83.
[36] G. Farrar to Folks, August 11, 1965.
[37] Asindi et al., "Brutality."

doesn't hurt now. The government furnishes drugs for T.B. patients, so she will be around for a long time to come and everyone's pet. The nurses are teaching her English. The next is another patient with spinal T.B. which is very common here, and we see many hunchbacks from it. Cornelius will be in his cast for about a year all the time receiving drugs and injections for his T.B. and vitamins and milk for his malnutrition. And so I could go on down the whole ward each one making a very heart-touching story.[38]

This portrayal of the medical and social situation of each child in her letters revealed Grace Farrar's desire to showcase the COC team's work to US family. Her and Patti Bryant's frequent use of first-person pronouns reflected their deep sense of identity as mission team members,[39] and the children's stories highlighted both the patient care by COC medical professionals and Grace's facilitative home management and teaching work. These individuals and others like them were why she had come to Nigeria. Their stories coupled with her in-hospital Bible class represented missionary success in filling a healthcare gap in the name of Jesus. Like 1950s COC women before her and 1960s contemporaries, she seized the opportunity to reach out to the most vulnerable.

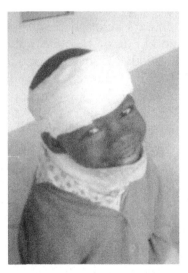

Photograph 32.2 Patience. Nigerian Christian Hospital. 1967.

---

[38]G. Farrar to Johnson, March 5, 1967.
[39]Bryant, *Divine*, 208; G. Farrar letters 1964–1967.

"The Nurses" Leave

Iris Hays left Onicha Ngwa abruptly on March 14, two weeks before planned, after the US Consulate sent word that her brother, who worked in Saudi Arabia, was ill. She hoped to see him before she traveled home to Texas and managed to get the rare, last-minute seat on a PH-to-Lagos plane. This left Matron Petty alone to hand over NCH to capable NRN-midwives, as well as to collect the US nurses' tickets and travel papers and pack their belongings.[40] The Consulate's communication reassured Grace Farrar that emergency messages could still reach them in the midst of Nigeria's political turmoil.[41]

As it happened, Hays got only as far as Lagos. A Muslim holiday made it impossible to get a Saudi flight or visa, and Petty counseled Hays not to return to Onicha Ngwa. Airplanes from PH were full of expatriates fleeing Nigeria's ongoing instability, and Hays might not be able to leave again. Hays took her advice and for two weeks waited as a guest of J.D. and Icy Thomas in Lagos until Nancy Petty and Mike King could join her.[42]

Meanwhile, Nancy Petty made the painful decision to leave Virginia in Nigeria. Believing this was in Ginny's best interest, she rehoused her in Aba with COC missionaries Gid and Ruth Walters and preschool son Alan until Virginia grew enough to rejoin her Igbo father. "I will miss Virginia," Petty jotted ten days before departure to her sister, "but Ruth & Gid are taking such good care of her. She is almost 8 months old and 21 pounds...A very beautiful baby." In that same letter, Petty wished that she could hand off her work to nurse Charley Bridges and hoped that undescribed "major problems with the nurses" were resolved—a kerfuffle perhaps triggered by transitioning to the Petty-designed auxiliary scarves in place of caps. While still downplaying any personal danger to herself, Petty confided that political violence might disrupt her March 30 Lagos departure, cautioned her sister that communications might be interrupted, and instructed her not to share this information with their mother "unless we (Nigeria) get in the news."[43] The departing COC John and Dottie Beckloff family carried Petty's letter overland by taxi to Lagos

---

[40]Petty-Kraus, Interview 2.

[41]Farrar, *Stand*, 155.

[42]Hays-Savio and Petty-Kraus, Interview.

[43]Petty to Spann, March 20, 1967.

after they tried unsuccessfully to persuade her to leave with them before political unrest closed her own exit.[44]

Petty and King left PH airport as planned on March 29. A crowd of missionaries saw them off, and they reunited with Hays in Lagos. As soon as they arrived at the Thomases' home for the night, however, an exhausted Petty realized that she had left her purse with all their travel papers and her money in the now-closed Lagos airport. There was nothing to do but wait until morning. A physically drained Petty, who had worked solidly for the preceding two days and nights at NCH, slept, while distressed King and Hays prayed for the purse and papers. Early the next morning at the airport, Petty's purse and all its contents were returned to her along with what she acknowledged was a well-deserved rebuke from the cleaning man who found them. "Madam," he asked, "Why were you so careless?" A grateful Petty gave him all her Nigerian currency, and the three US travelers left as scheduled for sightseeing through Egypt, the Middle East, and Europe.[45] NCH nursing was now fully in Nigerian hands.

Like so many things between the two nurses, their reasons for future plans differed. Hays's plans to return to NCH within months were motivated by compatible missionary coworkers, a missionary identity, and her family situation at home. Challenges of long hours, insects, and snakes were overshadowed by the gratitude of patients and the lives she preserved.[46] In contrast, Petty's intentions to remain in the US were supported by a reversal of life priorities, as her deep love of home and family overtook her Nigerian call. Petty left the country confident that the two nurses had completed all they planned to do—along with things they never imagined.[47] Too, she adored Virginia and cherished Nigerian and US friendships formed in the field. The nurses were now intimate confidantes and lifelong friends, and Henry Farrar, a respected and respectful mentor. And so while Petty happily abandoned her Matron paperwork, she, like Hays, was changed.[48]

---

[44]Author's recollection; Beckloff, Interview, June 6, 2014; G. Farrar to Johnson, March 20, 1967; Farrar and Petty-Kraus, Interview.

[45]Petty-Kraus, Interview 2; Petty to Spanns, March 31, April 3, April 5, April 11, April 14, April 20, 1967 (2), and April 21, 1967 (travel postcards).

[46]Hays-Savio, Interview.

[47]Petty to Corlew, June 6, 1966; Petty to Spann, March 20, 1967; Petty-Kraus, Presentation to Keen-Agers.

[48]Farrar and Petty-Kraus, Interview; Petty-Kraus, Interview 1.

East "On the Brink"

Meanwhile, Nigeria's political situation grew "continually...more gloomy." Grace Farrar still hoped that a visiting physician could give her husband a few weeks respite to recover from the combined effects of a sinus infection, malaria, and asthma.[49] Dr. Farrar had worked without a day off since the opening of inpatient units almost eight months prior, and now his missionary nurse support was gone. The Farrars hoped that Dr. Paul Spray, an orthopedic surgeon with CARE (Cooperative for American Relief Everywhere) might provide relief, but Spray canceled his planned three-month visit to NCH on the advice of Enugu officials concerned about political volatility.[50]

By the time Hays, Petty, and King left, Nigeria's East seemed set on secession. The region assembled an army, hired a public relations firm, prepared the airport for siege, halted railroad traffic from the rest of the country, and witnessed daily pro-secession street demonstrations. Nigeria's federal military leader, Gowon, reversed his earlier support of Northern secession and warned that he would use force if necessary to maintain the country's unity,[51] while the East became "like that of a nation on the brink of war."[52] The Eastern region's leadership saw no reason to accept any pretense of a unified Nigeria and was in no mood to turn over its oil revenues to a federal government that neither protected all its citizens nor sent resources to deal with the 1.8 million refugees who fled to Eastern homelands.[53]

COC missionaries hoped for peace but planned for heightened conflict, and the Farrars bought extra food and gasoline. Embassy officials told them that the US was not worried but had prepared evacuation plans if needed. Taking their statements as her cue, Grace reassured US family that the situation was an ethnic conflict, not an "anti-white" one and that the sometimes "skittish" Peace Corps maintained hundreds of personnel in the East.[54] "So never fear!" she penned. "Uncle Sam is here all around us."[55]

---

[49]G. Farrar to G.B. Farrars, March 26, 1967.

[50]G. Farrar to Johnsons, April 9, 1967; Spray, *Nigeria Orthopedic Project*.

[51]G. Farrar to G.B. Farrars, March 26, 1967; Garrison, "Eastern Nigeria;" Garrison, "Eastern Area."

[52]Garrison, "Eastern Nigeria."

[53]G. Farrar to G.B. Farrars, March 26 and April 9, 1967; Garrison, "Time."

[54]G. Farrar to Mrs. Henry Farrar [sic], March 25, 1967 (intended and sent to Johnson).

[55]G. Farrar to G.B. Farrars, March 26, 1967.

As anticipated, the East refused to relinquish oil revenue due to Lagos on April 1, and the federal government promptly shut down all flights to and from the East. Petty and King's March 29 flight was the last from PH,[56] and the Curry missionary family departed Enugu for scheduled furlough by chartered taxi. "Only God knows" what will happen, Grace Farrar wrote. Without a relief physician, she saw no "prospects for coming home" in 1967, and national tensions made Nigerian vacation sites inaccessible. Their oil company friends living in PH had not attended Onicha Ngwa church services for two weeks, and she assumed their companies forbade them to travel.[57] She could no longer buy vegetables from the North,[58] and the garden that she started for relaxation and exercise became "part of a serious effort to live off the land."[59] At the same time, the Farrar children remained so happy that they did not want to return to the US except to see family. Their days were full of Scouting, their pet genet, books from the Ikot Ekpene library, local bicycling adventures, soccer, a missionary children's track and field day, and homeschool.[60]

New missionaries were still en route. Nurse Bridges waited only on her visa,[61] and Vanderbilt medical student John Crothers wrote optimistically of coming to NCH for six weeks in June.[62] Dr. Lloyd and family from Indiana planned to relieve Dr. Farrar during August,[63] and Dr. Ken Yearwood remained enthusiastic about arriving in January 1968.[64] A second new medical school graduate, Dr. David Wilbanks, intended to join Yearwood;[65] Brenda Adams, RN, from Minneapolis, Minnesota,[66] too, had decided to come, and Dr. J.D. Cochrum from Austin, Texas, was considering NCH.[67] Additionally, M.N. and Inez Norwood from Marion,

---

[56]Petty-Kraus, Interview 2.

[57]Farrar, *Stand*, 159; G. Farrar to Johnsons, April 9, 1967.

[58]G. Farrar to Morgans, November 5, 1966; Farrar to Johnsons, April 16, 1967.

[59]Farrar, *Stand*, 160.

[60]Author's recollection; G. Farrar to Johnsons, April 9 and 16, 1967; G. Farrar to E. Farrar, April 13, 1967; G. Farrar to Mrs. H.C. Farrar, April 13, 1967; M. Farrar to B. Farrar, March 30, 1967.

[61]G. Farrar to Johnsons, April 9 and 16, 1967.

[62]G. Farrar to E. Farrar, April 13, 1967.

[63]G. Farrar to Johnsons, May 1, 1967; G. Farrar to Petty and Hays, May 1, 1967.

[64]G. Farrar to Mrs. H.C. Farrar, April 13, 1967.

[65]G. Farrar to G.B. Farrars, May 25, 1967; Yearwood and Wilbanks, quoted in Coleman, "Challenge."

[66]Adams to Elders, April 29, 1967, W-COC file; Adams to Bergstrom, May 22, 1967, W-COC file.

[67]Farrar to Mission Committee, May 16, 1967, *WEV*.

North Carolina, prepared for Ukpom work,[68] and Grace Farrar eagerly anticipated the arrival of Norwoods' shipped barrels that included much-needed Farrar family clothing.[69] Local tailor attempts at American-style outfits frustrated her.[70]

Mail and money for the Hospital continued to arrive. Among contributors were M. Norvel and Helen Young, the parents of Matt Young, who had worked at NCH in summer 1966; he had convinced them to spend $300 on NCH construction instead of a new color television.[71] US mail came overland from Lagos, and Grace warned her family: If letters stop, "don't worry." Hundreds of US citizens remain, and "Uncle Sam is prepared."[72]

Conclusion

Although COC missionaries successfully stepped between warring villages, they could not do the same between warring regions. Tensions over oil revenue only added fuel to raging, centuries-old, ethnic fires. The Hausa–Fulani pogrom against Igbo "strangers" that generated predictable Igbo flight and revenge killings,[73] also shut down Nigerian transit of goods and people and brought "the landlocked North…to the verge of economic breakdown."[74] The prospect of civil war loomed, and fears spread in the Western press: If Nigeria could not maintain unity, how could poorer African countries?[75]

Igbo confidence in their country's government failed, while American confidence in their own rose. COC missionaries came, went, and worked largely unimpeded. Grace Farrar's personal history of faith, hard work, and thrift stood her well, while Nancy Petty invested fully and fearlessly until she left NCH, bolstered by childhood lessons from her father: Don't be afraid, finish what you start, you have a responsibility to meet

---

[68]G. Farrar to Johnsons, April 9, 1967; G. Farrar to G.B. Farrars, March 26, 1967.

[69]G. Farrar to G.B. Farrars, March 26 and April 9, 1967; Norwood to Mrs. H.C. Farrar, March 31, 1967.

[70]G. Farrar to E. Farrar, April 13, 1967.

[71]G. Farrar to Mrs. H.C. Farrar, April 13, 1967.

[72]G. Farrar to E. Farrar, April 13, 1967.

[73]Garrison, "Wave."

[74]Ibid.; Garrison, "Railroads."

[75]*Chicago Defender*, "Crisis."

your neighbor's needs, hard work won't hurt you, and you don't control much.[76]

---

[76]Farrar and Petty-Kraus, Interview; Kraus, "On Daddy's Knee;" Petty-Kraus, Interview 1.

33

Walking Away: End of Their Beginnings

(April–July 1967)

Things have never looked better for us and the hospital, or worse for Nigeria.
—Grace Farrar

The Farrars traveled to Enugu for two days in late April, while Dr. Ud-ofia Udo "Edward" Akpabio,[1] a Seventh Day Adventist Ibibio physician, covered NCH responsibilities. In Enugu Henry Farrar asked regional officials to do for NCH what they were already doing for other missions: Send a government-salaried physician from among those fleeing other parts of the country. Farrar asked specifically for Akpabio, who was sympathetic with the Igbos and wanted to work with NCH, but officials initially refused his reassignment from Ogoja. Still, Grace Farrar was pleased that her husband experienced a brief holiday, and the family enjoyed the zoo, swimming, and seeing missionary friends. Too, Grace stocked up on meat and vegetables no longer available in Aba.[2]

"Things have never looked better for us and the hospital or worse for Nigeria," she wrote.[3] Missionaries anticipated an "abundance of good water," from NCH's completed well,[4] funds on hand were enough to finish the men's ward, and W-COC members sent money to buy much-needed clothes for the growing Farrar children.[5] NCH outpatient load rose again to 150 to 175 per day, and US physician and nurse replace-

---

[1] Akpabio, *He Dared*, 232, 267–68.
[2] Farrar to Mission Committee, August 11, 1967, *WEV*; G. Farrar to Johnsons, May 1, 1967; G. Farrar to Petty and Hays, May 1, 1967.
[3] Farrar, *Stand*, 164.
[4] G. Farrar to G.B. Farrars, May 25, 1967.
[5] G. Farrar to Mrs. H.C. Farrar, April 13, 1967.

ments were expected.[6] Nonetheless, in the context of his heavy workload Dr. Farrar lamented, "We really miss Iris and Nancy."[7]

At the same time, the missionaries' mail began "getting strayed and delayed,"[8] and they cabled Rees Bryant not to mail US donations but instead to deposit them in the bank for withdrawal in Nigeria. The only certainty about Nigeria's future seemed its uncertainty, and rumors abounded. True was that the US was sending no new Peace Corps or USAID personnel.[9] False was that British troops had arrived to support Nigeria's federal government. While Grace Farrar earlier assumed the inevitability of civil war, now on the eve of secession she expected "no fighting" if the East proclaimed itself an independent country.[10] Many expatriates agreed that "Nigerians palaver long, but fight seldom."[11]

Republic of Biafra

The Farrars were right about secession and wrong about war. On May 27, Easterners demanded that their military leader Lt. Col. C. Odumegwu Ojukwu declare independence from Nigeria. Ojukwu's choice was either to lead secession or be deposed so another could, and on May 30, 1967, he declared sovereignty of the East as the new Republic of Biafra under "Almighty God" and in affirmation of the "inalienable rights" of all. Ojukwu asserted that among many negative federal actions, the timing of violence against Igbos on May 29, July 29, and September 29, 1966, demonstrated Nigeria's premeditated rejection of the East. Under the pretext of maintaining unity, he noted, Northern soldiers had moved into Lagos, resuming the North's historical, explicitly articulated intentions of a "conquest to the sea" that was interrupted only by British colonizers.[12]

---

[6]G. Farrar to G.B. Farrars, May 25, 1967; H. Farrar to Mrs. H.C. Farrar, May 20, 1967.

[7]Farrar to Mission Committee, May 16, 1967, *WEV*.

[8]G. Farrar to G.B. Farrars, May 25, 1967.

[9]G. Farrar to Johnsons, May 1, 1967; G. Farrar to Petty and Hays, May 1, 1967.

[10]G. Farrar to G.B. Farrars, May 25, 1967.

[11]Farrar, *Stand*, 167.

[12]Ojukwu, *Biafra*, 147–48, 176–96; *New York Times*, "Man in News;" Reuters, "Lagos."

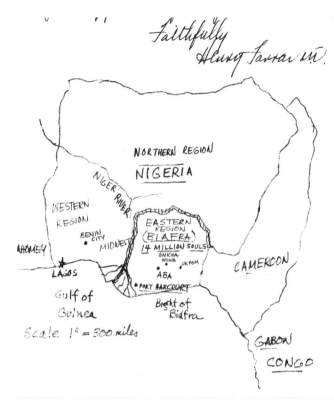

Map 3: Republic of Biafra, hand drawn by Henry Farrar, in Farrar to Mission Committee, August 11, 1967, *WEV*. (Author collection. Scale altered for print).

In the East jubilant crowds interrupted Ojukwu's speech with cheering and dancing,[13] while in Lagos federal leader Gowon ordered an immediate full communications and commerce blockade of Biafra.[14] Ojukwu ascended to "His Excellency" as military ruler of Biafra, and Gowon rose to Major General in Nigeria. Each British-educated leader was determined: Ojukwu to establish peaceful civilian rule in Biafra and Gowon to keep Nigeria unified. Each seemed lionized by their own supporters and vilified by others.[15] The *New York Times* portrayed both as "prisoners of political and tribal possessions that neither can fully control—both men…symbols rather than innovators of the country's tragic disunity."[16]

---

[13]Farrar, *Stand*, 166; Author's recollections.

[14]Reuters, "Lagos."

[15]Farrar, *Stand*, 166; Meisler, "Mood;" *New York Times*, "Man in News;" *New York Times*, "Nigeria's Military Ruler."

[16]*New York Times*, "Man in News."

Igbo Ojukwu proclaimed a commitment to govern the new Republic on behalf of all Eastern people.[17]

Rumors of impending war spread through expatriate communities. COC missionaries at Ukpom, except for Eno and LaVera Otoyo, turned their school over to Nigerians and surprised Onicha Ngwa colleagues with their sudden June 4 exodus. The next day, the alarmed Farrars traveled to PH where they learned that the US Ambassador had advised companies in the East to evacuate dependents aboard US-chartered, PH-to-Lagos flights from the otherwise closed PH airport. Planes would depart three times daily for five days during the first week of June only, confronting missionaries with an abrupt choice: Leave while their government provided a way out or stay and take their chances on potential war. NCH was nearing completion, and the situation was so fluid that each COC family decided for itself what to do. Recently arrived Kees and Tarbets could not bear to return to the US, and Grace Farrar wanted to stay, but her husband's perspective prevailed. If war came, Henry argued, he could more easily "sneak through the bush or get a boat down the river" on his own. The Aba bank was refusing withdrawals, and the Farrars had just spent all their cash for groceries that would last longer for a solo Dr. Farrar. In Lagos, Grace Farrar could access money and continue homeschooling. If calm returned to the East, so could she. If it did not, she and the children could wait for Dr. Farrar in Rome or the US.[18]

That night in Onicha Ngwa the Farrars feasted on expensive canned ham and strawberries that they no longer needed to save for a special occasion. Each, except Henry, packed a suitcase to the 44-pound limit with schoolbooks and treasured possessions,[19] and Grace Farrar took comfort in her faith that God would protect what was most important to her: her family. She went to sleep "determined" to use events to teach her children the relative unimportance of possessions.[20]

The next day, June 6, Grace Farrar kissed her husband goodbye and boarded a PH-to-Lagos flight with their five children, having directed the $175 per seat airline bill to W-COC. They had no cash for the flight, and Dr. Farrar wrote her a $1,000 check from his working fund in case she needed to evacuate further to Sierra Leone.[21] She remembered looking

[17]Ojukwu, *Biafra*.
[18]Associated Press, "Lagos;" G. Farrar, *Stand*, 166–68; Farrar to McInteers, June 17, 1967; G. Farrar, quoted in Bryant and Massey to Brethren, *Nigerian Evangelism*, Meadow COC, August 1, 1967, W-COC; Reuters. "Lagos."
[19]Farrar, *Stand*, 168; G. Farrar to G.B. Farrars, July 22, 1967.
[20]Farrar, *Stand*, 168.
[21]G. Farrar to Brethren, June 8, 1967, W-COC file.

back from the doorway of the plane "at a tearful Henry—both of us wondering when, if ever, we would see each other again."[22] The Farrars' life together in the Republic of Biafra had lasted one week. The futures of Nigeria, Biafra, and NCH were veiled, and COC missionaries put their trust in each other, God, and Uncle Sam.

Solidarity

An hour later, the Red Cross greeted evacuees at the US Embassy in Lagos, and Grace Farrar watched as oil company limousines transported other wives and children to safety. Meanwhile, she tried unsuccessfully all day to phone her only Lagos contact, Ted Greer, a US COC member and United Geophysical employee. The Greers and Farrars had never met, and as evening descended, only her family remained in the Embassy. She had no money and no idea where to go. As she later wrote of that moment,

> Loneliness swept over me. How comforting it must be to rest in the long arms of some oil company and hear, "You belong to us. We will take care of you. Tomorrow you will be at home in America." [Then] suddenly it dawned on me. What was I thinking! I work for the One who owns all the oil.[23]

Moments later, a US official reached Ted Greer by walkie-talkie with the message that a woman with five children waited at the Embassy for him. Greer's welcoming response was swift, and soon the Farrars, too, were whisked away in their own limousine into the comforting arms of the COC community with the unspoken message, "You belong to us. We will take care of you." Ted and Ada Greer greeted the Farrars warmly with a meal, a driver, and housing in the luxury condominium of furloughing J.D. and Icy Thomas, where the Bryants, Petty, King, and Hays previously stayed.[24] Other COC members, too, aided the Farrars during the weeks to come. Leslie Diestelkamp, who remained opposed to medical missions, twice visited to offer help,[25] and from the US Jim Massey made his Nigerian bank account available to Grace Farrar. Additionally, she obtained visas for the Cameroon and Sierra Leone, the latter at the invita-

---

[22]Farrar, *Stand,* 168.
[23]Ibid., 169–70.
[24]Ibid.
[25]G. Farrar to Johnson, June 24, 1967.

tion of missionary Paul Dillingham in Freetown in case she needed to wait out the situation there.[26] The "long arms"[27] of COC solidarity proved a supportive family of faith for the Farrars—the church's relational counterpart to oil companies' business obligations to employees.

For about six weeks, Grace Farrar hesitated in Lagos. Likely concerned that her husband could not get mail out to W-COC, she took the unusual step of writing them herself, including information from Henry's letters to her, summarizing family, local, and national situations for them[28] and emphasizing the Farrars' current safety. She reiterated to W-COC that the Nigerian upheaval was unlike the Congo's anti-white one. Meanwhile, she and her husband corresponded around army lines through various channels, including a PH friend, blockade runners for both the Peace Corps and Aba textile mill, and Cameroonian, COC member D.N. Elangwe in Kumba.[29] Mail delivery was erratic, but Grace Farrar watched and waited, fearing that she might lose all contact with her husband if she left.[30]

Meanwhile, in Onicha Ngwa, Dr. Farrar still could not justify leaving NCH without a physician on site. By June 10, he dismissed nonessential Hospital employees, raised patient fees, and accessed his working fund to support himself and NCH during the blockade. He still preached in multiple churches on Sundays and opened the men's ward the week of June 19, making NCH fully operational with hundreds of outpatients and an estimated ten surgical cases weekly.[31] The team appointed Miss Solomon NRN as Acting Matron and hired two more NRNs, Mrs. Nwaji and Miss Udo Affia.[32] The generally pessimistic, lonely Henry Farrar hoped that his wife might be able to return within a month, but the generally optimistic, practical Grace Farrar remained doubtful. Until banking and mail services were restored in Biafra, she thought it unwise to go back. If the situation "dragged on," she wanted their children to enter US schools in

---

[26]Dillingham to G. Farrar, June 15, 1967; G. Farrar to McInteers, June 17, 1967; G. Farrar to Johnson, June 24, 1967; G. Farrar to Brethren, July 14, 1967, W-COC file.
[27]Farrar, *Stand*, 169.
[28]G. Farrar to Mission Committee, June 8, June 18, June 27, and July 14, 1967, W-COC file.
[29]G. Farrar to McInteers, June 17, 1967; G. Farrar to Johnsons, July 5, 1967; G. Farrar to Brethren, July 14, 1967, W-COC file; H. Farrar to G. Farrar, June 20 and 22, 1967; Farrar to Mission Committee, July 11, 1967, W-COC file.
[30]G. Farrar to Johnsons, June 29, 1967.
[31]Ibid.; G. Farrar to Johnson, June 24, 1967; G. Farrar to Petty, June 10, 1967.
[32]H. Farrar to G. Farrar, June 20 and June 22, 1967.

the fall. Both were skeptical that civil war would come, given Igbo determination and federal limitations.[33]

Blockade Crossings

The Tarbets discovered that John Freeman, a friend and US drilling supply contractor in PH, would exchange missionaries' American checks for Nigerian currency.[34] Nonetheless, a lonely Dr. Farrar discharged inpatients, closed NCH for two weeks, and headed for Lagos, where he expected to obtain cash, see his family, gain a better picture of the political situation, and rest. If he deemed it unsafe to bring his family back, he promised Onicha Ngwa missionaries that he would return with money.[35]

Dr. Farrar taxied through the East, where friendly Biafran soldiers stopped him at frequent checkpoints. Once he crossed the Niger River into Nigeria alongside the hundreds of Africans traversing it back and forth by boat,[36] less welcoming federal soldiers demanded to know why he was helping Biafra. Farrar explained that he was a physician and reminded them of Gowon's instructions not to interfere with medical personnel. As a follow-up, he inquired about their health and handed out medications that he carried for just such goodwill purposes.[37] These strategies facilitated his safe arrival in Lagos on June 30 after one day's travel.[38]

In Lagos, he learned of seriously ill US relatives, and the Farrars decided that their obligation to family superseded that to NCH. They resolved to return briefly to Onicha Ngwa for packing and a more orderly exit.[39] Those plans did not last. In a July 6 military escalation that began the Nigeria-Biafra war, federal troops attacked the town of Ogoja just inside Biafra's border.[40] Mindful of rising tensions, but probably unaware of the meaning of July 6 events, Dr. Farrar started back to Biafra alone on July

---

[33]G. Farrar to Petty, June 10, 1967; H. Farrar to G. Farrar, June 11, 1967; G. Farrar to McInteers, June 17, 1967; G. Farrar to Johnson, June 24 and 29, 1967; G. Farrar to Mission Committee, June 27, 1967, W-COC.

[34]H. Farrar to G. Farrar, June 20 and June 22, 1967.

[35]G. Farrar to Johnsons, July 5 and July 11, 1967; H. Farrar to Brethren, July 2, 1967, W-COC file; Farrar and Farrar, Interview.

[36]H. Farrar to Brethren, July 2, 1967, W-COC file.

[37]Farrar and Farrar, Interview.

[38]Ibid.; Farrar, *Stand*, 172.

[39]G. Farrar to Johnsons, July 5 and July 11, 1967; G. Farrar to G.B. Farrars, July 15, 1967; Farrar to Mission Committee, July 11, 1967, W-COC file.

[40]Baxter, *Biafra*, 18.

13; he returned only because he had promised missionaries to do so.[41] Once there he planned to organize family belongings, find a local physician not drafted into Biafra's army, and then rejoin his family for departure to the US. The African physician would be salaried at NCH and work under administrator Windle Kee in order to maintain COC control of the Hospital.[42]

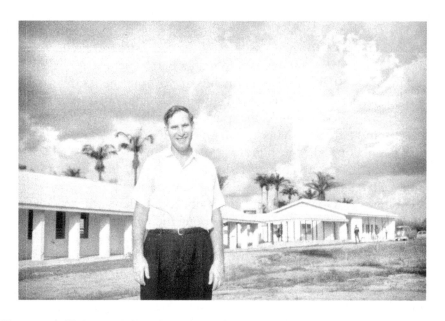

Photograph 33. Henry C. Farrar Jr., MD, in front of Nigerian Christian Hospital women and children's 30-bed ward with maternity ward and delivery suite to right. Water tower in background. To far right and outside of photograph is Aba-Ikot Ekepene Road. ca. 1967. (Author collection).

With Nigerian currency hidden in his Bible and a "supply of [Christian] tracts, malaria medicine and aspirin,"[43] Henry Farrar traveled back through the blockade. At numerous army checkpoints soldiers searched him from shirt to socks, and many picked up his Bible but never opened it. If soldiers got too close, Farrar offered medicines for common ailments. When asked his business, Farrar began answering, "Doctor," after one set of alarmed federal soldiers mistook his answer of "missionary"

---

[41]Farrar and Farrar, Interview.
[42]G. Farrar to Johnsons, July 11, 1967; G. Farrar to G.B. Farrars, July 15, 1967; Farrar to Mission Committee, July 11, 1967, W-COC file.
[43]Farrar, *Stand*, 173.

for "mercenary." When asked his destination, Farrar named the next Nigerian-controlled city—Benin, then Asaba, then the next. Once at the Niger River he hired a dugout powered by a Chrysler car engine to ferry him upriver and across to surprised and welcoming Biafran solders on the Eastern bank. From there he taxied through roadblocks to Onitsha, then Owerri, then Aba, then Onicha Ngwa. Checkpoints slowed his return trip to two days, and he spent a miserable intervening night on the concrete floor of a mosquito-infested village hall.[44] Then only two days after his return, on July 16, the US Embassy abruptly gave all Americans a last-chance choice: Exit Biafra now with our help or stay at your own peril.[45] It is unlikely that Dr. Farrar had time to reopen NCH.[46]

Walking Away

Meanwhile in Lagos, Nigerian news filled with reports of the federal "liberation" of Nsukka and anti-Igbo rioting in Ogoja,[47] and soon Grace Farrar encountered evacuating Peace Corps volunteers. Their departure from the East signaled to her that Dr. Farrar would be close behind, and she should not return to Onicha Ngwa. Moreover, anti-British and anti-American sentiment rose as Nigeria's government accused oil companies of favoring Biafra over Nigeria after companies made a partial payment to the East.[48] An angry Gowon announced that he would march on Biafra's capital of Enugu. Skirmishes increased,[49] "explosions...rocked" Lagos, tribal riots spread, and Grace was constantly "stopped and searched."[50]

On Friday, July 17, Grace Farrar and children fled a second time, now from Lagos to Rome, using six tickets that she obtained from Alitalia Airlines with only her promise that W-COC would cover the cost.[51] She left messages for her husband at the Embassy, with the Greers, and in two detailed instruction-filled, final letters sent to him at Onicha Ngwa

---

[44]Farrar and Farrar, Interview.

[45]G. Farrar to G.B. Farrars, July 22, 1967; Kee, *African*, 87–88.

[46]Kee, *African*, 89.

[47]Friendly, "Nigeria Reports;" Massey and R. Bryant to Brethren," August 1, 1967, W-COC file.

[48]G. Farrar to G.B. Farrars, July 15 and July 22, 1967; G. Farrar to Johnsons, July 11, 1967.

[49]G. Farrar to Johnsons, July 11, 1967.

[50]G. Farrar to G.B. Farrars, July 22, 1967. Dr. Akpabio's views in H. Farrar to G. Farrar, June 17, 1967.

[51]Farrar, *Stand*, 173.

through differing routes. Still focused on the practical, Grace Farrar directed Henry Farrar about what to bring, what to leave, and what to give to household staff: "testimonials" (recommendation letters), clothes, and money.[52] COC missionary Keith Robinson in Rome made local hotel reservations for the Farrars at Grace's cabled request.[53]

At the same time, Henry Farrar, Hazel Buice, the three Tarbets, four Kees, three Walters and hundreds of other expatriates readied to flee Biafra and Nigeria. Within two hours of receiving the July 16 US warning, COC missionaries began filling their luggage to the 44-pound allowance each.[54] The Walters returned baby Virginia to her Igbo family.[55] Missionaries left behind papers on desks and food in refrigerators and handed NCH keys to J.O. Akandu, Friday Onukafor, or possibly Moses Oparah. The task of finding a physician was left with hastily designated new NCH administrator Oparah.[56] They gave house keys to Mark Apollos, parked their three cars at the gated Aba textile mill—vehicles soon co-opted by Biafra's military[57]— and sent a few treasured possessions to Ukpom with the Otoyos. The Farrars' dog "would have to find his own food or be food." NCH moved to Biafran hands.[58]

As news spread of missionaries' imminent departure, heavily armed Igbos with machetes donned war paint and demanded a meeting; Chief Ebere came with shotgun. A translating Akandu cautioned missionaries to speak carefully,[59] and yet the reason for this first-ever, Igbo threat of violence against the missionaries still remains unclear. The crowd may have wanted to prevent Dr. Farrar's departure[60] or believed that he was deserting Biafra for Nigeria. Perhaps they suspected that he planned to deliver NCH into the hands of their political or tribal enemies, or they were troubled by some other issue. Locals knew he had closed NCH and traveled to Lagos and may have seen him return with Nigerian money. They also knew that he established COCs among their Annang enemies, who sided with Nigeria against Biafra. Whatever their reasons, the angry Biafran mob designated one of their number to kill Farrar and others to murder Moses Oparah, Anthony Agali, and Friday Onukafor.[61]

[52]G. Farrar to H. Farrar, July 15 and July 17, 1967.

[53]Farrar, *Stand*, 173.

[54]Buice, "Report," attached to McInteer letter, October 13, 1967, W-COC file.

[55]G. Farrar to Petty and Hays, May 1, 1967.

[56]"Biographical Sketches" (Oparah), 205–26; Farrar, *Stand*, 174–75.

[57]Farrar and Farrar, Interview.

[58]Ibid.; Farrar, *Stand*, 174–75.

[59]Farrar and Farrar, Interview.

[60]G. Farrar to G.B. Farrars, July 22, 1967.

[61]Farrar, "Dr. Farrar's Account," 52; Farrar and Farrar, Interview.

Eno Otoyo, who was loading Farrars' possessions into his vehicle for safekeeping, overheard the Igbos' violent plans and fled to his Ukpom home, stopping only to send police from the nearby Nwaigwe station. Frightened, ashen police controlled the mob long enough for the missionaries to escape to PH, Agali ran for his life to his Asaba home 200 miles away, and how Oparah and Onukafor remained safe is unknown. Igbo compound staff saved Dr. Farrar's life by persuading him to take a different path to NCH than his usual one, where they knew (but he did not) that an assassin waited, and Farrar departed directly from NCH for PH[62] through thirteen roadblocks in those fifty miles.[63]

He and the others assumed they would depart PH by air.[64] Instead, they waited three days in PH for the Isonzo, a last-chance, US-chartered, Italian freighter.[65] They could not afford a PH hotel, and drilling company friend John Freeman gave them his staffed and food-stocked apartment, as well as blankets for the boat.[66] He also handed over his personal credit card to Dr. Farrar, who used it to purchase supplies for the trip: cheese, crackers, candy bars, instant coffee, and a metal cup and a candle to heat water.[67] Finally, on July 20, COC missionaries boarded the Isonzo for their thirty-hour journey from PH across the Atlantic Ocean's Bight of Biafra to Lagos. The freighter was built for twelve passengers, but now carried roughly six hundred evacuees; men slept on the rain-soaked deck, while women stayed below on bed springs without mattresses.[68] On deck the next morning, Dr. Farrar made coffee for each of his colleagues—one metal cup at a time. After a tense freighter handover from Biafran to Nigerian soldiers at sea, followed by evacuees' disembarkation in Lagos, Farrar learned from the Greers that his family was in Rome. There they were reunited on July 22 through a series of events that they described as a remarkable story of God's care.[69] Henry Farrar still carried a gracious Freeman's credit card.[70]

---

[62]Farrar and Farrar, Interview; Farrar, "Dr. Farrar's Account," 52–53; "Biographical Sketches" (Agali), 190; Hank Farrar, personal communications, n.d. and August 26, 2018.

[63]Buice, "Report," W-COC file; Kee, *African*, 89.

[64]Ibid.

[65]Farrar, *Stand*, 175; Farrar and Farrar, Interview; Kee, *African*, 89–94.

[66]Kee, *African*, 89.

[67]G. Farrar to G.B. Farrars, July 22, 1967.

[68]Buice, "Report," W-COC file; Kee, *African*, 91–94.

[69]Farrar, *Stand*, 166–78; G. Farrar to G.B. Farrars, July 22, 1967; Kee *African*, 91–94. Per Barbara Kee, Facebook Messenger to author, August 13, 2017, the Walters returned home to Star, Arkansas, where Gid preached for decades.

[70]Farrar and Farrar, Interview.

That day, from the safety of Italy, Grace Farrar wrote to George Farrar, Henry's brother and W-COC elder, of an exhausted Henry and her own palpable relief at being out of tumultuous Nigeria. "I feel as if I had been released from prison," she penned. "I never realized how all the turmoil...affected me."[71]

The Farrars rested in Rome and then returned to Nashville, Tennessee, on July 26, 1967, exactly three years to the day that they had arrived in Onicha Ngwa.[72] The Walters also returned to the US, while Buice and the Kee and Tarbet families planted a new COC mission work in the neighboring Federal Republic of Cameroon. The missionary diaspora from Onicha Ngwa did not shrink COC missions; it expanded them.[73]

Conclusion

In September 1966, when Grace Farrar had declared that the missionaries' goal at NCH was "to train the local people so well that they can carry on without us someday,"[74] none realized how soon "someday" would come. Now in July 1967 as COC missionaries from Onicha Ngwa scattered, the future of the Hospital, in which they and supporters had invested years of blood, sweat, and treasure, was hidden from them all. Yet, their efforts were not undone, as a willing and able West African staff emerged to take up NCH's work of caring for the most important persons in the hospital: the patients. From the small seed of missionary nurse beginnings, an Iroko grew.

---

[71]G. Farrar to G.B. Farrars, July 22, 1967.
[72]Farrar, *Stand*, 176–77.
[73]Farrar, "1966–1970," 49; Kee, *African*.
[74]G. Farrar to Johnsons, September 6, 1966.

Epilogue[1]

COC missionary nurses' constructive work in Nigeria lasted roughly thirteen years; the Nigeria-Biafra conflict's destruction lasted two and a half. The first brought healing; the second, death to an estimated 100,000 military personnel and 500,000–3,000,000 Biafran civilians—mostly from starvation. Hospital walls survived, and the conflict ended in reunification of Nigeria under federal military rule on January 15, 1970, exactly four years after the first coup d'état.

During the war, Iris Hays's love of missions and Nancy Petty's love of Nigeria drove them into missionary nursing in Nigeria's neighbor: the Republic of Cameroon. There, in spring 1968, the two worked alongside nurse Charley Bridges and missionary physicians David (and Kathryn) Wilbanks and Ken (and Lola) Yearwood to provide care from a four-wheel-drive Christian Mobile Clinic, a work established in consultation with a visiting Dr. Henry Farrar and with support from F.F. Carson and Southside COC in California.[2] Missionaries intended to drive the Clinic across the border to ameliorate postwar devastation in Nigeria, but as the Nigeria-Biafra conflict dragged on, that plan never materialized. Instead, Hays and Petty often stood outside their Cameroonian home, only a few hundred miles from NCH, listening to supply planes flying into Biafra from Sao Tome and crying for the people they loved.[3] Sadly, baby Virginia died; details are scant; food shortages were severe and thousands of children perished.[4]

Throughout the conflict, the nurses' Canadian friend, nurse Dianne North, continued at QEH,[5] the Otoyos remained in Ukpom, and Rees Bryant made two relief trips. Bryant's first foray was into "liberated Nigeria" with Howard Horton, and the second was into Biafra with Jim Massey. Bryant and Massey traveled via a DC-3 military supply plane that landed on the darkened "Uli Airstrip," a section of the Onitsha-Owerri highway. They brought much-needed, one-time financial aid and visited

---

[1]This epilogue rests on many author recollections alongside documented sources.
[2]Carson, "Meeting;" Farrar, "Chronology;" Farrar, "1966–1970;" Farrar, "Nigeria;" Farrar to Mission Committee, November 5, 1968.
[3]Farrar and Petty-Kraus, Interview.
[4]Petty-Kraus, personal communication, July 16, 2012.
[5]Kotlarsky, "From Canada."

churches and refugee camps.[6] F.F. Carson at Southside COC and Green-lawn COC continued to send NCH and Kumba mobile clinic funds to Henry Farrar[7] possibly through the African Christian Schools Foundation (formerly NCSF) with assistance from the Otoyos; the Hospital board was not yet incorporated.

NCH functioned under African leadership from summer 1967 onward. I do not know the story well, but some during the conflict were Moses Oparah and/or Friday Onukafor as administrators, Mabel Solomon NRN as matron followed by translator Rhoda Udogwu as lay matron and midwife,[8] and Dr. Edward Akpabio as government-salaried physician, Biafran sympathizer, and the Otoyos' friend.[9] At some point during the conflict, British physician Derek Belgrave along with three (probably ex-patriate) Red Cross nurses ran a feeding station and maternity and outpa-tient clinic from NCH.[10] One of these volunteers from the UK, Sally Abel, visited the Hospital after the war.[11]

In 1969 Iris Hays married her neighbor in Cameroon, Giuseppe Savio, and later in 1981 she briefly visited NCH with Petty. In 1992, the Savios moved from Cameroon to his home in Tollegno, Italy, and they main-tained other residences in Texas and Alaska. She and Petty remained best friends, calling each other weekly until Hays-Savio's unexpected death in 2012 while she visited family in Texas. She is buried in Resthaven Memo-rial Park in Rockwall, Texas[12] and survived by her husband, beloved nephews and nieces, other family, and many friends. In 2018 Petty and Hays (posthumously) received the Henry and Grace Farrar Service Award from the International Health Care Foundation/African Christian Hospitals (IHCF/ACH).

After evacuating Nigeria, the Farrars first maintained a permanent US residence in Dickson, Tennessee (1967–1969), where daughter Samantha was born, then in Searcy, Arkansas (1969–1982), and finally Lebanon, Tennessee (1983–2013); Henry continued surgical practice in each loca-

---

[6]Bryant, Interview, January 1, 1971; Farrar, "Dr. Farrar's Account;" Massey, "Former;" Massey, "Demanding;" Massey and Bryant, *Former*.

[7]Farrar to Mission Committee, September 26, 1967, *WEV*; Farrar to Carson, March 7, 1968; *Nigerian Informer*, February–July, 1967.

[8]G. Farrar, Interview.

[9]Akpabio to Farrar, September 20, 1967; Farrar, "1966–1970;" Farrar, "Dr. Farrar's Account;" Farrar to Mission Committee, August 11 and September 26, 1967, *WEV*; H. Farrar, Interview 1; Farrar and Farrar, Interview; Onukafor to Farrar, September 12, 1967, W-COC file; Otoyos to H. Farrar, July 31, 1967.

[10]Farrar, "Christian Hospital;" Farrar, "Dr. Farrar's Description."

[11]G. Farrar to author, July 12, 2010.

[12]"Iris Fay Hays Savio," September 13, 2012, findagrave.com no. 97014106.

tion. By the time the bitter Nigeria-Biafra conflict ended, NCH was gutted—even the wiring in the walls was gone—and only its bullet-riddled walls still stood on a final battleground. Dr. Farrar returned to PH in fall 1970 with support from USAID and the Kaiser Foundation International in Oakland, California.[13] On weekdays, he rehabilitated PH General Hospital, and on weekends he worked with Moses Oparah and others to resurrect NCH, using funds donated from the Christian Council of Nigeria.[14] In 1971 expatriate families were allowed into the area, and the Farrar family moved to PH then back to Onicha Ngwa with their younger four children, while the author and older brother Paul attended Harding College in the US. The Farrars furloughed in 1973, followed by forty-five years of almost annual Nigeria missionary service. During those years, Dr. Farrar recruited and mentored countless physicians, nurses, and students, while Rees Bryant and others raised thousands of US dollars for NCH. Henry and Grace Farrar's final multiweek trip to Nigeria was in spring 2009.[15]

Dr. Farrar remained a member of both the West African and the American Colleges of Surgeons. Additionally, the couple received chieftaincy titles of Dibia Oha 1 and Akanri Dibia Oha 1 of Susana Homes in Obuzor, Nigeria (2004). They also served ten months at Chimala Hospital in Tanzania (1979–1980) and twelve months at the Shenyang Medical College, People's Republic of China (1982–1983). Grace Farrar also spent three weeks with Barbara Kee in Cameroon, where she taught community health workers (1996). Moreover, at College Hills COC in Lebanon, Tennessee, she translated COC services into American Sign Language and began a crisis pregnancy center. Individually and together the couple received numerous service recognition awards from diverse groups, such as the Igbo Union of Tennessee, IHCF/ACH, Harding University, Nashville Baha'i Center, Pepperdine University, Power for Today, Tennessee Hospital Association, and the University of Tennessee. Healing Hands International named their Volunteer Center after the couple, and Harding University's Henry and Grace Farrar Health Sciences Center was dedicated in 2010—the same year that Grace received the Outstanding Alumnus Award from Harding's College of Nursing. Both Farrars were active in local US COC leadership. Henry died in February 2010; Grace, in January 2013. They are buried in Ames Chapel

---

[13]Farrar, "Christian Hospital;" Farrar, "Chronology;" Farrar, *Stand*, 179; Farrar, personal photograph collection.

[14]Farrar, "Christian Hospital;" H. Farrar, Interview 1; Farrar, "Biographical Sketches" (Oparah), 205–06.

[15]Author's recollection.

Cemetery in Paoli, Indiana, and survived by their six children and families and other extended family, and friends on five continents.[16]

Nancy Petty's love for the Nigerian people never faded, and in 1973 she yielded to Dr. Farrar's pleas for help at NCH.[17] The Farrars furloughed within days of Petty's arrival, and she oversaw all aspects of NCH for two years while enacting an expanded clinical practice. During that tour, Nigeria became "home" for Petty. In 1984, she married artist Harold Kraus in the US and visited Onicha Ngwa with him briefly in 1987. They reside in Nashville, Tennessee, where they were active members at West End (W-COC) and now at Charlotte Avenue COC. Petty has said that she never felt more welcomed, more loved and less judged than by Nigerians; she would return if she could.[18]

In the US Rees Bryant taught, preached, and pursued graduate studies, and the Bryants returned to teach in northern Nigerian schools in 1981. Bryant earned a doctorate of missiology from Fuller Theological Seminary, and Patti Bryant taught elementary through college classes and completed a master's in theology/philosophy at Lincoln Christian Seminary.[19] They reside in Florida, and in 2016 were honored by IHCF/ACH with the Henry and Grace Farrar Service Award.

Many other expatriates came to NCH after the war, and some of their stories are included in Farrar and Hood's *Bandaging the Brokenhearted*. I ask for forgiveness from those whose names I do not remember here, and I acknowledge the many remarkable family members and Nigerians who worked beside these individuals. NCH administrators included Jacob Achinefu, Bob Bentley, Joe Cross, Brent Magner, Samuel Okpolor, and Lucien Palmer; Sonny Parkhill and Don Thompson became invaluable handymen. Among the Registered Nurses were Janice Bingham, Lola Bowen (Nation), Linda Ferguson, Gem Spence, Lynne Harris, Jonnie Hood, Nancy Leslie (O'Brien), Becky Smith, Lori Sutherland, Michele Tritt, Deanna Womack, and Patty Woods (Wilson). Resident physicians included Drs. Henry Farrar, Maurice Hood, Robert Mahaffey, Viktor

---

[16]Farrar, "Chronology;" "Grace Angeline Johnson Farrar," March 28, 2014, findagrave.com no. 127059782.

[17]Petty-Kraus, Farrar, and Farrar Interview.

[18]Petty-Kraus, Presentation to Keen-Agers; Petty-Kraus, personal communication, June 30, 2008.

[19]Bryant, *Divine*, 323-28.

Vadney, and Robert "Bob" Whitaker from Wales; others made shorter visits.[20] Dr. Brian Camazine went often. Notably Dr. Whitaker lived and worked at NCH from the 1970s until after his 2009 violent kidnapping, including gunshot injury and imprisonment. After his release and treatment in the US, he and wife Annette began a new COC medical mission work in Swaziland, now the Kingdom of eSwatini.

At the time of this writing, COC-affiliated NCH is fully staffed and led by Nigerians, including Israel Jombo MD, as chief medical officer, Jacob Nwachi as chaplain, Vine China NRN, as matron, and Nnamdi Awaziema as chief security officer. A Nigerian Policy Board, including the Matron and one representative from IHCF/ACH (now Dr. Whitaker), provides on-site NCH governance. Throughout NCH history, Nigerian chaplains from Agharanya alongside nurse Sermanoukian to Nwachi today have taught and baptized NCH outpatients and inpatients. NCH is also affiliated with Abia State University in Aba and serves as a training site for Nigerian nurses and physicians.

*

The histories of many NCH staff and Hays-educated nursing auxiliaries are difficult to trace. Petty saw most of the auxiliaries after the war, but knew of none who become NRNs. Male auxiliaries were added,[21] and NCH rehired all interested Hays-educated auxiliaries during postwar years.[22] In the 1970s, anesthesiologist Dr. Howard Ausherman of Florida, taught lay Friday Nwagwugwu and Eunice Uzuegbu Uche to deliver general anesthesia during NCH surgeries.[23]

Eunice Ukegbu, possibly the longest-serving of Hays's graduates, worked at NCH for almost fifty years. After retirement, she was invited back to assist short-term surgical missionaries in the operating room, where her skills were lauded by many, including internationally recognized neurosurgeon Dr. Charles Branch Sr.[24] As Nigerians say, Eunice went to her reward in 2014.

---

[20]Boyd, "Overview;" Farrar and Hood, *Bandaging.*
[21]"Biographical Sketches" (Nwagu), 203; "Biographical Sketches" (Nwagwugwu), 203–04.
[22]Petty-Kraus, Interview 1.
[23]"Biographical Sketches" (Nwagwugwu), 203–204; Hood to Whom It May Concern, November 12, 1984, Eunice Uche collection, AUTH.
[24]Author's recollection.

Retired Rose Ngwakwe from Hays's second cohort, now in her eighties, loved her nursing work at NCH and speaks highly of both preaching by Dr. Farrar and healthcare delivered by Hays, Petty, and Farrar. Rose learned professional skills from NCH midwife colleagues, and she was especially proud of saving one premature baby, now a grown man and only child of his mother. Henry Farrar always called on Rose for help in difficult patient situations, but she was unhappy with the limited career prospects at NCH and missionaries' unwillingness or inability to fund her NRN education, and so she left NCH for a second successful career as secondary school teacher and administrator.[25] One of my great joys was re-meeting and hearing stories from the very accomplished Rose in 2018 in Obuzor.

Rachel Akwarandu married longtime NCH administrator Samuel Okpulor and worked many years at NCH; Petty saved the lives of Rachel and her newborn in 1978 during childbirth.[26] Hays and Petty's translators, Rhoda Udogwu and Comfort Eguzo, functioned as NCH nurses during and after the war, including work with the Red Cross.[27] Comfort later became the nurse at a school built for NCH staff children,[28] and my recollection is that she was also NCH librarian.

Moses Oparah served as NCH administrator for several years, leaving the position in January 1974. Following that time, the (IHCF)/ACH Board appointed as Hospital administrator first US evangelist Joe Cross and then Joseph Nwaoguegbe.[29] Friday and Grace Onukafor and family remained welcome friends in missionary homes. Lab technicians Sylvanus Nwagbara and Peter Uhiara worked at NCH before and after the Biafra War, with Uhiara continuing until his death years later.[30]

*

The African Christian Hospitals Foundation (now International Health Care Foundation/ACH) was officially incorporated on July 20, 1972, and its first meeting to follow was September 7, 1972. Charter members of the incorporated board were F.W. Mattox, Jesse Paul, Henry Farrar, Maurice Hood, Thomas Johnson, and Rees Bryant. Rees Bryant became ACH

---

[25]Ngwakwe, Interview.

[26]"Biographical Sketches" (Okpular), 204–205.

[27]G. Farrar, Interview; Hays-Savio, Interview.

[28]G. Farrar, Interview; G. Farrar, personal communication, July 2, 2010.

[29]Mitchell, "Position Paper."

[30]G. Farrar, personal communication, n.d.

President and Patti Bryant, secretary, from 1972 to 1981.[31] Rees was followed by ACH presidents/executive directors Dr. H. Glenn Boyd, Frank Black MD, Josiah Tilton, Tom Carr, and currently Kevin Linderman.

Although the IHCF/ACH board initially played a hands-on oversight role for NCH,[32] it now serves in a more advisory and fund-raising capacity for seven facilities across Africa, including the Palmer Hospital in Ikot Usen. Its headquarters are in Searcy, Arkansas. Currently, its thirty-plus Board members include these: Henry C. Farrar III, MD, as chairperson; Jerry Canfield, JD, as immediate past chairperson; member Martha "Marty" Farrar Highfield, PhD, RN (author) and many missionary nurses and physicians. In 1993, IHCF/ACH12 launched a successful scholarship program for preparing Nigerian COC nurses and physicians, and many of its graduates worked for a time at NCH or Palmer Hospital.

"And so they went from village to village,
proclaiming the good news and healing people everywhere."

—1st century physician, Luke[33]

---

[31]Ibid.
[32]Mitchell, "Position Paper."
[33]Luke 9:6, New International Version.

Works Cited
Manuscript Sources Summary

Key Correspondence
Copies or originals in author collection

- Bryant, Rees, and Patti Bryant. Correspondence 1958–1967, unpublished.

- Farrar, Henry & Grace. Correspondence 1959–1967, unpublished.

- Petty, Nancy Corinne. Correspondence 1965–1967, unpublished.

Libraries

- Center for Restoration Studies, Abilene Christian University Special Collections, ACU

- Delmar T. Oviatt Library, California State University/Northridge

Collections
Photographs, personal papers, and other materials

- Author (AUTH)
- Rees and Patti Bryant (RPB)
- Jane Doe (JD)
- Henry and Grace Farrar (HGF)
- John R. Morgan (JRM)
- Rose Ngwakwe (RN)
- Betty Jo Peden (BJP)
- Nancy Petty-Kraus (NPK)
- Mission Study Committee Files, West End Church of Christ (W-COC file)

Interviews and Recordings

Beckloff, Dottie. Interview: Beckloff Nigeria Years. By Author. June 6, 2014. Digital recording, Nashville, TN. (lost)

Bryant, Rees. "Interview of Rees Bryant: Updates from Nigeria." By Evertt Huffard, *Harding College Living History of Mission*s 2, no. 7. (January 1, 1971). scholarworks.harding.edu/missions-history/18/.

Bryant, Rees, and Patti Bryant. Interview: Bryants and NCH. By Author. July 19, 2010. Digital recording, Kissimmee, FL. Transcript. AUTH.

Doe, Jane, and CeLeste Fraga. Interview: History of Nurse Mary Kelton. By Author. November 9, 2019. Digital recording, San Anselmo, CA. (Name withheld by request.) AUTH.

Ekwenye-Hendricks, Chi, Interview 1: Nursing History of NCH. By Author. May 4, 2017. Digital recording, Agoura Hills, CA. AUTH.

———. Interview 2: Nursing History of NCH. By Author. October 11, 2017. Digital recording, Lagos, Nigeria, (via WhatsApp). AUTH.

Farrar, Grace. Interview: Nursing History of NCH. By Author. June 8, 2009. Digital recording, Lebanon, TN. Transcript. AUTH.

———, and Nancy Petty-Kraus. Interview: Petty Nigeria Experiences. By Author. June 30, 2008. Digital recording, Nashville, TN. Transcript. AUTH.

Farrar Jr., Henry. "Heroes of Medical Missions: Dr. Henry Farrar." By O'Neal Tankersley (producer). Center for World Missions, Harding University, Accessed February 22, 2010. *youtube.com/watch?v=hy-ZLOSFzP90*.

———. Interview 1: NCH History. By Author. June 9, 2009. Digital recording, Lebanon, TN. Transcript. AUTH.

———. Interview 2: NCH History. By Author. October 18, 2009. Digital recording, Lebanon, TN. AUTH.

———, and Grace Farrar. Interview: Farrars' NCH History. By Author. June 10, 2009. Digital recording, Lebanon, TN. AUTH.

Hays-Savio, Iris. Interview: Hays Nigeria Experiences. By Author. July 17–18, 2009. Digital recording, Rockwall, TX. Transcript. AUTH.

———, and Nancy Petty-Kraus. Interview: Hays and Petty Nigeria Experiences. By Author. May 16, 2012. Digital recording, Rockwall, TX. AUTH.

Morgan, John, Donna Morgan, and Grace Farrar. Interview: Morgans' Nigeria Experiences. By Author. June 8, 2011. Digital recording, Lebanon, TN. AUTH.

Ngwakwe, Rose. Interview: Ngwakwe NCH Experiences. By Author. March 3, 2018. Digital recording, Obuzor, Nigeria. AUTH.

Peden, Betty Jo. Interview: Nurse Glenna Peden, Missionary. By Author. June 8, 2017. Digital recording, Nashville, TN. AUTH.

Petty-Kraus, Nancy. Interview 1: Petty Nigeria Experiences. By Author. June 11, 2009. Digital recording Nashville, TN. Transcript. AUTH.

———. Interview 2: Petty 1967 Exit from Nigeria. By Author. June 9, 2017. Digital recording, Nashville, TN. AUTH.

———. Presentation to Keen-Agers. N.d. Digital recording, West End COC, Nashville, TN. HGF.

———, Henry Farrar, and Grace Farrar. Interview: NCH History. By Author. June 12, 2009. Digital recording, Lebanon, TN. AUTH.

Robinson, Edward J. "A Conversation with Edward J. Robinson." By Lynn McMillon. February 1, 2009. christianchronicle.org/article/a-conversation-with-edward-j-robinson.

Publications & Documents

Abilene Christian University. "Experiences." *ACU Today: The Alumni Magazine of Abilene Christian University.* (Spring-Summer 2014): 77.

Achebe, Chinua. *There Was a Country.* New York: Penguin, 2012.

———. *Things Fall Apart.* New York: Penguin, 1959/1994/2017. Kindle edition.

Agbasiere, Joseph Thérèse. *Women in Igbo Life and Thought.* New York: Routledge, 2000.

Akpabio, Offonmbuk C. *He Dared: The Story of Okuku Udo Akpabio, The Great Colonial African Ruler.* Self-published: Xlibris, 2011.

Andrews High School Yearbook Staff. *The Mustang.* 1959. Savio private collection.

Asindi, A.A., M. Young, I. Etuk, and J.J. Udo. "Brutality to Twins in South-eastern Nigeria: What is the Existing Situation?" *West African Journal of Medicine* 12, no. 3 (July–September 1993): 148–52.

Associated Press. "Lagos Orders Blockade." *Herald*, May 31, 1967. HGF.

Ayandele, E.A. *Nigerian Historical Studies.* London: Frank Cass, 1979.

Barnes, Kenneth J. *A Rough Passage: Memories of Empire*, vol.1. New York: St. Martin's, 2007.

Basden, George Thomas, *Niger Ibos*. London: Frank Cass, 1966.

———. *Among the Ibos of Nigeria: An Account of the Curious and Interesting Habits, Customs and Beliefs*. Philadelphia: J.B. Lippincott, 1921.

Baxter, Peter. *Biafra: The Nigerian Civil War, 1967–1970*. Vol. 16 of *Africa@War*. West Midlands, England: Hellion, 2015.

Benson, George S. "A Real Opportunity." *Gospel Advocate* 107, no. 26, July 1, 1965.

"Biographical Information: Myles Thomas Tune." *Old Paths Archive® Electronic Library*. Accessed May 3, 2018. oldpaths.com/Archive/Tune/Myles/Thomas/1929/bio.html.

"Biographical Sketches: Teamwork." In *Bandaging the Brokenhearted*, edited by Farrar and Hood, 189–210.

Bohrer, Stanley P. "Narration: Nigeria, Farabale." *Journal of the American Medical Association* 197 (August 15, 1966): 228–232. HGF.

Boyd, H. Glenn. "A Historical Overview of Medical Evangelism among Churches of Christ in Africa." In *100 Years of African Missions*, edited by Granberg, 187–213.

———. "An Overview of the Work of African Christian Hospitals Foundation During My Tenure, 1981–2000." In *Bandaging the Brokenhearted*, edited by Farrar and Hood, 135-50.

Brewer, Charles R., ed. *A Missionary Pictorial*. 3rd ed. Nashville, TN: World Vision, 1968.

Broom, Betty. "A Typical Day in Nigeria." *The Gospel Guardian* 7, (April 19, 1956): wordsfitlyspoken.org/gospel_guardian/v7/v7n49p6a.html.

Bryant, Patti. *Gently Led: An Autobiography*. 5 books. Unpublished, 2009. RPB.

———. *Divine Choreography*. Self-published, 2012.

Bryant, Rees. "Bloody Tribal Dispute Causes Nigeria Strife." *Christian Chronicle*, February 3, 1967. Tennessee Valley Edition.

———. "Nigerian Highlights–1959." Transcribed by P.Bryant. RPB.

———. "Reflections on the Beginnings of the Nigerian Christian Hospital." In *Bandaging the Brokenhearted*. edited by Farrar and Hood, 20–29.

Bryant, Rees, and Douglas Lawyer. "Opportunities in Nigeria." N.d. Unpublished. RPB.

Bryant, Sara Jo. "The Diary of Sara Jo Bryant: A Young MK's Experience of Missionary Life in Nigeria (1964–1967)." Transcribed by P. Bryant. Unpublished. RPB.

Burger, Wayne. "God's Providence, Nigeria, and C.A.O. Essien: Churches of Christ Restored in Nigeria." *Undenominational Christianity* (blog), N.d. Accessed December 10, 2017. https://undenominationalchristianity.wordpress.com/2016/04/03/gods-providence-nigeria-and-c-a-o-essien/.

"Capping Ceremony [Program], Nigerian Christian Hospital." February 15, 1967. AUTH (from NPK).

Carson, F.F. "Meeting the Great Challenge." *The Nigerian Informer* 4, no. 6, June 1969. HGF.

Choate, Julian Ernest. *Roll Jordan Roll: A Biography of Marshall Keeble.* Nashville, TN: Gospel Advocate, 1974.

Chicago Defender. "Crisis in Nigeria." April 15, 1967. National Edition. ProQuest Historical Newspapers (HNP_68419_19670415_0070).

———. "Nigeria On Right Road." February 26, 1966. National Edition. ProQuest Historical Newspapers (HNP_68419_19660226_0096).

Christian Chronicle. "1–35,000 Ratio Face M.D. Serving in Nigeria Today." November 12, 1965. Central Oklahoma Edition.

———. "99-Year Lease Signed for Nigeria Hospital." November 12, 1965. Central Oklahoma Edition.

———. "Hospital planned: Nigeria—'Phenomenal' results in '65." January 7, 1966. Central Oklahoma Edition.

———. "Otoyos Are Holding Key Positions in Nigeria." November 12, 1965. Central Oklahoma Edition.

———. "Three Facets Highlight Nigeria Break-Through." November 19, 1965. International Edition.

Chronicle News. "Bryants Leave Nigeria To Work in Lubbock, Tex; Diestelkamp Replaced by McKee." *Christian Chronicle,* August 11, 1961. RPB.

———. "Month-long Evangelism Adds Over 450 Nigerians." *Christian Chronicle,* September 2, 1966. International Edition.

Chuku, Gloria. *Igbo Women and Economic Transformation in Southeastern Nigeria, 1900–1960.* New York: Routledge, 2005.

Church of Christ Nigeria, Ibiaku Itam II. "Church History." Accessed March 2, 2016 (discontinued). cocibiakuitam2.org/about/church-history. AUTH (copy).

Coleman, F.B. "The Challenge for Physicians." *Action* 31, no. 6, June 1966. HGF.

Commercial Appeal. "Myra Louise Wade Underwood: 1931-2019." March 21, 2019. www.legacy.com/obituaries/commercialappeal/obituary-print.aspx?n=myra-louise-wade-underwood&pid=191879400.

Cook, Edward Tyas. *The Life of Florence Nightingale (1820-1861)*, Vol. 1. London: Macmillan, 1923/2012. Project Gutenberg, Ebook. gutenberg.org/files/40057/40057-h/40057-h.htm.

Daily Defender. "Nigeria's School Problem." October 20, 1960. Daily Edition. ProQuest Historical Newspapers (68422).

Dickson County Herald. "Miss Nancy Petty Now on Foreign Soil." April 29, 1965. AUTH (copy).

Dixon, O. "Graduate of Nursing School: Miss Iris Hays Soon Will Reach Goal as Missionary to Nigeria." *Lubbock Avalanche-Journal*, September 20, 1964. AUTH (copy).

Echols, Eldred. "The Beginning of the Church in Nigeria." In *Bandaging the Brokenhearted*, edited by Farrar and Hood, 7–11.

———. *Beyond the Rivers of Cush.* Winona, MS: J.C. Choate, 2000.

———. "1950 Nigerian Diary." *Stone Campbell Books.* 193. digitalcommons.acu.edu/crs_books/193.

Eichman, Phillip. *Medical Missions Among the Churches of Christ.* 2nd ed. Self-published, 2001.

Ellah, Francis J. *Nigeria and States Creation: Based on "The Unfinished Motion."* Port Harcourt: Chief J.W. Ellah, 1983.

"Evangelist fund." N.d. Unpublished slide script. RBP:N.

Farrar, Grace. "Chronology of the Henry & Grace Farrar Family." N.d. Unpublished. HGF.

———. "A Letter Written by Grace Farrar." In *Bandaging the Brokenhearted*, edited by Farrar and Hood, 45.

———. "My Spiritual Journey." N.d. Unpublished. HGF.

———. *Stand By and See What the Lord Will Accomplish: The Story of One Family Serving the Lord in Nigeria 1964 to 1967.* Fort Worth, TX: Star Bible, 2002.

———. Untitled book manuscript. N.d. Unpublished. HGF.

Farrar, Henry. "1966–1970 Transitions of the Nigerian Christian Hospital and Onicha Ngwa Bible Training College." In *Bandaging the Brokenhearted*, edited by Farrar and Hood, 49.

———. "Christian Hospital Serves 75,000 Nigerians." *Christian Chronicle*, July 5, 1971.

———. "Dr. Farrar's Account of the War." In *Bandaging the Brokenhearted*, edited by Farrar and Hood, 52-53.

———. "Dr. Farrar's Description of the Same Period: January to December 1970 at NCH." In *Bandaging the Brokenhearted*, edited by Farrar and Hood, 57.

———. "Nigeria." *Action*, August 1968.

———. "The Story of Henry and Grace Farrar." In *Bandaging the Brokenhearted*, edited by Farrar and Hood, 41–44.

Farrar, Henry, and R. Maurice Hood. "The Beginning of the Church in Nigeria." In *Bandaging the Brokenhearted*, edited by Farrar and Hood, 5–6.

———, eds. *Bandaging the Brokenhearted: A Pictorial History of the Nigerian Christian Hospital*. Self-published, 2003.

Farrar, Martha Ellen. "Travel Collins Diary." Unpublished. AUTH.

"Former CHS Student is Program Guest for Future Homemakers." N.p, n.d. NPK.

Frankl, Victor E., *Man's Search for Meaning: An Introduction to Logotherapy*. New York: Pocket Books, Simon and Schuster, 1959/1984.

Friendly Jr., Alfred. "Nigeria Reports Capture of Town: Says Eastern Rebels Flee Nsukka in Disarray." *New York Times*, July 16, 1967. ProQuest Historical Newspapers (03624331).

"F.W. Mattox to Visit Nigeria." [unknown source], October 1964. RPB.

Garrison, Lloyd. "Army Units Back Nigeria Regime." *New York Times*, January 18, 1966. ProQuest Historical Newspapers (117498721).

———. "The Crisis in Nigeria: Regional Riots Put Nation to Biggest Test Thus Far." *New York Times*, June 1, 1966. ProQuest Historical Newspapers (116864367).

———. "Eastern Area Warned by Leader of Nigeria." *New York Times*, March 15, 1967. ProQuest Historical Newspapers (117750494).

———. "Eastern Nigeria in Tension's Grip: Mood Like That of a Nation on the Brink of War." *New York Times*, March 12, 1967. ProQuest Historical Newspapers (118121197).

———. "Head of Eastern Nigeria Calls for Independence." *New York Times*, May 27, 1967. ProQuest Historical Newspapers (117736214).

———. "Idealistic Views Voiced in Nigeria." *New York Times*, January 30, 1966. ProQuest Historical Newspapers (117157176).

———. "New Cry in Nigeria Is 'Down With Ironsi.'" *New York Times*, June 5, 1966. ProQuest Historical Newspapers (116861988).

———. "A New Dynamism Sweeping Nigeria: Young Army Leaders Bring Dedication and Discipline." *New York Times*, February 18, 1966. ProQuest Historical Newspapers (117121911).

———. "Nigeria Outwardly Placid but Killings Increase: Unity Apparently Shattered in Hausa Take-Over—Ironsi Reported To Be Dead." *New York Times*, August 4, 1966. ProQuest Historical Newspapers (117322726).

———. "Nigeria Peaceful in Wake of Strife: North, Rent by Tribal Riots, Calmed by Ironsi Pledge." *New York Times*, July 23, 1966. ProQuest Historical Newspapers (117258339).

———. "Nigeria to Name Civilian Advisors: Ruler Planning Committee—Frees 15 More Politicians." *New York Times*, August 5, 1966. ProQuest Historical Newspapers (117533937).

———. "Nigeria: Wounds Too Deep?." *New York Times*, August 14, 1966. ProQuest Historical Newspapers (117687462).

———. "Political Breakup Looms in Nigeria as Ibos Challenge Regime." *New York Times*, August 3, 1966. ProQuest Historical Newspapers (117278509).

———. "Power Struggle Rages in Nigeria." *New York Times*, January 19, 1966. ProQuest Historical Newspapers (1095368214).

———. "Railroads Halt in North Nigeria: Tie-up Caused by Exodus of Eastern Workers." *New York Times*, September 25, 1966. ProQuest Historical Newspapers (117411227).

———. "Rioting Renewed in North Nigeria: Lagos Flies Police to Area—Pressure on Ironsi Grows." *New York Times*, June 6, 1966. ProQuest Historical Newspapers (116845788).

———. "A Time Bomb Ticks in Nigeria." *New York Times*, March 19, 1967. ProQuest Historical Newspapers (117750827).

———. "Wave of Rumors Tears at Nigeria: While Nation Fights for Life, They Deepen Antagonisms." *New York Times*, October 1, 1966. ProQuest Historical Newspapers (117376330).

Goff, Reda C. *The Great Nigerian Mission*. Nashville, TN: Nigerian Christian Schools Foundation, 1964.

———. "There Stood a Man of Nigeria–Calling." *Christian Chronicle*, November 12, 1965. Central Oklahoma Edition.

Golightly, Annie. "Medicine Woman: Out of Africa to NE Campus." *Tarrant County Junior College Newspaper*, n.d. Private collection.

Granberg, Stanley, ed. *100 Years of African Missions: Essays in Honor of Wendell Broom*. Abilene, TX: Abilene Christian University, 2001.

———. "Wendell Broom: A Biography." In *100 Years of African Missions*, edited by Granberg, 3–26.

Green Lawn Church of Christ. *Nigerian Evangelism: Broadened Through Medical Benevolence*. Lubbock, TX: Green Lawn Church of Christ, n.d. AUTH.

Harp, Scott, comp. "Batsell Barrett Baxter." In *History of the Restoration Movement*. 2016. www.therestorationmovement.com/_states/tennessee/baxter,bb.htm.

———. "Calvin Leonard Johnson." In *History of the Restoration Movement*. 2016. www.therestorationmovement.com/_states/alabama/johnson,cl.htm.

———. "Henry Clyde Hale." In *History of the Restoration Movement*. 2016. www.therestorationmovement.com/_states/tennessee/hale,hc.htm.

———. "Howard Patrick Horton." In *History of the Restoration Movement*. 2016. www.therestorationmovement.com/_states/alabama/horton.htm.

———. "James Richard Massey." In *History of the Restoration Movement*. 2016. www.therestorationmovement.com/_states/florida/massey,jr.htm.

———. "Marion Douglas Lawyer." In *History of the Restoration Movement*. 2016. www.therestorationmovement.com/_states/oklahoma/lawyer.htm.

Hillsboro Church of Christ. "Dr. Henry Farrar is Medical Missionary in Nigeria." *Sunday Bulletin* 22, August 2, 1964. AUTH.

———. "Report from Nigeria." *Sunday Bulletin* 25, no. 5, March 13, 1966. AUTH.

———. "Dr. Henry Farrar." *Sunday Bulletin* 25, no. 38, November 6, 1966. AUTH.

———. "Dr. Farrar," *Sunday Bulletin* 26, no. 17, June 11, 1967. AUTH.

Hooper, Robert E. *A Distinct People: A History of the Churches of Christ in the 20th Century*. West Monroe, LA: Howard, 1993.

Huffard, Henry. "Christian Education in Africa ('Teach Us'": The Lineage and Development of African Christian Schools Foundation)." In *100 Years of African Missions*, edited by Granberg, 215–227.

Huntsville Times, "Ralph Underwood Obituary." Obituaries & Guestbooks. Accessed September 10, 2016. obits.al.com/obituaries/huntsville/obituary.aspx?pid=139701329.

Indenture of Lease. 18th October 1965. Registered as No. 88 at page 88 in Volume 421 of the Lands Registry, Enugu. Drawn up by A. Ijoma Aseme & Co., Solicitors, Aba. HGF (copy).

Inwood, Michael. *A Hegel Dictionary.* In *The Blackwell Philosopher Dictionaries.* Malden, MA: Blackwell, 1992.

Kaplan, Carol Farrar. "Memories of Our Farrar Family." March 2012. Unpublished. AUTH.

Kee, Barbara Oteka. *African Treks I've Taken: Part One.* Wichita Falls, TX: Self-published, 2010.

Kelton, Tom. *More Than a Conqueror: The Ups and Downs of a Christian Manic Depressive.* Fayetteville, AR: Gospel Tracts International, 2012.

Kennedy, Levi. "Greetings." *Action* 31, no. 6, June 1966. HGF.

Korieh, Chima J. *The Land Has Changed: History, Society, and Gender in Colonial Nigeria.* University of Calgary, 2016.

———, ed. *"Life Not Worth Living": Nigerian Petitions Reflecting an African Society's Experiences During World War II.* African World Series, edited by Toyin Falola. Durham, NC: Carolina Academic, 2014.

———. "May it please your honor": Letters of Petition as Historical Evidence in an African Colonial Context." *History in Africa* 37 (2010): 88–106.

Kotlarsky, Carol. "From Canada to Biafra." *The Canadian Nurse* 66, no. 3 (2007): 39–42.

Kraus, Nancy Petty. "On Daddy's Knee." *Christian Woman* 9 (May/June 1993): 27.

Lawyer, Charla. "Doug Lawyer, Early Missionary to Nigeria." IHCF African Christian Hospitals, Nigerian Christian Hospital, n.d. Accessed April 20, 2018 (discontinued). ihcf.net. AUTH (copy).

Lawyer, Douglas. "Narrative of Douglas Lawyer," In *Bandaging the Brokenhearted,* edited by Farrar and Hood, 37–39.

———. Untitled article. *Nigerian Newsletter* 7, no. 1 (November 1963). RPB:N.

Lawyers, The. "The Douglas Lawyers Arrive in Nigeria." *Nigerian News-letter* 5, no.1 (December 3, 1960). RPB:N.

Liggin, O. Fred, "Is Preaching the Gospel Enough?" *Truth Magazine* 9, no. 4 (January 1965): 7–10. truthmagazine.com/archives/volume9/TM009030.htm.

Livingstone, W.P. *Mary Slessor of Calabar: Pioneer Missionary.* N.p., 1918/2005. Project Gutenberg, EBook #8906. gutenberg.org/cache/epub/8906/pg8906-images.html.

Lovell, James L. "An Editorial." *Action* 31, no. 6, June 1966. HGF.

Lubbock Avalanche. "Peace Seen for Nation: Missionary for Church of Christ Writes of Nigeria," October 16, 1960. RPB:N.

Madiebo, Alexander A. *The Nigerian Revolution and the Biafran War.* Enugu, Nigeria: Fourth Dimension, 1980.

Martin, Glenn. "Nigeria Missionaries Convert 650 in Three-Week Series." *Christian Chronicle* 20, no. 8, November 23, 1962.

Massey, Jim. "The Demanding Challenge in Biafra." *Christian Chronicle* 27, no 4, January 26, 1970: 1, 4, 6.

———. "Former Nigerian Missionaries Fly the Biafran Blockade." *Gospel Advocate* 112, no. 6, February 5, 1970. HGF.

———. "Rees Bryants Return from Nigeria." ca.1961. RPB.

———. "Green Lawn to Oversee Nigerian Hospital Construction." *The Bulletin: Green Lawn Church of Christ*, n.d. AUTH.

———. "Nigerian Disturbance Unlikely to Affect Brethren." *Weekly Bulletin: Church of Christ* 16, January 27, 1966. RPB.

———, and Rees Bryant. *Former Nigerian Missionaries Return to Biafra with Aid for Starving Brethren.* N.p. January 9, [1970]. RPB.

Mattox, F.W. "Nigerian Hospital." *Gospel Advocate* 107, no. 48, December 2, 1965. AUTH.

McDaniel, Ken. "Nigeria and Henry Farrar, M.D.: A Special Report by Rees Bryant." *West End Visitor* 23 no. 22, April 3, 1967.

Medical Missionaries of Mary Congregation. "Milestones: The Second Decade." 2013. mmmworldwide.org.

Meisler, Stanley. "Mood in Biafra Blends Ugliness, Playfulness: War Infatuation Breeds Casual Cruelty in Secessionist Eastern Area of Nigeria." *Los Angeles Times*, June 5, 1967. ProQuest Historical Newspapers (155754069).

Mitchell, Carl. "Position Paper for the African Christian Hospitals Foundation." Paper presented to the Foundation Board, January 3, 1984. Unpublished. IHCF/ACH.

Morgan, John R. "Nigeria: Summer 1965." Color slide collection. Photographer Morgan. 1965. AUTH (copy).

————. "John's Nigerian Journal." June–August 1965. Unpublished. AUTH (copy).

————. "Memories of a Three Month Visit." In *Bandaging the Brokenhearted*, edited by Farrar and Hood, 40.

————. "Report of SKF Fellow on Summer in Nigeria." Vanderbilt Medical School, Nashville, TN. Unpublished manuscript presented to the Association of American Medical Colleges and Smith Kline & French Laboratories, n.d. AUTH (copy).

"Mrs. Mary Kelton Wofford, Obituary." Bluebonnet Hills Funeral Home and Memorial Park. Accessed February 29, 2016. tributes.com/show/95154275.

Nau, Henry. *We Move Into Africa: The Story of the Planting of the Lutheran Church in Southeastern Nigeria.* St. Louis, MO: Concordia, 1945.

New York Times. "Man In the News: Ojukwu Leads Ibo Tribe Out of Nigerian Federation." May 31, 1967. HGF.

————. "Nigeria's Military Ruler: Yakubu Dan Yumma Gowon." June 3, 1967. ProQuest Historical Newspapers (117367815).

Nicks, Bill/J.W. "The Boy With a 'Popeye'." In *Short Stories*, edited by Nicks and Nicks, 70-76.

————. "Doctoring the Witch Doctor." In *Short Stories*, edited by Nicks and Nicks, 120-23.

————. "Familiarity Breeds Contempt?" In *Short Stories*, edited by Nicks and Nicks, 9-11.

————. "Fellow Workers in the Lord." In *Short Stories*, edited by Nicks and Nicks, 12-21.

————. "The 'Healing Prophet'." In *Short Stories*, edited by Nicks and Nicks, 44-46.

————. "Our First Missionaries." In *Short Stories*, edited by Nicks and Nicks, 6-8.

————. *Missions and the Message of the Master.* Winona, MS: J.C. Choate, 1987.

―――. "Narrative of J.W. Nicks." In *Bandaging the Brokenhearted*, edited by Farrar and Hood, 19.

―――. "Rees Bryants Returning to States for Leave." N.d. RPB:N.

―――. "'Okorobeke,' Son of a White Man." In *Short Stories,* edited by Nicks and Nicks, 22-27.

―――, and Gerry Nicks, eds. *Short Stories of West Africa Long Remembered.* Winona, MS: J.C. Choate, 1997.

Nicks, Gerry. "An Unexpected Opportunity." In *Short Stories,* edited by Nicks and Nicks, 77-79.

―――. "Why Have Servants If You're Not Rich?" In *Short Stories*, edited by Nicks and Nicks, 67–69.

Nigerian Christian Schools Foundation. "Two too late?" *Newsletter* 2, no. 2, September/October 1965. RPB:N.

"Nigerian Evangelism to Be Broadened Through Medical Benevolence," *Action* 31, no. 6, June 1966. HGF.

Nnadi, Eucharia F., and Hugh F. Kabat. "Nigerians' Use of Native and Western Medicine for the Same Illness." *Public Health Report* 99 (January–February 1984): 93–98.

Ojukwu, C. Odumegwu. *Biafra: Selected Speeches and Random Thoughts of C. Odumegwu Ojukwu, General of the People's Army.* New York: Harper and Row, 1969.

Ottuh, John Arierhi. "The Church and Community Development in Nigeria: The Church in Etinan as an Illustration." *Research on Humanities and Social Sciences* 4, no. 6 (2014): 2225–0484 (online). Accessed February 5, 2018. http://iiste.org/Journals/index.php/RHSS/article/viewFile/11880/12246.

Owolabi, Biodun. *The New Testament Church in Reality: A Historical Assessment of the Restoration Movement in Nigeria.* N.p.: Devangell Te Ventures, 2009.

Palmer, Ida. "Memories of Lucien and Ida Palmer While They Served the Lord Through Christian Education in Nigeria and Briefly Assisted Nigerian Christian Hospital." In *Bandaging the Brokenhearted*, edited by Farrar and Hood, 16-17.

―――. "A Narrative of Ida and Lucien Palmer's Experiences on Their First Trip to Nigeria." In *Bandaging the Brokenhearted*, edited by Farrar and Hood, 12–15.

Peden, Betty Jo. "Chronology: Glenna Jean Shifflett Peden." June 8, 2017. Unpublished. AUTH.

Pollock, David C., and Ruth E. Van Reken. *Third Culture Kids: Growing Up Among Worlds.* Boston: Nicholas Brealey, 2009.

Proctor Street Church of Christ. "The Bill Currys Leaving January 26," *Nigerian Newsletter* 6, no. 1, January 25, 1962. RPB:N.

"Programme for the Opening of the First In-Patient Units of the Nigerian Christian Hospital, on the Land Donated by the Villages of Ntigha Onicha Ngwa, Nlagu and Umuwoma." August 23, 1966. AUTH.

Reese, Boyd, and Eldred Echols. *Report on Nigeria.* Nashville, TN: Lawrence Avenue Church of Christ, 1950.

Reuters. "Lagos Orders Blockade of Seceded East: General Mobilization Begins in Nigeria." *Herald,* May 31, 1967. HGF.

———. "Nigeria Army Chief Heads a Provisional Government." *New York Times,* January 17, 1966. ProQuest Historical Newspapers (117158393).

Robinson, Edward J., ed. *A Godsend to His People: The Essential Writings and Speeches of Marshall Keeble.* Knoxville, TN: University of Tennessee, 2008.

Savio, Iris Hays. "The Nigerian Christian Hospital." In *Bandaging the Brokenhearted,* edited by Farrar and Hood, 46–48.

Shannon, Don. "Indefinite Military Rule Predicted for Nigeria." *Los Angeles Times,* January 27, 1966. ProQuest Historical Newspapers (155392969).

Silvey, Billie. "Richmond's F.F. Carson." *Pacific Church News* 7 (Fall 1987): 7.

Snyder, Al. "Western Africa: National Impetus." *Christianity Today* 8 (July 31, 1964): 8–9.

Southside Church of Christ, "Financial Report," *The Nigerian Informer* 2, no. 4, April 1967, and no. 7, July 1967. HGF.

Spray, Paul. *Nigeria Orthopedic Project History—1962–1967.* Washington, D.C.: Medico Orthopaedics Overseas Division, ca. June 1967. HGF.

Special. "Army Aid Takes Power in Nigeria: Chief of Staff Announces He Heads Regime—Fate of Ironsi Still Uncertain." *New York Times,* August 2, 1966. ProQuest Historical Newspapers (117223583).

———. "Weekend Rioting in North Nigeria Leaves 64 Dead." *New York Times,* May 31, 1966. ProQuest Historical Newspapers (117004759).

Star Reporter. "Keesee to Join Forces With Nigeria." April 1964. Star Bible.

Summerlin, M.I. "An Elder's Evaluation: Nigerian Christians Flourish as New Mission Fields Ripen." *Christian Chronicle* 20, no. 8, November 23, 1962.

Talley, Wanda Nell. "Bonnie Elizabeth Ramsey." In *In the Kitchen with Bonnie: A Tribute to Our Mothers and Bonnie, Our Grandmother,* edited by Iris Savio and Jerry Lipham. Kearney, NE: Morris Press Cookbooks, 2003, 48930-vm 2–10.

Tennessean. "Don't Quote Me: Miss Green, Mr. Lanham Are Married." *Nashville Tennessean,* January 3, 1965. Sunday Morning Edition.

Time Magazine. "Nigeria: The Model Breaks Down." January 8, 1965.

———. "The World. Nigeria: The Men of Sandhurst." January 28, 1966.

Umeora, O.U.J., S.O. Onuh, and M.C. Umeora. "Socio-Cultural Barriers to Voluntary Blood Donation for Obstetric Use in a Rural Nigerian Village." *African Journal of Reproductive Health* 9 (December 2005): 72–76.

Walker, Bill. "Summary of Our Trip to Nigeria." In *Short Stories,* edited by Nicks and Nicks, 168–73.

Wall, Barbara Mann. "Changes in Nursing and Mission in Post-Colonial Nigeria." In *A History of Colonial and Post-Colonial Nursing,* edited by Helen Sweet and Sue Hawkins, 188-207.

Washington Street Church of Christ. "Glenna Jean Shifflett Peden." *Ladies Newsletter,* June 1999. Fayetteville, TN: Washington Street Church of Christ. AUTH (copy).

Williams, Newell E., Douglas Allen Foster, and Paul M. Blowers, eds. *The Stone-Campbell Movement: A Global History.* Danvers, MA: Chalice, 2013. Kindle Edition.

Wilson, Patty Woods. "Biography of Mark Ugwunna." In *Mark's Cookbook.* 2nd ed. Edited by Patty W. Wilson and Lola B. Nation. Self-published, 2001.

Wofford, Mary. "Resume of Mary Wofford," n.d. Unpublished. AUTH (copy).

Index

Abilene Christian College, x, xviii, 25, 30, 81–2

African Christian Hospital Board (see International Health Care Foundation)

African Christian Schools Foundation (see Nigerian Christian Schools Foundation)

African National Church, 240, 240n.22

Agali, Anthony, 58, 114, 166, 169, 208, 298–9

Aguiyi-Ironsi, Maj. Gen. Johnson T.U., 212–3, 220, 243

Akandu, Josiah O./Abigail, 120, 200, 246, 265–6, 277, 298

Akpabio, Dr. Udofia Udo "Edward," 103, 103n.30, 289, 297n.50, 302

Akpakpan, Monday John, 211, 249

Amobi, Dr., 54–5

Annang (also Anaangs or Anangs), 1n.6, 114, 275–6, 275n.2, 276n.7, 298

Apollos, Mark (see Ugwunna)

Backdoor clinics, iii, 10, 12–3, 15, 20, 24, 26–8, 36, 39, 41, 43, 53, 69, 109–11, 175, 211

Bales, J.D., 44n.4

Bawcom, Burney/Louanna, 23–4, 28

Baxter, Batsell Barrett, 36

Beckloff, John/Dottie, 130, 202, 210, 246, 282

Benson, George S., 108, 108n.23

Bent, Matron Ann, 146–50, 152

Biafra, Republic of, iv, xxi, 160, 216n.6, 290–1, 293–9, 301–3, 306

Bible classes/teaching: children, 18–9, 90, 125, 145–6, 165, 217, 280–1; NCH, 173, 181, 222, 239, 280–1; women (incl. domestic skills), 18–9, 24, 35, 90, 133–4, 165, 233–4

Bible Training College (BTC): Onicha Ngwa, x, 34, 37–9, 45n.10, 47, 66, 99, 102–3, 109–10, 113–4, 120, 123, 129n.21, 141n.58, 146, 158, 158n.55, 165, 170, 176, 191, 199–200, 205, 211, 218, 221–2, 236, 242, 250–2, 265, 277; Ukpom, x, xix, 17, 33–4, 37, 134, 205

Blood bank, 215, 248, 250–1, 253, 279

Boyd, Glenn, 307

Braide, Dr. M.T.D., 245–6

Braun, Anna-Maria, 1–3, 3n.11

Bridges, Charley, 268, 268n.8, 282, 285, 301

Broom, Wendell/Betty, 17n.55, 23–4, 26–9, 31, 33, 54

Buice, Hazel, 258–9, 258n.23, 298, 300

Burton, A.M. and Elizabeth, 227

Calabar, 3, 71

Cameroon, Republic of, 130, 258n.23, 293–4, 300–3

Carson, Francis Frank ("F.F."), 203–5, 218, 301–2

Catholic missions, Roman, 11–2, 41, 239 (see also Medical Mission of Mary)

Cayce, John S., 49, 55, 57n.20, 107n.18, 237

Christian Council of Nigeria, 303

Churches of Christ (COC): Andrews (Andrews, TX), 86; Bay Shore (Long Island, NY), 82, 258n.23; Charlotte Avenue, 304; Chisolm Hills (Florence, AL), 257; Creswell Street (Shreveport, LA), 73; Figueroa (Los Angeles, CA), 204; Green Lawn (Lubbock, TX), 65, 70, 88, 202–5, 207, 228, 233, 259; Hillsboro Avenue (Nashville, TN), 36, 269; Lawrence Avenue (Nashville, TN), x, 1–6, 6n.38, 14–5, 23–4, 26, 50n.41, 81, 83, 165; Meadow, 268, 268n.8; Michigan Avenue/Sheldon Heights (Chicago, IL), 203, 203n.27; Onicha Ngwa Campus, 112; Proctor Street (Port Arthur, TX), 33, 36, 47, 50, 57, 65–6, 71, 99, 102, 237; Sherrod Avenue (Florence, AL), 65; Sixth Street (Port Arthur, TX), 7; South Park (Beaumont, TX), 51, 73, 167; Southside (Odessa, TX), 26; Southside (Richmond, CA), 203–5, 301–2; Sunset Ridge (San Antonio, TX), 24; Tenth and Francis Street (Oklahoma City, OK), 23; Thomas Boulevard (Port Arthur, TX), 44; Tripoli (Libya) 50, 61; University (Nashville, TN), 77–8, 83; Vanleer (Vanleer, TN), 75, 77, 83–4, 89, 124; Vultee (Nashville, TN), 205; Walnut Hill (Cincinnati, OH), 56; Walnut Street (Dickson, TN), 83; West End (Nashville, TN), x–xi, 49–50, 55, 57, 69–70, 73, 83, 100–1, 105, 107, 110, 113–4, 125, 155, 167, 174, 193–6, 202–3, 202n.21, 207–8, 213, 218, 220, 227, 232, 237, 261, 268n.8, 269–71, 289, 292, 294, 297, 300, 304

Coleman, F.B., 228, 238

"Conquest for Christ," 96n.15

"Conquest to the sea," 290

Cross, Joe/Dorothy, 26, 28–30, 304, 306

Curry, Bill/MaryLou, 71, 73, 102, 107n.15, 196, 260, 285

Cussick, Lorraine, 255

David Lipscomb College, 6

Dedman, John, 207–8, 216–7

Derr, Harold/Jane, 103n.26

Diestelkamp, Leslie/Sarah, xix, 43–5, 63–4, 69–70, 293

Dillingham, Paul, 294

Diseases/common health issues, 4–5, 10–3, 23–4, 27, 35, 37–41, 47, 51, 58, 109–11, 111n.48, 134, 139, 146, 155, 171, 174–6, 182, 187, 191, 193–5, 216, 218–9, 231–5, 241, 247–8, 250, 260, 263, 271, 279–81 (see also Female circumcision and Twins)

Dunn, Phil & family, 104, 130

Echols, Eldred, xviii, 4–6, 6n.34, 6n.38, 16, 18, 29, 234

Efik (see Ibibio)

Elangwe, D.N., 294

Ellah, Francis J., 107, 107n.21

Enugu, 27n.24, 29, 54, 67, 73, 100, 102, 107, 111–3, 130, 167, 196, 200, 210, 216, 219, 232, 243, 255–6, 260, 284–5, 289, 297

Essien, C.A.O./Nwa A. Ukpong, 2–7, 3n.11, 6n.34, 18–20, 75, 265

Exodus movement (See Bayshore Church of Christ)

Ezell, Houston/Mabel, 205, 207–8, 216–7, 227, 256, 259

Ezerie, Sunday, 103

Farrar, George/Evelyn, xi, 213, 270, 300

Female circumcision, 110, 134, 155

Finney, James/Mary Louise, xix, 26, 34, 36, 38, 43–4

First-aid classes, 158–60, 194

Florida Christian College, 25

Formby, Adrian, 108

Freeman, John, 239, 239n.18, 295, 299

Fulani (see Hausa/Fulani)

Gowon, Major General Yakubu "Jack," 243, 284, 291, 295, 297

Greer, Ted/Ada, 293, 297, 299

Hale, Henry Clyde, 77–8, 80, 82

Hall, Sewell/Caneta, xix–xx, 26, 43–4, 45n.10, 63–4, 260n.35

Harding College, 44n.4, 50, 56, 80–1, 107n.15, 108, 108n.23, 303

Harrison, Don/Joyce Huffard, 18, 129, 130n.28, 232

Hausa/Fulani, 94, 211, 220–1, 286

Hobbs, June, 23–4, 26–8, 33, 89

Horton, Howard/Mildred, xviii–xix, 2, 6, 9–11, 18–20, 27–8, 33, 143, 301

Hospitals, near NCH: government hospitals, 51, 68, 109; Itu Leprosarium, 109, 193; Medical Mission of Mary, x, 27, 37–9, 41, 48, 51, 240, 248–9; Medico, 216; Nigeria Baptist mission hospital, 107; Qua Iboe Hospital, 54, 109, 167; Queen Elizabeth Hospital (QEH), x, 63, 70, 109–10, 120, 122–3, 145–9, 152, 197, 215–6, 219, 232, 235–6, 240, 301; Shell Oil Hospital/Delta Clinic, 99, 109, 194, 232

Huffard, Elvis/Emily, xviii–xix, 17–9, 27–8, 130n.28

Ibe, Tom, 140, 249

Ibibio/Ibibioland, 1–2, 1n.6, 2, 12–5, 19, 19n.66, 33, 51, 114, 143, 155, 170, 275–6, 275n.2, 276n.7, 280, 289

Igbo (Ibo): 33n.1, 46; conflict/war, 114, 155, 211–2, 220–3, 243, 255, 275–7, 286, 289–92, 295, 297–9; culture/beliefs, i, 48, 51, 94, 110, 134, 136, 138, 140n.48, 175, 182, 187–92, 277, 280; gender, 14, 133, 141–3, 141n.58, 156–7; Igbo-missionary relationships, 34, 105, 107, 110, 114, 134–6, 135n.15, 138–40, 143, 151–2, 170, 183–4, 187–92, 200, 214, 221–2, 240–2, 251–2, 254, 265–6, 277–8, 282, 298–9; Igbo Union, 303; Igboland, 33, 38, 114; language, 51, 134, 136–7, 170, 280

Ikot Ekpene, iv, 34, 51, 114, 276, 285

Immigration quota, 45, 54, 62, 72, 92, 99–100, 103–5, 103n.26, 133, 239, 256, 270, 278

Independence Day, Nigeria, xx, 183–4, 211–2

International Health Care Foundation/ACH, x, xxi, 53, 258–60, 260n.35, 269, 302–7

Irondi "Tailor," 163, 257

Johnson, Elva and Martha, xi, 55, 265

Johnson, Jimmy/Rosa Lee & Pamela, xviii–xix, 2, 6, 10–1, 10n.9, 18–9, 28, 233

Johnson, Leonard Calvin/Bernice & Janice, 24, 26–8, 33, 36, 38, 233

Jos, 233–4

Juju or "witch" doctors (see Native doctors)

Kaiser Foundation International, 303

Keasling, Janice, 81

Kee, Windle/Barbara, 256–7, 259, 271, 273, 278, 292, 296, 298, 300, 303

Keeble, Marshall, 205–6, 222

Keesee, Dayton/Ruth, 73, 112, 196, 219

Kelton, Tom/Mary, xii, xviii–xix, 24–31, 36, 38

Kennedy Jr., Levi, 203–5

King, Mike, 217, 227, 232, 267, 282–85, 293

Kola nut, 170, 200, 253

Laboratory, NCH: 147, 164, 253, 258; lay technicians, 156–7, 171–3, 245, 258–9, 306; Registered Medical Technologist, 99, 103 (also see Buice)

Lanham, Ray/Charlotte, 217, 232, 241

Lawyer, Douglas/Charla, xx, 46, 50, 53, 57–9, 63–4, 66–7, 71–2, 99–102, 107n.15, 110, 112, 121–2, 127, 129n.21, 130–1, 137, 165, 174, 199–200, 200n.8, 208, 270

Leprosarium (see Itu Leprosarium)

Lewis, J.R., 238–9

Lubbock Christian College, x, xx, 49, 86–90, 279

Manning, Preston, 147, 147n.7

Maps: Biafra, 291; Nigeria, xvi; Onicha Ngwa mission compound, 126

Martin, Glenn/Dee, 54

Martin, Damon, 227–8, 269

Massey, Jim/Joyce, xx, 50–1, 57–8, 66–7, 71–3, 90, 95, 100, 107n.15, 137, 199, 213, 222, 233, 237–8, 244, 260, 268, 293, 301

Mattox, F.W./Mildred, xi, 49, 70, 91, 106, 107n.15, 110, 181n.13, 202, 204, 207–8, 237–8 259–60, 268–9, 306

Mattox, Joe, 233–8

Methodist Hospital School of Nursing: Dallas, xviii, 25; Lubbock, xx, 87, 91

Mid-State Baptist Nursing School, xx, 76

Mitchell, Carl, 260

Mobile Clinic, Christian (Cameroon), 301–2

Morgan, John/Donna, 127, 132, 154, 165–6, 169–70, 172, 172n.23, 193–4, 199, 204, 216, 228

Muslim/Islam, 214, 220–2, 255, 282

Native (juju) doctors, 14, 35, 40, 48, 58, 108, 190–1, 218, 222, 222n.44, 250

Native treatments/care, 12, 40, 51, 139, 171, 176, 181–3, 190–1, 202, 218, 231

Ndiakata, 102, 102n.21, 106, 114

Newberry, Cathy, 255–6

Nicks, J.W. "Bill"/Gerry, x, xix–xx, 26, 33–6, 38–41, 44n.4, 45, 47–8, 50, 51n.48, 52–4, 66, 73, 80, 83n.46, 101, 114, 120, 199, 227

Nigerian Christian Hospital (incl. Clinic): administrators, 257, 261, 271, 296, 298, 302, 304, 306; architectural blueprints, 108, 110–2, 147, 163–4, 167, 196–7, 199–200, 215; clinic buildings, 163–4; funding, 24, 43, 69–70, 105–8, 107n.18, 112, 114, 202–4; 207–8; 216–8, 228, 237–8, 249, 258–61, 270, 279, 289–90, 303; government approval (see also architectural plans), 105, 107, 111–3, 152, 166–7, 196–7, 199–200, 212, 226, 245; grand openings, xxi, 165, 169–70, 226, 245–7; Hospital fully open, 294; land acquisition, xxi, 54, 105–6, 111–2, 114, 133, 143, 151, 153, 155, 157–9, 161, 199–202, 200n.8, 202n.17; water and electrical supply, 107, 111, 114, 163, 165–7, 169, 237–9, 249, 259, 264, 275, 277–8, 289, 296

Nigerian Christian Schools Foundation (NCSF), x, 24, 259, 302

Nigerian Christian Secondary School (NCSS), x, 24, 153, 207–8, 211, 259

Nlagu, 201, 245

North, Diane, 123, 147, 232, 301

Ntigha, 34, 201, 245

Nurse Auxiliaries: applicant selection, 153–6, 166, 225–26; baptisms, 239; classes, xx–xxi, 152, 158, 171, 179–82, 197, 245, 261, 271n.33, 273; graduation, xxi, 251–4, 271–3; names, 155, 173, 226, 258, 272; top students, 181–2, 253, 272; uniforms, 163, 172–3, 172n.23, 180, 247, 251–2, 257, 272, 282; work, 174, 226, 258, 263, 273, 305–6

Nurses, Registered: Nigerian (NRN), xxi, 148, 152, 156, 180, 216, 227, 245, 248, 254, 257, 261, 282, 294, 302, 305–6; US (RN) prewar, xii; US (RN) postwar, 304

Obudu Cattle Ranch & Rest House, 130, 219, 234

Ojukwu, Chukwuemeka Odumegwu, 212–3, 243, 290–2

Omenai, H.O., 104

Onukafor, Friday, 101, 146, 160, 174, 252, 264, 272, 298–9, 302, 306

Oparah, Moses/Comfort, 190, 221–2, 222n.44, 276–7, 298–9, 302–3, 306

Otoyo, Eno/LaVera, 130, 153, 201, 203, 246, 292, 298–9, 301–2

Palmer, Lucien/Ida, xix, 11–2, 18, 20, 24, 26, 28, 33–4, 37–8, 205, 304

Palmer Hospital, 307

Peace Corps, 87, 100, 213, 215, 265, 279, 284, 290, 294, 297

Peden, Glenna/Eugene, iii, vii, xii, xviii–xix, 1–2, 7, 9–15, 17–21, 23, 26, 28, 35–9, 42, 56, 75, 77–8, 81, 95, 199, 233, 268

Pepperdine University, 303

Petitionary letters, 134–6, 153, 265–6, 269

Petty, Albert/Kitty, 75–80, 83–4, 124, 275

Pharmacy/technicians, NCH: 147, 156–7, 164, 171, 173–5, 182, 197, 245, 253

Polygamy, 16, 123, 142–3

Port Harcourt (PH), x, 1, 5, 10–2, 10n.9, 18, 33–4, 39, 62, 67, 71, 83, 99, 106, 109, 114, 117–9, 121–2, 129, 145, 166, 194, 210, 220, 232, 238–9, 244, 246, 255–6, 258, 278, 282–3, 285, 292, 294–5, 299, 303

Reese, Boyd, xviii, 4–5, 16, 18, 29, 234

Red Cross, xxi, 159, 293, 302, 306

Registered Trustees of Churches of Christ (Nigeria), 45, 71, 99, 201, 266

Registrar of NCH (Joseph Nwaoguegbe), 157, 164, 171, 173–4, 187–8, 306

Robinson, Keith, 298

Sanders, Doug, 256, 259

School Nurse: Abilene, 25, 81; Florida Christian, 25; Harding, 56, 108n.23; Onicha Ngwa, 110

Sermanoukian, Letty, xii, xx, 50, 61–74, 81, 95, 114, 120, 305

Seventh Day Adventists, 239–40, 239n.18, 289

Sinclair, Bruce D. "Jack," 57, 57n.20

Southwestern Christian College, 203

Spray, Dr. Paul, 216n.6, 284

Sudan Interior Mission (SIM), 234

Sweetham, Rosemary, 147, 219

Tarbet, Gaston/Jan, 256, 272, 276–8, 292, 295, 298, 300

Taylor, Lawrence, 50, 61–2, 66–8

Thieves, 140n.48, 189–90, 222, 278

Thomas, J.D. & Icy, 278, 278n.22, 282–3, 293

Translators: 137; auxiliaries as, 151, 171, 176, 180; Agharanya, 65–6, 305; Akandu, 298; Eguzo and Udogwu, 135–7, 141, 143, 158, 302, 306; G. Farrar, 303; Nwa Essien, 19; Okoronkwo, 51; Onukafor, 146, 252, 272; Oparah, 276; records as, 280; staff, 35, 51, 241; Uyo, 39; Wycliffe, 120

Turner, George, 3

Twins, traditional beliefs, 13, 134, 280

Ugwunna, Mark Apollos, 34, 101–2, 121–2, 127, 129, 131–2, 183, 190, 210, 218, 298

Umuwoma, 201, 245

Underwood, R. David/Myra, 131, 199, 201, 208, 210, 219–20, 229, 231, 235–6, 244, 246, 256–7

USAID, x, 229, 238, 290, 303

Village schools, 4, 17–8, 24, 53, 205

Virginia (Petty's foster daughter), 241–2, 246, 265, 282–3, 298, 301

Walters, Gid/Ruth, 256, 272, 282, 298, 299n.69, 300

Well-baby clinic, 189, 233

Whitaker, Robert/Annette, 305

Wilbanks, David/Kathryn, 285, 301

Yearwood, Ken/Lola, 227–8, 269, 285, 301

Yoruba, 94, 211

Young, M. Norvel/Helen and Matt, 233, 286

About the Author

Martha F. Highfield PhD RN is Professor Emeritus of Nursing at California State University/Northridge and Advisor for the Research Fellowship Magnet Program at Providence Holy Cross Medical Center in Mission Hills, California. She has authored numerous peer-reviewed publications and serves on the Board of the International Health Care Foundation/African Christian Hospitals.

If you enjoyed this book, please consider leaving an online review. The author would appreciate reading your thoughts.

About the Publisher

Sulis International Press publishes select fiction and nonfiction in a variety of genres under four imprints: Riversong Books, Sulis Academic Press, Sulis Press, and Keledei Publications.

For more, visit the website at
https://sulisinternational.com

Subscribe to the newsletter at
https://sulisinternational.com/subscribe/

Follow us on social media
https://www.facebook.com/SulisInternational
https://twitter.com/Sulis_Intl
https://www.pinterest.com/Sulis_Intl/
https://www.instagram.com/sulis_international/

Made in the USA
Columbia, SC
17 June 2021